ESAP™ 2021

Endocrine Society's
Endocrine Self-Assessment Program
Questions, Answers, and Discussions

Lisa R. Tannock, MD, Program Chair
Professor of Medicine
Chief, Division of Endocrinology
and Molecular Medicine
University of Kentucky and
Department of Veterans Affairs

Barbara Gisella Carranza Leon, MD
Assistant Professor of Medicine
Division of Diabetes, Endocrinology,
and Metabolism
Vanderbilt University Medical Center

Alice Y. Chang, MD, MSc
Assistant Professor
Division of Endocrinology,
Diabetes, and Nutrition
Mayo Clinic

Dima Lutfi Diab, MD
Associate Professor of Clinical Medicine
University of Cincinnati

Nazanene H. Esfandiari, MD
Associate Professor
University of Michigan

Mathis Grossmann, MD, PhD, FRACP
Professor of Medicine
University of Melbourne
Austin Health

**Mark Gurnell, MBBS, MA
(Med Ed), PhD, FRCP**
Professor of Clinical Endocrinology
& Clinical SubDean
University of Cambridge,
Wellcome Trust-MRC Institute
of Metabolic Science &
School of Clinical Medicine

Steven B. Magill, MD, PhD
Associate Clinical Professor of Medicine
Endocrinology, Diabetes, and Metabolism
Medical College of Wisconsin

Sarah E. Mayson, MD
Associate Professor of Medicine
Director of the Endocrinology
Fellowship Program
Division of Endocrinology,
Metabolism, and Diabetes
University of Colorado School of Medicine

Kevin M. Pantalone, DO, FACE
Staff Endocrinologist
Director of Diabetes Initiatives
Department of Endocrinology
Cleveland Clinic

Deepika Reddy, MD
Associate Professor of Medicine
Division of Diabetes, Endocrinology,
and Metabolism
University of Utah Healthcare

Roberto Salvatori, MD
Professor of Medicine
Medical Director,
Johns Hopkins Pituitary Center
Johns Hopkins University

Aniket Sidhaye, MD
Assistant Professor of Medicine
Johns Hopkins University

Savitha Subramanian, MD
Associate Professor of Medicine
University of Washington

Anand Vaidya, MD, MMSC
Associate Professor of Medicine
Brigham and Women's Hospital
Harvard Medical School

Thomas J. Weber, MD
Associate Professor of Medicine
Division of Endocrinology,
Metabolism, and Nutrition
Duke University Medical Center

Abbie L. Young, MS, CGC, ELS(D)
Medical Editor

Endocrine Society
2055 L Street NW, Suite 600, Washington, DC 20036
1-888-ENDOCRINE • www.endocrine.org

ENDOCRINE
SOCIETY

Hormone Science to Health

ENDOCRINE
SOCIETY
Hormone Science to Health

The Endocrine Society is the world's largest, oldest, and most active organization working to advance the clinical practice of endocrinology and hormone research. Founded in 1916, the Society now has more than 18,000 global members across a range of disciplines. The Society has earned an international reputation for excellence in the quality of its peer-reviewed journals, educational resources, meetings, and programs that improve public health through the practice and science of endocrinology.

Visit us at:
education.endocrine.org
endocrine.org

Other Publications:
endocrine.org/publications

For updates to the professional development books between editions:
https://www.endocrine.org/bookupdates

The statements and opinions expressed in this publication are those of the individual authors and do not necessarily reflect the views of the Endocrine Society. The Endocrine Society is not responsible or liable in any way for the currency of the information, for any errors, omissions, or inaccuracies, or for any consequences arising therefrom. With respect to any drugs mentioned, the reader is advised to refer to the appropriate medical literature and the product information currently provided by the manufacturer to verify appropriate dosage, method and duration of administration, and other relevant information. In all instances, it is the responsibility of the treating physician or other health care professional, relying on independent experience and expertise, as well as knowledge of the patient, to determine the best treatment for the patient.

ISBN: 978-1-879225-93-0

Library of Congress Control Number: 2020947880

On the Cover: @ Freepik. Doctor wearing white robe and stethoscope (by Racool_studio).

OVERVIEW

The Endocrine Self-Assessment Program (ESAP™) is a self-study curriculum aimed at physicians wanting a self-assessment and a broad review of endocrinology. The ESAP Reference Edition consists of 120 brand-new multiple-choice questions in all areas of endocrinology, diabetes, and metabolism. There is extensive discussion of each correct answer, a comprehensive syllabus, and references. ESAP is updated annually with new questions.

The ESAP reference book is intended primarily for consultation and self-assessment of knowledge relating to endocrinology. As a reference book, educational credits are not available upon completion of the multiple-choice questions included. For information on educational products that include educational credit, please visit endocrine.org/store.

LEARNING OBJECTIVES

ESAP 2021 will allow learners to assess their knowledge of all aspects of endocrinology, diabetes, and metabolism.

Completion of this educational activity enables learners to accomplish key objectives:

- Recognize clinical manifestations of endocrine and metabolic disorders and select among current options for diagnosis, management, and therapy.
- Identify risk factors for endocrine and metabolic disorders and develop strategies for prevention.
- Evaluate endocrine and metabolic manifestations of systemic disorders.
- Use existing resources pertaining to clinical guidelines and treatment recommendations for endocrine and related metabolic disorders to guide diagnosis and treatment.

TARGET AUDIENCE

ESAP is a self-study curriculum aimed at physicians seeking initial certification or recertification in endocrinology, program directors interested in a testing and training instrument, and clinicians simply wanting a self-assessment and broad review of endocrinology.

STATEMENT OF INDEPENDENCE

The Endocrine Society has a policy of ensuring that the content and quality of this educational activity are balanced, independent, objective, and scientifically rigorous. The scientific content of this activity was developed under the supervision of the Endocrine Society's ESAP Faculty Working Group.

DISCLOSURE POLICY

The faculty, committee members, and staff who are in position to control the content of this activity are required to disclose to the Endocrine Society and to learners any relevant financial relationship(s) of the individual or spouse/partner that have occurred within the last 12 months with any commercial interest(s) whose products or services are related to the CME content. Financial relationships are defined by remuneration in any amount from the commercial interest(s) in the form of grants; research support; consulting fees; salary; ownership interest (eg, stocks, stock options, or ownership interest excluding diversified mutual funds); honoraria or other payments for participation in speakers' bureaus, advisory boards, or boards of directors; or other financial benefits. The intent of this disclosure is not to prevent CME planners with relevant financial relationships from planning or delivering content, but rather to provide learners with information that allows them to make their own judgments of whether these financial relationships may have influenced the educational activity with regard to exposition or conclusion. The Endocrine Society has reviewed all disclosures and resolved or managed all identified conflicts of interest, as applicable.

The following faculty reported relevant financial relationship(s): **Alice Y. Chang, MD, MSc,** is a site investigator and on the advisory board for clinical trial for Millendo Therapeutics. She is also on the national advisory board for Corcept Therapeutics. **Roberto Salvatori, MD,** receives grant funds from Roche, and he is on the advisory board of Pfizer and NovoNordisk. He serves as a clinical trial investigator for Novartis, Chiasma, OPKO, Strongbridge Biopharma, Corcept Therapeutics, and Crinetics Pharmaceuticals. **Savitha Subramanian, MD,** serves on the advisory board for Sanofi. **Anand Vaidya, MD, MMSC,** is a consultant for Selenity Therapeutics, HRA Pharma, and Orphagen Pharmaceuticals. **Thomas J. Weber, MD,** is a consultant for Ultragenyx Pharmaceutical and Pharmacosmos, He is also a primary investigator for Ultragenyx Pharmaceutical. His spouse is an editor for Nivalis Therapeutics and a primary investigator for AstraZeneca. **Kevin M. Pantalone, DO,** is a consultant for AstraZeneca, Bayer, Corcept Therapeutics, Eli Lilly, Merck, and Novo Nordisk and a speaker for AstraZeneca, Merck, and Novo Nordisk. He has received research support from Bayer, Merck, and Novo Nordisk.

The following committee members reported no relevant financial relationships: **Lisa R. Tannock, MD; Barbara Gisella Carranza Leon, MD; Dima Lutfi Diab, MD; Nazanene H. Esfandiari, MD; Mathis Grossmann, MD, PhD, FRCP; Mark Gurnell, MBBS, MA (Med Ed), PhD; Steven B. Magill, MD, PhD; Deepika Reddy, MD; Aniket Sidhaye, MD; Sarah E. Mayson, MD.**

The medical editor for this program, **Abbie L. Young, MS, CGC, ELS(D),** reported no relevant financial relationships.

The Endocrine Society staff associated with the development of content for this activity reported no relevant financial relationships.

DISCLAIMERS

The information presented in this activity represents the opinion of the faculty and is not necessarily the official position of the Endocrine Society.

USE OF PROFESSIONAL JUDGMENT:

The educational content in this self-assessment test relates to basic principles of diagnosis and therapy and does not substitute for individual patient assessment based on the health care provider's examination of the patient and consideration of laboratory data and other factors unique to the patient. Standards in medicine change as new data become available.

DRUGS AND DOSAGES:

When prescribing medications, the physician is advised to check the product information sheet accompanying each drug to verify conditions of use and to identify any changes in drug dosage schedule or contraindications.

POLICY ON UNLABELED/OFF-LABEL USE

The Endocrine Society has determined that disclosure of unlabeled/off-label or investigational use of commercial product(s) is informative for audiences and therefore requires this information to be disclosed to the learners at the beginning of the presentation. Uses of specific therapeutic agents, devices, and other products discussed in this educational activity may not be the same as those indicated in product labeling approved by the Food and Drug Administration (FDA). The Endocrine Society requires that any discussions of such "off-label" use be based on scientific research that conforms to generally accepted standards of experimental design, data collection, and data analysis. Before recommending or prescribing any therapeutic agent or device, learners should review the complete prescribing information, including indications, contraindications, warnings, precautions, and adverse events.

ACKNOWLEDGMENT OF COMMERCIAL SUPPORT

This activity is not supported by educational grant(s) or other funds from any commercial supporter.

PUBLICATION DATE: March 2021

Laboratory Reference Ranges

Reference ranges vary among laboratories. The listed reference ranges should be used when interpreting laboratory values presented in ESAP™. Conventional units are listed first with SI units in parentheses.

Lipid Values

High-density lipoprotein (HDL) cholesterol

    Optimal -------------------------------- >60 mg/dL (SI: >1.55 mmol/L)

    Normal ---------------------- 40-60 mg/dL (SI: 1.04-1.55 mmol/L)

    Low ------------------------------------- <40 mg/dL (SI: <1.04 mmol/L)

Low-density lipoprotein (LDL) cholesterol

    Optimal ---------------------------- <100 mg/dL (SI: <2.59 mmol/L)

    Low ---------------------- 100-129 mg/dL (SI: 2.59-3.34 mmol/L)

    Borderline-high ---------- 130-159 mg/dL (SI: 3.37-4.12 mmol/L)

    High ---------------------- 160-189 mg/dL (SI: 4.14-4.90 mmol/L)

    Very high ------------------------ ≥190 mg/dL (SI: ≥4.92 mmol/L)

Non-HDL cholesterol

    Optimal ------------------------- <130 mg/dL (SI: <3.37 mmol/L)

    Borderline-high ---------- 130-159 mg/dL (SI: 3.37-4.12 mmol/L)

    High --------------------------- ≥240 mg/dL (SI: ≥6.22 mmol/L)

Total cholesterol

    Optimal ------------------------- <200 mg/dL (SI: <5.18 mmol/L)

    Borderline-high ---------- 200-239 mg/dL (SI: 5.18-6.19 mmol/L)

    High --------------------------- ≥240 mg/dL (SI: ≥6.22 mmol/L)

Triglycerides

    Optimal ------------------------- <150 mg/dL (SI: <1.70 mmol/L)

    Borderline-high ---------- 150-199 mg/dL (SI: 1.70-2.25 mmol/L)

    High ---------------------- 200-499 mg/dL (SI: 2.26-5.64 mmol/L)

    Very high ------------------------ ≥500 mg/dL (SI: ≥5.65 mmol/L)

Lipoprotein (a) --------------------------- ≤30 mg/dL (SI: ≤1.07 μmol/L)

Apolipoprotein B -------------------- 50-110 mg/dL (SI: 0.5-1.1 g/L)

Hematologic Values

Erythrocyte sedimentation rate -------------------------- 0-20 mm/h

Haptoglobin --------------------- 30-200 mg/dL (SI: 300-2000 mg/L)

Hematocrit ------------------------------ 41%-50% (SI: 0.41-0.51) (male);

    35%-45% (SI: 0.35-0.45) (female)

Hemoglobin A_{1c} ----------------------- 4.0%-5.6% (20-38 mmol/mol)

Hemoglobin ---------------- 13.8-17.2 g/dL (SI: 138-172 g/L) (male);

    12.1-15.1 g/dL (SI: 121-151 g/L) (female)

International normalized ratio -------------------------------- 0.8-1.2

Mean corpuscular volume (MCV) --------- 80-100 μm³ (SI: 80-100 fL)

Platelet count ---------------- 150-450 × 10³/μL (SI: 150-450 × 10⁹/L)

Protein (total) --------------------------- 6.3-7.9 g/dL (SI: 63-79 g/L)

Reticulocyte count --- 0.5%-1.5% of red blood cells (SI: 0.005-0.015)

White blood cell count -------- 4500-11,000/μL (SI: 4.5-11.0 × 10⁹/L)

Thyroid Values

Thyroglobulin --------- 3-42 ng/mL (SI: 3-42 μg/L) (after surgery and radioactive iodine treatment: <1.0 ng/mL [SI: <1.0 μg/L])

Thyroglobulin antibodies ------------------ ≤4.0 IU/mL (SI: ≤4.0 kIU/L)

Thyrotropin (TSH) ------------------------------------- 0.5-5.0 mIU/L

Thyrotropin-receptor antibodies (TRAb) ------------------ ≤1.75 IU/L

Thyroid-stimulating immunoglobulin -------- ≤120% of basal activity

Thyroperoxidase (TPO) antibodies -------- <2.0 IU/mL (SI: <2.0 kIU/L)

Thyroxine (T_4) (free) ---------- 0.8-1.8 ng/dL (SI: 10.30-23.17 pmol/L)

Thyroxine (T_4) (total) ------- 5.5-12.5 μg/dL (SI: 94.02-213.68 nmol/L)

Free thyroxine (T_4) index ------------------------------------- 4-12

Triiodothyronine (T_3) (free) ------ 2.3-4.2 pg/mL (SI: 3.53-6.45 pmol/L)

Triiodothyronine (T_3) (total) ----- 70-200 ng/dL (SI: 1.08-3.08 nmol/L)

Triiodothyronine (T_3), reverse ---- 10-24 ng/dL (SI: 0.15-0.37 nmol/L)

Triiodothyronine uptake, resin --------------------------- 25%-38%

Radioactive iodine uptake - 3%-16% (6 hours); 15%-30% (24 hours)

Endocrine Values

Serum

Aldosterone ---------------------- 4-21 ng/dL (SI: 111.0-582.5 pmol/L)

Alkaline phosphatase ------------- 50-120 U/L (SI: 0.84-2.00 μkat/L)

Alkaline phosphatase (bone-specific) --------- ≤20 μg/L (adult male);

    ≤14 μg/L (premenopausal female);

    ≤22 μg/L (postmenopausal female)

Androstenedione -- 65-210 ng/dL (SI: 2.27-7.33 nmol/L) (adult male);

    30-200 ng/dL (SI: 1.05-6.98 nmol/L) (adult female)

Antimullerian hormone ------- 0.7-19.0 ng/mL (SI: 5.0-135.7 pmol/L)

    (male, >12 years);

    0.9-9.5 ng/mL (SI: 6.4-67.9 pmol/L) (female, 13-45 years);

    <1.0 ng/mL (SI: <7.1 pmol/L) (female, >45 years)

Calcitonin ----------------- <16 pg/mL (SI: <4.67 pmol/L) (basal, male);

    <8 pg/mL (SI: <2.34 pmol/L) (basal, female);

    ≤130 pg/mL (SI: ≤37.96 pmol/L) (peak calcium infusion, male);

    ≤90 pg/mL (SI: ≤26.28 pmol/L) (peak calcium infusion, female)

Carcinoembryonic antigen --------------- <2.5 ng/mL (SI: <2.5 μg/L)

Chromogranin A ---------------------------- <93 ng/mL (SI: <93 μg/L)

Corticosterone --- 53-1560 ng/dL (SI: 1.53-45.08 nmol/L) (>18 years)

Corticotropin (ACTH) ------------- 10-60 pg/mL (SI: 2.2-13.2 pmol/L)

Cortisol (8 AM) ----------------- 5-25 μg/dL (SI: 137.9-689.7 nmol/L)

Cortisol (4 PM) -------------------- 2-14 μg/dL (SI: 55.2-386.2 nmol/L)

C-peptide ----------------------- 0.9-4.3 ng/mL (SI: 0.30-1.42 nmol/L)

C-reactive protein -------------- 0.8-3.1 mg/L (SI: 7.62-29.52 nmol/L)

Cross-linked N-telopeptide of type 1 collagen -----------------------

    5.4-24.2 nmol BCE/mmol creat (male);

    6.2-19.0 nmol BCE/mmol creat (female)

Dehydroepiandrosterone sulfate (DHEA-S)

Patient Age	Female	Male
18-29 years	44-332 μg/dL	89-457 μg/dL
	(SI: 1.19-9.00 μmol/L)	(SI: 2.41-12.38 μmol/L)
30-39 years	31-228 μg/dL	65-334 μg/dL
	(SI: 0.84-6.78 μmol/L)	(SI: 1.76-9.05 μmol/L)

Patient Age	Female	Male
40-49 years	18-244 µg/dL	48-244 µg/dL
	(SI: 0.49-6.61 µmol/L)	(SI: 1.30-6.61 µmol/L)
50-59 years	15-200 µg/dL	35-179 µg/dL
	(SI: 0.41-5.42 µmol/L)	(SI: 0.95-4.85 µmol/L)
≥60 years	15-157 µg/dL	25-131 µg/dL
	(SI: 0.41-4.25 µmol/L)	(SI: 0.68-3.55 µmol/L)

Deoxycorticosterone ------ <10 ng/dL (SI: <0.30 nmol/L) (>18 years)

1,25-Dihydroxyvitamin D₃----- 16-65 pg/mL (SI: 41.6-169.0 pmol/L)

Estradiol --------------- 10-40 pg/mL (SI: 36.7-146.8 pmol/L) (male);
  10-180 pg/mL (SI: 36.7-660.8 pmol/L) (follicular, female);
  100-300 pg/mL (SI: 367.1-1101.3 pmol/L) (midcycle, female);
  40-200 pg/mL (SI: 146.8-734.2 pmol/L) (luteal, female);
  <20 pg/mL (SI: <73.4 pmol/L) (postmenopausal, female)

Estrone --------------- 10-60 pg/mL (SI: 37.0-221.9 pmol/L) (male);
  17-200 pg/mL (SI: 62.9-739.6 pmol/L) (premenopausal female);
  7-40 pg/mL (SI: 25.9-147.9 pmol/L) (postmenopausal female)

α-Fetoprotein --------------------------------<6 ng/mL (SI: <6 µg/L)

Follicle-stimulating hormone (FSH) ----------------------------------
  1.0-13.0 mIU/mL (SI: 1.0-13.0 IU/L) (male);
  <3.0 mIU/mL (SI: <3.0 IU/L) (prepuberty, female);
  2.0-12.0 mIU/mL (SI: 2.0-12.0 IU/L) (follicular, female);
  4.0-36.0 mIU/mL (SI: 4.0-36.0 IU/L) (midcycle, female);
  1.0-9.0 mIU/mL (SI: 1.0-9.0 IU/L) (luteal, female);
  >30 mIU/mL (SI: >30 IU/L) (postmenopausal, female)

Free fatty acids ----------------- 10.6-18.0 mg/dL (SI: 0.4-0.7 nmol/L)

Gastrin----------------------------------- <100 pg/mL (SI: <100 ng/L)

Growth hormone (GH) --0.01-0.97 ng/mL (SI: 0.01-0.97 µg/L) (male);
  0.01-3.61 ng/mL (SI: 0.01-3.61 µg/L) (female)

Homocysteine -------------------------≤1.76 mg/L (SI: ≤13 µmol/L)

β-Human chorionic gonadotropin (β-hCG)---------------------------
  <3.0 mIU/mL (SI: <3.0 IU/L) (nonpregnant female);
  >25 mIU/mL ----(SI: >25 IU/L) indicates a positive pregnancy test

β-Hydroxybutyrate -------------------<3.0 mg/dL (SI: <288.2 µmol/L)

17-Hydroxypregnenolone ------ 29-189 ng/dL (SI: 0.87-5.69 nmol/L)

17α-Hydroxyprogesterone <220 ng/dL (SI: <6.67 nmol/L) (adult male);
  <80 ng/dL (SI: <2.42 nmol/L) (follicular, female);
  <285 ng/dL (SI: <8.64 nmol/L) (luteal, female);
  <51 ng/dL (SI: <1.55 nmol/L) (postmenopausal, female)

25-Hydroxyvitamin D ---- <20 ng/mL (SI: <49.9 nmol/L) (deficiency);
  21-29 ng/mL (SI: 52.4-72.4 nmol/L) (insufficiency);
  30-80 ng/mL (SI: 74.9-199.7 nmol/L) (optimal levels);
  >80 ng/mL (SI: >199.7 nmol/L) (toxicity possible)

Inhibin B -------------------------- 15-300 pg/mL (SI: 15-300 ng/L)

Insulinlike growth factor 1 (IGF-1)

Patient Age	Female	Male
18 years	162-541 ng/mL	170-640 ng/mL
	(SI: 21.2-70.9 nmol/L)	(SI: 22.3-83.8 nmol/L)
19 years	138-442 ng/mL	147-527 ng/mL
	(SI: 18.1-57.9 nmol/L)	(SI: 19.3-69.0 nmol/L)
20 years	122-384 ng/mL	132-457 ng/mL
	(SI: 16.0-50.3 nmol/L)	(SI: 17.3-59.9 nmol/L)

Patient Age	Female	Male
21-25 years	116-341 ng/mL	116-341 ng/mL
	(SI: 15.2-44.7 nmol/L)	(SI: 15.2-44.7 nmol/L)
26-30 years	117-321 ng/mL	117-321 ng/mL
	(SI: 15.3-42.1 nmol/L)	(SI: 15.3-42.1 nmol/L)
31-35 years	113-297 ng/mL	113-297 ng/mL
	(SI: 14.8-38.9 nmol/L)	(SI: 14.8-38.9 nmol/L)
36-40 years	106-277 ng/mL	106-277 ng/mL
	(SI: 13.9-36.3 nmol/L)	(SI: 13.9-36.3 nmol/L)
41-45 years	98-261 ng/mL	98-261 ng/mL
	(SI: 12.8-34.2 nmol/L)	(SI: 12.8-34.2 nmol/L)
46-50 years	91-246 ng/mL	91-246 ng/mL
	(SI: 11.9-32.2 nmol/L)	(SI: 11.9-32.2 nmol/L)
51-55 years	84-233 ng/mL	84-233 ng/mL
	(SI: 11.0-30.5 nmol/L)	(SI: 11.0-30.5 nmol/L)
56-60 years	78-220 ng/mL	78-220 ng/mL
	(SI: 10.2-28.8 nmol/L)	(SI: 10.2-28.8 nmol/L)
61-65 years	72-207 ng/mL	72-207 ng/mL
	(SI: 9.4-27.1 nmol/L)	(SI: 9.4-27.1 nmol/L)
66-70 years	67-195 ng/mL	67-195 ng/mL
	(SI: 8.8-25.5 nmol/L)	(SI: 8.8-25.5 nmol/L)
71-75 years	62-184 ng/mL	62-184 ng/mL
	(SI: 8.1-24.1 nmol/L)	(SI: 8.1-24.1 nmol/L)
76-80 years	57-172 ng/mL	57-172 ng/mL
	(SI: 7.5-22.5 nmol/L)	(SI: 7.5-22.5 nmol/L)
>80 years	53-162 ng/mL	53-162 ng/mL
	(SI: 6.9-21.2 nmol/L)	(SI: 6.9-21.2 nmol/L)

Insulinlike growth factor binding protein 3 --------------2.5-4.8 mg/L

Insulin------------------------- 1.4-14.0 µIU/mL (SI: 9.7-97.2 pmol/L)

Islet-cell antibody assay------- 0 Juvenile Diabetes Foundation units

Luteinizing hormone (LH)--- 1.0-9.0 mIU/mL (SI: 1.0-9.0 IU/L) (male);
  <1.0 mIU/mL (SI: <1.0 IU/L) (prepuberty, female);
  1.0-18.0 mIU/mL (SI: 1.0-18.0 IU/L) (follicular, female);
  20.0-80.0 mIU/mL (SI: 20.0-80.0 IU/L) (midcycle, female);
  0.5-18.0 mIU/mL (SI: 0.5-18.0 IU/L) (luteal, female);
  >30 mIU/mL (SI: >30 IU/L) (postmenopausal, female)

Metanephrines (plasma fractionated)
  Metanephrine -----------------------<99 pg/mL (SI: <0.50 nmol/L)
  Normetanephrine ----------------- <165 pg/mL (SI: <0.90 nmol/L)

75-g oral glucose tolerance test blood glucose values---------------
  60-100 mg/dL (SI: 3.3-5.6 mmol/L) (fasting);
  <200 mg/dL (SI: <11.1 mmol/L) (1 hour);
  <140 mg/dL (SI: <7.8 mmol/L) (2 hour); between 140-200 mg/dL
  (SI: 7.8-11.1 mmol/L) is considered impaired glucose tolerance or
  prediabetes. Greater than 200 mg/dL (SI: 11.1 mmol/L) is a sign
  of diabetes mellitus.

50-g oral glucose tolerance test for gestational diabetes -----------
  <140 mg/dL (SI: <7.8 mmol/L) (1 hour)

100-g oral glucose tolerance test for gestational diabetes ----------
  <95 mg/dL (SI: <5.3 mmol/L) (fasting);
  <180 mg/dL (SI: <10.0 mmol/L) (1 hour);
  <155 mg/dL (SI: <8.6 mmol/L) (2 hour);
  <140 mg/dL (SI: <7.8 mmol/L) (3 hour)

Osteocalcin ---------------------- 9.0-42.0 ng/mL (SI: 9.0-42.0 µg/L)

Parathyroid hormone, intact (PTH) ---- 10-65 pg/mL (SI: 10-65 ng/L)

Parathyroid hormone–related protein (PTHrP) -----------<2.0 pmol/L

Progesterone --------------------≤1.2 ng/mL (SI: ≤3.8 nmol/L) (male);

    ≤1.0 ng/mL (SI: ≤3.2 nmol/L) (follicular, female);

    2.0-20.0 ng/mL (SI: 6.4-63.6 nmol/L) (luteal, female);

    ≤1.1 ng/mL (SI: ≤3.5 nmol/L) (postmenopausal, female);

    >10.0 ng/mL (SI: >31.8 nmol/L) (evidence of ovulatory adequacy)

Proinsulin -------------------- 26.5-176.4 pg/mL (SI: 3.0-20.0 pmol/L)

Prolactin ------------------ 4-23 ng/mL (SI: 0.17-1.00 nmol/L) (male);

    4-30 ng/mL (SI: 0.17-1.30 nmol/L) (nonlactating female);

    10-200 ng/mL (SI: 0.43-8.70 nmol/L) (lactating female)

Prostate-specific antigen (PSA) -------------------------------------

    <2.0 ng/mL (SI: <2.0 µg/L) (≤40 years);

    <2.8 ng/mL (SI: <2.8 µg/L) (≤50 years);

    <3.8 ng/mL (SI: <3.8 µg/L) (≤60 years);

    <5.3 ng/mL (SI: <5.3 µg/L) (≤70 years);

    <7.0 ng/mL (SI: <7.0 µg/L) (≤79 years);

    <7.2 ng/mL (SI: <7.2 µg/L) (≥80 years)

Renin activity, plasma, sodium replete, ambulatory ----------------

    0.6-4.3 ng/mL per h

Renin, direct concentration ---------- 4-44 pg/mL (SI: 0.1-1.0 pmol/L)

Sex hormone–binding globulin (SHBG) --------------- 1.1-6.7 µg/mL

    (SI: 10-60 nmol/L) (male);

    2.2-14.6 µg/mL (SI: 20-130 nmol/L) (female)

α-Subunit of pituitary glycoprotein hormones ----------------------

    <1.2 ng/mL (SI: <1.2 µg/L)

Testosterone (bioavailable) ----- 0.8-4.0 ng/dL (SI: 0.03-0.14 nmol/L)

    (20-50 years, female on oral estrogen);

    0.8-10.0 ng/dL (SI: 0.03-0.35 nmol/L)

    (20-50 years, female not on oral estrogen);

    83.0-257.0 ng/dL (SI: 2.88-8.92 nmol/L) (male 20-29 years);

    72.0-235.0 ng/dL (SI: 2.50-8.15 nmol/L) (male 30-39 years);

    61.0-213.0 ng/dL (SI: 2.12-7.39 nmol/L) (male 40-49 years);

    50.0-190.0 ng/dL (SI: 1.74-6.59 nmol/L) (male 50-59 years);

    40.0-168.0 ng/dL (SI: 1.39-5.83 nmol/L) (male 60-69 years)

Testosterone (free) ----- 9.0-30.0 ng/dL (SI: 0.31-1.04 nmol/L) (male);

    0.3-1.9 ng/dL (SI: 0.01-0.07 nmol/L) (female)

Testosterone (total) ------- 300-900 ng/dL (10.4-31.2 nmol/L) (male);

    8-60 ng/dL (0.3-2.1 nmol/L) (female)

Vitamin B_{12} -------------------- 180-914 pg/mL (SI: 133-674 pmol/L)

Chemistry Values

Alanine aminotransferase ---------- 10-40 U/L (SI: 0.17-0.67 µkat/L)

Albumin---------------------------------3.5-5.0 g/dL (SI: 35-50 g/L)

Amylase -------------------------- 26-102 U/L (SI: 0.43-1.70 µkat/L)

Aspartate aminotransferase ------- 20-48 U/L (SI: 0.33-0.80 µkat/L)

Bicarbonate ---------------------- 21-28 mEq/L (SI: 21-28 mmol/L)

Bilirubin (total) ------------------- 0.3-1.2 mg/dL (SI: 5.1-20.5 µmol/L)

Blood gases

    P_{O_2}, arterial blood ------------ 80-100 mm Hg (SI: 10.6-13.3 kPa)

    P_{CO_2}, arterial blood ----------------35-45 mm Hg (SI: 4.7-6.0 kPa)

Blood pH---7.35-7.45

Calcium ----------------------- 8.2-10.2 mg/dL (SI: 2.1-2.6 mmol/L)

Calcium (ionized) -------------- 4.60-5.08 mg/dL (SI: 1.2-1.3 mmol/L)

Carbon dioxide ---------------------- 22-28 mEq/L (SI: 22-28 mmol/L)

CD_4 cell count---------------------- 500-1400/µL (SI: 0.5-1.4 × 10^9/L)

Chloride------------------------- 96-106 mEq/L (SI: 96-106 mmol/L)

Creatine kinase ------------------- 50-200 U/L (SI: 0.84-3.34 µkat/L)

Creatinine------------- 0.7-1.3 mg/dL (SI: 61.9-114.9 µmol/L) (male);

    0.6-1.1 mg/dL (SI: 53.0-97.2 µmol/L) (female)

Ferritin ----------------------- 15-200 ng/mL (SI: 33.7-449.4 pmol/L)

Folate -- ≥4.0 ng/mL (SI: ≥4.0 µg/L)

Glucose --------------------------- 70-99 mg/dL (SI: 3.9-5.5 mmol/L)

γ-Glutamyltransferase --------------- 2-30 U/L (SI: 0.03-0.50 µkat/L)

Iron ----------------------50-150 µg/dL (SI: 9.0-26.8 µmol/L) (male);

    35-145 µg/dL (SI: 6.3-26.0 µmol/L) (female)

Lactate dehydrogenase ------------ 100-200 U/L (SI: 1.7-3.3 µkat/L)

Lactic acid ---------------------- 5.4-20.7 mg/dL (SI: 0.6-2.3 mmol/L)

Lipase ----------------------------- 10-73 U/L (SI: 0.17-1.22 µkat/L)

Magnesium ---------------------- 1.5-2.3 mg/dL (SI: 0.6-0.9 mmol/L)

Osmolality --------------- 275-295 mOsm/kg (SI: 275-295 mmol/kg)

Phosphate ----------------------- 2.3-4.7 mg/dL (SI: 0.7-1.5 mmol/L)

Potassium ------------------------3.5-5.0 mEq/L (SI: 3.5-5.0 mmol/L)

Prothrombin time -- 8.3-10.8 s

Serum urea nitrogen---------------- 8-23 mg/dL (SI: 2.9-8.2 mmol/L)

Sodium ---------------------- 136-142 mEq/L (SI: 136-142 mmol/L)

Transferrin saturation -------------------------------------- 14%-50%

Troponin I -------------------------------- <0.6 ng/mL (SI: <0.6 µg/L)

Tryptase -------------------------------- <11.5 ng/mL (SI: <11.5 µg/L)

Uric acid --------------------- 3.5-7.0 mg/dL (SI: 208.2-416.4 µmol/L)

Urine

Albumin------------- 30-300 µg/mg creat (SI: 3.4-33.9 µg/mol creat)

Albumin-to-creatinine ratio -------------------------- <30 mg/g creat

Aldosterone---------------------- 3-20 µg/24 h (SI: 8.3-55.4 nmol/d)

    (should be <12 µg/24 h [SI: <33.2 nmol/d] with oral sodium

    loading—confirmed with 24-hour urinary sodium >200 mEq)

Calcium ----------------------- 100-300 mg/24 h (SI: 2.5-7.5 mmol/d)

Catecholamine fractionation

    Normotensive normal ranges:

        Dopamine--------------------<400 µg/24 h (SI: <2610 nmol/d)

        Epinephrine ----------------------<21 µg/24 h (SI: <115 nmol/d)

        Norepinephrine -----------------<80 µg/24 h (SI: <473 nmol/d)

Citrate --------------------320-1240 mg/24 h (SI: 16.7-64.5 mmol/d)

Cortisol ------------------------- 4-50 µg/24 h (SI: 11-138 nmol/d)

Cortisol following dexamethasone suppression test (low-dose:

    2 day, 2 mg daily) ------------------ <10 µg/24 h (SI: <27.6 nmol/d)

Creatinine------------------------ 1.0-2.0 g/24 h (SI: 8.8-17.7 mmol/d)

Glomerular filtration rate (estimated) ------->60 mL/min per 1.73 m^2

5-Hydroxyindole acetic acid----- 2-9 mg/24 h (SI: 10.5-47.1 µmol/d)

Iodine (random)--- >100 µg/L

17-Ketosteroids ---- 6.0-21.0 mg/24 h (SI: 20.8-72.9 µmol/d) (male);

    4.0-17.0 mg/24 h (SI: 13.9-59.0 µmol/d) (female)

Metanephrine fractionation

  Normotensive normal ranges:

    Metanephrine -------- <261 µg/24 h (SI: <1323 nmol/d) (male); <180 µg/24 h (<913 nmol/d) (female)

    Normetanephrine -------------------- age and sex dependent

    Total metanephrine ------------------ age and sex dependent

Osmolality ------------- 150-1150 mOsm/kg (SI: 150-1150 mmol/kg)

Oxalate ----------------------------- <40 mg/24 h (SI: <456 mmol/d)

Phosphate -------------------- 0.9-1.3 g/24 h (SI: 29.1-42.0 mmol/d)

Potassium ---------------------- 17-77 mEq/24 h (SI: 17-77 mmol/d)

Sodium ----------------------40-217 mEq/24 h (SI: 40-217 mmol/d)

Uric acid ----------------------------<800 mg/24 h (SI: <4.7 mmol/d)

Saliva

Cortisol (salivary), midnight ------------<0.13 µg/dL (SI: <3.6 nmol/L)

Semen

Semen analysis ---------------- >20 million sperm/mL; >50% motility

Abbreviations

ACTH --corticotropin

ACE inhibitor--------------- angiotensin-converting enzyme inhibitor

ALT -- alanine aminotransferase

AST ------------------------------------- aspartate aminotransferase

BMI --- body mass index

CNS--- central nervous system

CT--computed tomography

DHEA ------------------------------------- dehydroepiandrosterone

DHEA-S-------------------------- dehydroepiandrosterone sulfate

DNA -------------------------------------- deoxyribonucleic acid

DPP-4 inhibitor ----------------------dipeptidyl-peptidase 4 inhibitor

DXA ------------------------------ dual-energy x-ray absorptiometry

FDA ------------------------------------Food and Drug Administration

FGF-23 ------------------------------------ fibroblast growth factor 23

FNA---fine-needle aspiration

FSH ------------------------------------- follicle-stimulating hormone

GH --- growth hormone

GHRH------------------------ growth hormone–releasing hormone

GLP-1 receptor agonist----- glucagonlike peptide 1 receptor agonist

GnRH ----------------------------gonadotropin-releasing hormone

hCG ---------------------------------- human chorionic gonadotropin

HDL---high-density lipoprotein

HIV-- human immunodeficiency virus

HMG-CoA reductase inhibitor ---------- 3-hydroxy-3-methylglutaryl coenzyme A reductase inhibitor

IGF-1------------------------------------- insulinlike growth factor 1

LDL ---low-density lipoprotein

LH --- luteinizing hormone

MCV --mean corpuscular volume

MIBG----------------------------------- meta-iodobenzylguanidine

MRI ----------------------------------- magnetic resonance imaging

NPH insulin --------------------- neutral protamine Hagedorn insulin

PCSK9 inhibitor---- proprotein convertase subtilisin/kexin 9 inhibitor

PET ------------------------------------positron emission tomography

PSA -------------------------------------- prostate-specific antigen

PTH ---parathyroid hormone

PTHrP------------------------parathyroid hormone–related protein

SGLT-2 inhibitor -----------sodium-glucose cotransporter 2 inhibitor

SHBG -------------------------------- sex hormone–binding globulin

T_3 --- triiodothyronine

T_4 --- thyroxine

TPO antibodies ------------------------- thyroperoxidase antibodies

TRH------------------------------ thyrotropin-releasing hormone

TRAb ---------------------------------------TSH-receptor antibodies

TSH --- thyrotropin

VLDL----------------------------------- very low-density lipoprotein

ENDOCRINE SELF-ASSESSMENT PROGRAM 2021

Part I

1   A 44-year-old woman with type 2 diabetes mellitus treated with insulin presents with worsening hirsutism. She has a history of polycystic ovary syndrome and was previously treated with an oral contraceptive and spironolactone with good control of hyperandrogenism. She stopped taking both of these medications 3 years ago. Type 2 diabetes was diagnosed 7 years ago and was initially treated with metformin. Two years ago, her hemoglobin A_{1c} level was documented to be 8.3% (67 mmol/mol), and a basal-bolus insulin regimen was started. Over the past year, despite doubling her insulin doses and good adherence to her insulin regimen, her hemoglobin A_{1c} level has risen to 9.6% (81 mmol/mol). Concomitantly, she has noticed worsening hair growth on her face and chest. In the past 2 months, she has also had worsening lower-extremity edema, amenorrhea, fatigue, and generalized weakness.

On physical examination, her blood pressure is 180/96 mm Hg and pulse rate is 79 beats/min. Her height is 64 in (162.5 cm), and weight is 250 lb (113.4 kg) (BMI = 43 kg/m²). She has moon facies and a dorsocervical hump. There are terminal hairs on her face and chest, mostly removed by shaving. She has thick violaceous striae on her abdomen, proximal muscle weakness, and diffuse ecchymoses scattered over her arms and legs.

Laboratory test results:
    Morning serum cortisol following overnight 1-mg dexamethasone = 37.8 µg/dL (SI: 1042.8 nmol/L)
    Urinary free cortisol = 1925 µg/24 h (<4-50 µg/24 h) (SI: 5313 nmol/d [11-138 nmol/d])
    Random ACTH = <5 pg/mL (10-60 pg/mL) (SI: <1.1 pmol/L [2.2-13.2 pmol/L])
    Total testosterone = 182 ng/dL (8-60 ng/dL) (SI: 6.3 nmol/L [0.3-2.1 nmol/L])
    DHEA-S = 1490 µg/dL (18-244 µg/dL) (SI: 40.38 µmol/L [0.49-6.61 µmol/L])

Which of the following is the most likely cause of this patient's current presentation?
    A.   Surreptitious use of exogenous glucocorticoids
    B.   Adrenocortical adenoma
    C.   Adrenocortical carcinoma
    D.   Neuroendocrine tumor
    E.   Primary pigmented nodular adrenocortical disease

2   A 72-year-old woman is referred for management of osteoporosis, which was diagnosed at age 68 years when she had a DXA scan revealing T-scores of −3.2 in the right femoral neck and −2.9 in the left total hip. She took alendronate for 1 year and stopped due to the development of osteonecrosis of the jaw. She has not tried any other medications. She went through natural menopause at age 40 years and has not taken estrogen. She has no history of fragility fractures, kidney stones, or parathyroid disease.

Physical examination reveals a 2-cm area of exposed yellow bone in the right upper maxilla.

Laboratory test results:
    Serum calcium = 8.6 mg/dL (8.2-10.2 mg/dL) (SI: 2.2 mmol/L [2.1-2.6 mmol/L])
    Serum phosphate = 3.0 mg/dL (2.3-4.7 mg/dL) (SI: 1.0 mmol/L [0.7-1.5 mmol/L])
    Serum creatinine = 0.9 mg/dL (0.6-1.1 mg/dL) (SI: 79.6 µmol/L [53.0-97.2 µmol/L])
    Glomerular filtration rate (estimated) = 72 mL/min per 1.73 m² (>60 mL/min per 1.73 m²)
    Serum intact PTH = 60 pg/mL (10-65 pg/mL) (SI: 60 ng/L [10-65 ng/L])
    Serum 25-hydroxyvitamin D = 26 ng/mL (30-80 ng/mL [optimal]) (SI: 64.9 nmol/L [74.9-199.7 nmol/L])
    Serum albumin = 3.5 g/dL (3.5-5.0 g/dL) (SI: 35 g/L [35-50 g/L])
    Serum alkaline phosphatase = 110 U/L (50-120 U/L) (SI: 1.84 µkat/L [0.84-2.00 µkat/L])

A second DXA scan reveals declining bone mineral density in both hips, with T-scores of −3.5 in the right femoral neck and −3.2 in the left total hip.

Which of the following should be recommended in addition to adequate calcium and vitamin D supplementation?

    A. Raloxifene

    B. Zoledronic acid

    C. Denosumab

    D. Romosozumab

    E. Teriparatide

3 An 83-year-old woman with a 25-year history of type 2 diabetes mellitus presents for follow-up. Her hemoglobin A_{1c} level was approximately 6.5% (48 mmol/mol) for many years. Over the past 12 months, it has risen to greater than 8.0% (>64 mmol/mol). The patient reports that her diet is poor. She eats cake and cookies, especially at bedtime, although this is not substantially different from what she has done for years. She reports being in her usual state of health except for fatigue, lightheadedness, occasional loose stool, and unsteadiness on her feet. Review of her medical record reveals a 20-lb (9.1-kg) weight loss over 3 years. Current medications for blood glucose control are sitagliptin and metformin.

On physical examination, she is a frail elderly woman who needs help with ambulation. Her blood pressure is 131/71 mm Hg, and pulse rate is 84 beats/min. Her height is 64 in (162.6 cm), and weight is 117.5 lb (53.4 kg) (BMI = 20 kg/m²). Examination findings are normal.

Laboratory test results:

    Hemoglobin A_{1c} = 8.4% (4.0%-5.6%) (68 mmol/mol [20-38 mmol/mol])

    Sodium = 132 mEq/L (136-142 mEq/L) (SI: 132 mmol/L [136-142 mmol/L])

    Potassium = 4.2 mEq/L (3.5-5.0 mEq/L) (SI: 4.2 mmol/L [3.5-5.0 mmol/L])

    Chloride = 96 mEq/L (96-106 mEq/L) (SI: 96 mmol/L [96-106 mmol/L])

    Carbon dioxide = 26 mEq/L (22-28 mEq/L) (SI: 26 mmol/L [22-28 mmol/L])

    Serum urea nitrogen = 16 mg/dL (8-23 mg/dL) (SI: 5.7 mmol/L [2.9-8.2 mmol/L])

    Creatinine = 0.62 mg/dL (0.6-1.1 mg/dL) (SI: 54.8 μmol/L [53.0-97.2 μmol/L])

    Glucose = 342 mg/dL (70-99 mg/dL) (SI: 19.0 mmol/L [3.9-5.5 mmol/L])

Which of the following is the best next step in this patient's management?

    A. Initiate insulin therapy

    B. Measure fructosamine

    C. Perform abdominal CT

    D. Add glimepiride

    E. Measure serum somatostatin

4 A 56-year-old woman is referred for cardiovascular risk management. She has a history of moderate hypercholesterolemia. Despite multiple attempts, she has been unable to take statins for many years because of muscle aches. She has no major concerns or other medical problems. Medications include ezetimibe, 10 mg daily, and aspirin, 81 mg daily. She does not smoke cigarettes or drink alcohol. Family history is notable for premature cardiovascular disease in her 49-year-old brother (nonsmoker) who underwent placement of 2 coronary stents. Her mother, who had a 40 pack-year history of cigarette smoking, had coronary bypass surgery at age 74 years.

On physical examination, she is an anxious-appearing woman in no acute distress. Her blood pressure is 132/84 mm Hg. Her height is 63 in (160 cm), and weight is 178 lb (80.9 kg) (BMI = 31.5 kg/m²). The rest of the examination findings are normal except for abdominal adiposity.

Laboratory test results (sample drawn while fasting):

Total cholesterol = 211 mg/dL (<200 mg/dL [optimal]) (SI: 5.46 mmol/L [<5.18 mmol/L])

Triglycerides = 130 mg/dL (<150 mg/dL [optimal]) (SI: 1.47 mmol/L [<1.70 mmol/L])

HDL cholesterol = 55 mg/dL (>60 mg/dL [optimal]) (SI: 1.42 mmol/L [>1.55 mmol/L])

LDL cholesterol = 130 mg/dL (<100 mg/dL [optimal]) (SI: 3.37 mmol/L [<2.59 mmol/L])

Non-HDL cholesterol = 156 mg/dL (<130 mg/dL [optimal]) (SI: 4.04 mmol/L [<3.37 mmol/L])

Lipoprotein (a) = 26 mg/dL (≤30 mg/dL) (SI: 0.93 μmol/L [≤1.07 μmol/L])

Hemoglobin A_{1c} = 5.2% (4.0%-5.6%) (33 mmol/mol [20-38 mmol/mol])

Creatinine = 0.84 mg/dL (0.6-1.1 mg/dL) (SI: 74.3 μmol/L [53.0-97.2 μmol/L])

TSH = 1.8 mIU/L (0.5-5.0 mIU/L)

She is unwilling to try statin therapy again. Using the American College of Cardiology/American Heart Association risk calculator, you calculate her 10-year cardiovascular risk to be 2.5%. However, based on her family history, you are concerned that this tool underestimates her risk.

Which of the following is the best next test in the evaluation of this patient's cardiovascular disease risk stratification?
- A. Apolipoprotein B measurement
- B. Apolipoprotein A-1 measurement
- C. Carotid intima media thickness
- D. Coronary artery calcium scoring
- E. Stress echocardiography

5 A 66-year-old man is referred for management of type 2 diabetes mellitus. He has had type 2 diabetes for 16 years, and his regimen was transitioned to multiple daily injections (U500 regular insulin) 4 years ago. The dosage of U500 has been titrated over the past few years, but despite 175 units of U500 regular insulin 3 times daily (total daily dose = 525 units), his blood glucose remains suboptimally controlled with a hemoglobin A_{1c} level of 9.7% (83 mmol/mol).

The patient's BMI is 57 kg/m², and he reports that his lifestyle is sedentary. His comorbidities include coronary artery disease status post coronary artery bypass grafting 8 years ago, obstructive sleep apnea, hypertension, hyperlipidemia, and stage 4 chronic kidney disease with microalbuminuria. His diabetes is complicated by neuropathy, which is currently well controlled with gabapentin. His wife reports that while he is adherent to his insulin regimen and point-of-care blood glucose checks, he does not follow the dietary recommendations he has received from nutrition counseling. He snacks frequently and generally consumes large portions of food, particularly carbohydrates.

Current medications are atorvastatin, U500 regular insulin, gabapentin, lisinopril, and amlodipine.

Laboratory test results:

Hemoglobin A_{1c} = 9.7% (4.0%-5.6%) (83 mmol/mol [20-38 mmol/mol])

Serum creatinine = 2.4 mg/dL (0.7-1.3 mg/dL) (SI: 212.2 μmol/L [61.9-114.9 μmol/L])

Estimated glomerular filtration rate = 27 mL/min per 1.73 m² (>60 mL/min per 1.73 m²)

Which of the following is the best next step in this patient's management?
- A. Add an SGLT-2 inhibitor
- B. Increase the dosage of U500 regular insulin
- C. Add pioglitazone
- D. Add a GLP-1 receptor agonist
- E. Add metformin

6   A 46-year-old man presents with gradual-onset fatigue, decreased libido, and erectile dysfunction over the last 12 months. He reports a significant alcohol history and consumes an average of 3 standard drinks per day. His father died of heart failure at age 63 years. He has 2 sons aged 23 and 18 years. On review of systems, he describes occasional joint pain in his hands and knees.

On physical examination, he has a tanned appearance. His height is 68 in (173 cm), and weight is 185 lb (83.9 kg) (BMI = 28 kg/m²). Waist circumference is 41 in (104 cm). Blood pressure is 152/85 mm Hg, and resting pulse rate is 70 beats/min. There is no evidence of arthropathy, and findings on cardiac examination are normal. His liver is palpable 2 cm below the right costal margin. There is no clinical visual field defect, and he has full range of eye movements. There is no palpable gynecomastia, and testes are 18 mL bilaterally.

Laboratory test results (sample drawn at 8 AM while fasting):
    Total testosterone = 167 ng/dL (300-900 ng/dL) (SI: 5.8 nmol/L [10.4-31.2 nmol/L])
    SHBG = 6.6 μg/mL (1.1-6.7 μg/mL) (SI: 59 nmol/L [10-60 nmol/L])
    LH = 3.5 mIU/mL (1.0-9.0 mIU/mL) (SI: 3.5 IU/L [1.0-9.0 IU/L])
    FSH = 2.9 mIU/mL (1.0-13.0 mIU/mL) (SI: 2.9 IU/L [1.0-13.0 IU/L])
    Hemoglobin = 16.9 g/dL (13.8-17.2 g/dL) (SI: 169 g/L [138-172 g/L])
    ALT = 54 U/L (10-40 U/L) (SI: 0.90 μkat/L [0.17-0.67 μkat/L])
    AST = 70 U/L (20-48 U/L) (SI: 1.17 μkat/L [0.33-0.80 μkat/L])
    γ-Glutamyltransferase = 84 U/L (2-30 U/L) (SI: 1.40 μkat/L [0.03-0.50 μkat/L])
    Hemoglobin A_{1c} = 6.6% (4.0%-5.6%) (49 mmol/mol [20-38 mmol/L])
    Serum electrolytes, normal
    Thyroid function, normal
    Prolactin, normal

A repeated total testosterone measurement 1 week later (sample drawn at 8 AM while fasting) is 150 ng/dL (SI: 5.2 nmol/L).

Which of the following is the most important test to order now?
    A. No further testing necessary, hypogonadism will improve with weight loss and alcohol abstinence
    B. Pituitary-directed MRI
    C. ACTH and cortisol measurements
    D. Iron studies
    E. Serum ACE measurement

7   An 82-year-old man is referred for evaluation and recommendations regarding a recent vertebral fracture. Approximately 3 weeks ago, he lost his balance and sat down severely onto his buttocks, which was immediately followed by acute onset of midline low back pain. Subsequent plain x-rays obtained by his primary care physician revealed a moderate (~35%) biconcave compression deformity at the second lumbar vertebrae. He has no other history of fractures as an adult. His medical history is notable for hypertension and hyperlipidemia. Family history is positive for osteoporosis in his mother based on history of vertebral fractures and kyphosis. His medications include benazepril, atorvastatin, and a multivitamin.

On physical examination, his blood pressure is 135/80 mm Hg and pulse rate is 95 beats/min. His height is 68 in (172.7 cm), and weight is 143 lb (64.8 kg) (BMI = 22 kg/m²). His current height is 3 in (7.6 cm) shorter than his self-reported adult maximum height. He has tenderness to palpation and percussion over the mid-lumbar spine. Mild midthoracic kyphosis is also noted. Rib-to-pelvis distance is diminished at 1 fingerbreadth bilaterally.

Laboratory test results (serum):
    Calcium = 9.5 mg/dL (8.2-10.2 mg/dL) (SI: 2.4 mmol/L [2.1-2.6 mmol/L])
    Phosphate = 3.5 mg/dL (2.3-4.7 mg/dL) (SI: 1.1 mmol/L [0.7-1.5 mmol/L])
    Creatinine = 1.6 mg/dL (0.7-1.3 mg/dL) (SI: 141.4 μmol/L [61.9-114.9 μmol/L])
    Albumin = 4.0 g/dL (3.5-5.0 g/dL) (SI: 40 g/L [35-50 g/L])
    Intact PTH = 70 pg/mL (10-65 pg/mL) (SI: 70 ng/L [10-65 ng/L])

25-Hydroxyvitamin D = 25 ng/mL (30-80 ng/mL [optimal]) (SI: 62.4 nmol/L [74.9-199.7 nmol/L])
Urinary calcium excretion = 300 mg/24 h (100-300 mg/24 h) (SI: 7.5 mmol/d [2.5-7.5 mmol/d])
Urinary creatinine excretion = 1.2 g/24 h (1.0-2.0 g/24 h) (SI: 10.6 mmol/d [8.8-17.7 mmol/d])

DXA documents the following values:
Lumbar spine T-score (excluding L2) = −1.6
Right femoral neck T-score = −2.2
Right total hip T-score = −1.8

Given these clinical findings, which of the following is the most appropriate treatment for this patient's metabolic bone disorder?
A. Supplemental calcium and vitamin D
B. Supplemental calcium and vitamin D and an oral bisphosphonate
C. Supplemental calcium and vitamin D and an intravenous bisphosphonate
D. Supplemental calcium and vitamin D and teriparatide
E. No treatment is required

8 A 30-year-old woman returns for continued management of type 1 diabetes mellitus and hypothyroidism. She feels well and has no concerns on review of systems. Diabetes was diagnosed at age 14 years. She has been treated with basal-bolus insulin for the last 14 years. She has had reasonable glycemic control, with hemoglobin A_{1c} levels ranging from 6.6% to 7.5% (49-58 mmol/mol) over the last 4 years. Diabetes-related microvascular complications include mild nonproliferative diabetic retinopathy and peripheral neuropathy.

Primary hypothyroidism was diagnosed 12 years ago and is treated with levothyroxine. The levothyroxine dosage was increased to 175 mcg daily 2 months ago. She takes her medication as directed, 60 minutes before eating breakfast, and never misses a dose. She has a history of anemia, which was treated with a 12-month course of iron, ending 1 year ago. She has 2 bowel movements per day and has no abdominal bloating. Her mother and sister have a history of hypothyroidism. Her mother has thalassemia major.

On physical examination, her height is 67 in (170.2 cm) and weight is 168 lb (76.4 kg) (BMI = 26.3 kg/m²). Blood pressure is 112/68 mm Hg, and pulse rate is 72 beats/min. There is a slight deficit in sensation to 10-g monofilament in each foot.

Laboratory test results:
Hemoglobin A_{1c} = 7.2% (4.0%-5.6%) (55 mmol/mol [20-38 mmol/mol])
Creatinine = 0.8 mg/dL (0.6-1.1 mg/dL) (SI: 70.7 μmol/L [53.0-97.2 μmol/L])
Fasting plasma glucose = 92 mg/dL (70-99 mg/dL) (SI: 5.1 mmol/L [3.9-5.5 mmol/L])
Calcium = 9.0 mg/dL (8.2-10.2 mg/dL) (SI: 2.3 mmol/L [2.1-2.6 mmol/L])
TSH = 10.1 mIU/L (0.5-5.0 mIU/L)
Free T_4 = 1.0 ng/dL (0.8-1.8 ng/dL) (SI: 12.9 pmol/L [10.30-23.17 pmol/L])
Hemoglobin = 11.2 g/dL (12.1-15.1 g/dL) (SI: 112 g/L [121-151 g/L])
Iron = 28 μg/dL (35-145 μg/dL) (SI: 5.0 μmol/L [6.3-26.0 μmol/L])
Mean corpuscular volume = 78 μm³ (80-100 μm³) (SI: 78 fL [80-100 fL])

Which of the following is the best next step in this patient's management?
A. Start iron sulfate to be taken separately from the levothyroxine
B. Increase the levothyroxine dosage to 200 mcg daily
C. Order hemoglobin electrophoresis
D. Order a celiac enteropathy panel
E. Switch the time levothyroxine is administered to bedtime

9 A 43-year-old woman is referred for a newly diagnosed pituitary macroadenoma. She developed amenorrhea 6 years ago and was told (without any hormonal evaluation) that she had early menopause. She has frequent headaches and has noted blurry vision that started 4 months ago. MRI shows a very large solid sellar mass (4.2 cm in maximal diameter) compressing the optic chiasm and most likely invading the left cavernous sinus (*see image*). On physical examination, she has bitemporal hemianopsia.

Laboratory test results:
  Prolactin = 37 ng/mL (4-30 ng/mL) (SI: 1.6 nmol/L [0.17-1.30 nmol/L])
  Free T$_4$ = 0.7 ng/dL (0.8-1.8 ng/dL) (SI: 9.0 nmol/L [10.30-23.17 pmol/L])
  TSH = 1.3 mIU/L (0.5-5 mIU/L)
  IGF-1 = 112 ng/mL (98-261 ng/mL) (SI: 14.7 nmol/L [12.8-34.2 nmol/L])
  Cortisol (8 AM) = 16.8 µg/dL (5-25 µg/dL) (SI: 463.5 nmol/L
    [137.9-689.7 nmol/L])

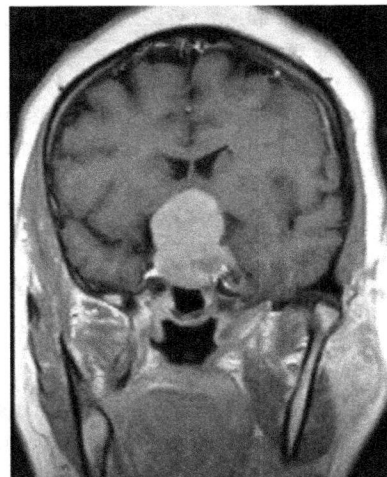

In addition to starting levothyroxine replacement therapy, which of the following is the best next step?
  A. Measure α-subunit
  B. Measure prolactin after dilution
  C. Measure macroprolactin
  D. Refer to radiation oncology
  E. Refer to neurosurgery

10 A 36-year-old man falls on ice and sustains a right hip fracture. DXA scan shows a Z-score of −3.5 in the spine and −2.7 in the left femoral neck. He reports multiple shoulder and knee dislocations as a child and adolescent. He also reports easy bruising. He has good dietary calcium intake and does not take any supplements or medications. He has normal libido. His mother is being treated for osteoporosis.

On physical examination, he has velvety skin and mild thoracolumbar scoliosis. His arm span to height ratio is 0.9.

Laboratory testing documents normal results from a complete metabolic panel (including calcium and phosphate) and serum 25-hydroxyvitamin D measurement.

Which of the following is this patient's most likely diagnosis?
  A. Osteogenesis imperfecta
  B. Ehlers-Danlos syndrome
  C. Marfan syndrome
  D. Hereditary hypophosphatemic rickets
  E. Hypophosphatasia

11 A 19-year-old woman with hypothyroidism presents for her yearly follow-up visit. She reports a left neck swelling and tenderness that has been present for 4 days. She has had no fever, chills, shortness of breath, dysphagia, or dysphonia. There is no history of radiation to her head and neck and no family history of thyroid cancer or laryngeal cancer. She currently takes levothyroxine, 112 mcg daily.

On physical examination, her blood pressure is 103/56 mm Hg and pulse rate is 90 beats/min. Her temperature is 98.6°F (37°C). There is a visible fullness on the left side of her neck (level II). On palpation, you feel a 3 × 2-cm, subcutaneous, mildly tender, fluctuant, somewhat mobile mass anterior to the sternocleidomastoid muscle and under the angle of the mandible. The overlying skin is not erythematous and the lesion is not fixed to the skin. The thyroid gland is not palpable, and there is no tracheal deviation. The rest of the examination findings are normal.

Laboratory test results:
 TSH = 1.4 mIU/L (0.5-5.0 mIU/L)
 Calcium = 9.0 mg/dL (8.2-10.2 mg/dL)
  (SI: 2.3 mmol/L [2.1-2.6 mmol/L])
 Complete blood cell count, normal

Neck CT is ordered (*see images*).

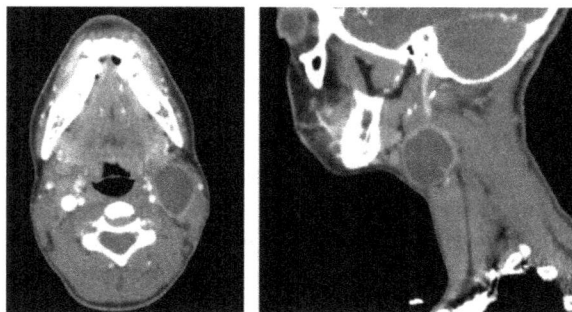

Which of the following is this patient's most likely diagnosis?
 A. Cervical lymphadenopathy
 B. Neck abscess
 C. Paraganglioma
 D. Thyroglossal duct cyst
 E. Branchial cleft cyst

12 A 40-year-old woman is referred for evaluation of worsening alopecia and hirsutism. She has a several-year history of cyclical symptoms. The most recent episode of hair loss is her primary concern because of the severity and lack of response to medication changes. Her medical history is notable for premature ovarian insufficiency diagnosed 2 years ago when she developed secondary amenorrhea. Concentrations of FSH and total testosterone were documented to be 65 mIU/mL (65 IU/L) and 61 ng/dL (2.1 nmol/L), respectively. At that time, she restarted oral contraceptives. Menarche was at age 11 years, and she initially had regular menses, occurring every 30 to 35 days. She conceived without difficulty at age 24 years.

On physical examination, her height is 62.5 in (158.8 cm) and weight is 149.5 lb (83 kg) (BMI = 27 kg/m^2). Her blood pressure is 113/59 mm Hg. Scalp demonstrates male-pattern hair loss without any patches of hair loss. She has no striae, facial plethora, or dorsocervical or supraclavicular fat pads. There is mild papular acne. Terminal hair growth is present on the chin only. She is able to rise and walk without difficulty. The rest of her examination findings are normal.

Laboratory test results on oral contraceptives:
 TSH = 1.4 mIU/L (0.5-5.0 mIU/L)
 Total testosterone = 92 ng/dL (8-60 ng/dL) (SI: 3.2 nmol/L [0.3-2.1 nmol/L])
 Prolactin = 13.1 ng/mL (4-30 ng/mL) (SI: 0.57 nmol/L [0.17-1.30 nmol/L])
 FSH = 24.5 mIU/mL (>30.0 mIU/mL [postmenopausal]) (SI: 24.5 IU/L [>30.0 IU/L])
 LH = 22.2 mIU/mL (>30.0 mIU/mL [postmenopausal]) (SI: 24.5 IU/L [>30.0 IU/L])
 DHEA-S = 70 µg/dL (31-228 µg/dL) (SI: 1.90 µmol/L [0.84-6.78 µmol/L])

Ovarian ultrasonography does not reveal a tumor; the right ovarian volume is 7.7 mL and the left ovarian volume is 2.2 mL.

Which of the following is the best next step in this patient's management?
 A. Start spironolactone
 B. Prescribe the combined oral contraceptive continuously to eliminate the placebo week
 C. Refer for ovarian/adrenal venous sampling
 D. Refer to gynecology for right oophorectomy
 E. Start leuprolide

13 A 36-year-old man with a 26-year history of type 1 diabetes mellitus presents for a visit. He reports that he underwent a coronary artery calcium study through his employer, as it was offered for free, and he brings the report for your interpretation. The coronary artery calcium score is 153, placing him at greater than or equal to the 75th percentile for his age.

He uses a multiple daily injection regimen for management of diabetes and takes no other medications. His regimen consists of insulin degludec, 18 units daily, and insulin aspart via a smart pen based on carbohydrate ratios. He is an avid cyclist and hiker. He does not smoke cigarettes, and he drinks 2 to 3 alcoholic beverages a week. There is no strong family history of atherosclerotic cardiovascular disease.

On physical examination, his height is 78 in (198 cm) and weight is 204.5 lb (93 kg) (BMI = 23.6 kg/m^2). His blood pressure is 106/77 mm Hg. There is vitiligo on his hands, but the rest of his examination findings are normal.

Laboratory test results (sample drawn while fasting):
Total cholesterol = 158 mg/dL (<200 mg/dL [optimal]) (SI: 4.09 mmol/L [<5.18 mmol/L])
Triglycerides = 82 mg/dL (<150 mg/dL [optimal]) (SI: 0.93 mmol/L [<1.70 mmol/L])
HDL cholesterol = 55 mg/dL (>60 mg/dL [optimal]) (SI: 1.42 mmol/L [>1.55 mmol/L])
LDL cholesterol = 87 mg/dL (<100 mg/dL [optimal]) (SI: 2.25 mmol/L [<2.59 mmol/L])
Non-HDL cholesterol = 103 mg/dL (<130 mg/dL [optimal]) (SI: 2.67 mmol/L [<3.37 mmol/L])
Lipoprotein (a) = 3 mg/dL (≤30 mg/dL) (SI: 0.11 μmol/L [≤1.07 μmol/L])
Hemoglobin A$_{1c}$ = 6.6% (4.0%-5.6%) (49 mmol/mol [20-38 mmol/mol])
Creatinine = 0.7 mg/dL (0.7-1.3 mg/dL) (SI: 61.9 μmol/L [61.9-114.9 μmol/L])
TSH = 2.8 mIU/L (0.5-5.0 mIU/L)
Urine albumin-to-creatinine ratio = 3 mg/g creat (<30 mg/g creat)

His American College of Cardiology/American Heart Association cardiovascular risk score is calculated to be 3.9%.

Which of the following is the best next step in this patient's management?
A. Refer to a dietician for counseling on a low-calcium diet
B. Start empagliflozin, 10 mg daily
C. Start atorvastatin, 20 mg daily
D. Start atorvastatin, 5 mg daily
E. Recommend no further therapy at this time

14 A 37-year-old white man presents for management of diabetes. He reports that type 1 diabetes mellitus was diagnosed when he was a child. He has had suboptimal glucose control most of his life, with a hemoglobin A$_{1c}$ level in the range of 9% to 11% (75-97 mmol/mol). His most recent hemoglobin A$_{1c}$ value is 10.5% (91 mmol/mol). He has neuropathy, stage 4 chronic kidney disease with macroalbuminuria, and uncontrolled hypertension.

He takes insulin lispro, 5 units at meals, plus supplemental insulin (1 unit per 50 mg/dL blood glucose >150 mg/dL [>8.3 mmol/L]) and 22 units of insulin glargine at bedtime.

He reports that his mother and 2 siblings also have diabetes. His mother is on insulin therapy, but he is not sure how long she has been receiving insulin or when she was diagnosed with diabetes. His mother told him that he was diagnosed with diabetes shortly after birth and that his 2 siblings were also diagnosed with type 1 diabetes in a similar timeframe.

On physical examination, his height is 67 in (170.2 cm), and weight is 142 lb (64.5 kg) (BMI = 22 kg/m^2). No lipohypertrophy is noted around the sites of insulin administration. Decreased sensation on the plantar aspect of both feet is appreciated with 10-g monofilament testing.

Hemoglobin A$_{1c}$ = 10.5% (4.0%-5.6%) (91 mmol/mol [20-38 mmol/mol])
Creatinine = 2.8 mg/dL (0.7-1.3 mg/dL) (SI: 247.5 μmol/L [61.9-114.9 μmol/L])
Random glucose = 275 mg/dL (70-99 mg/dL) (SI: 15.3 mmol/L [3.9-5.5 mmol/L])
C-peptide (drawn simultaneously with random glucose) = <0.2 ng/mL (0.9-4.3 ng/mL) (SI: <0.07 nmol/L [0.30-1.42 nmol/L])
Glutamic acid decarboxylase antibodies, undetectable
Islet-cell antibodies, undetectable

Ordering genetic testing for pathogenic variants in which of the following genes would most likely confirm this patient's diagnosis?
- A. *BSCL2*
- B. *HNF4A*
- C. *KCNJ11*
- D. *HNF1A*
- E. *AGPAT2*

15 An 18-year-old woman presents with worsening fatigue, sweating, and anxiety. She has a history of depression and anxiety and has been treated with venlafaxine, 37.5 mg daily, for the past year. Her mother describes her as always being a "sweaty child," even when she was younger.

On physical examination, her blood pressure is 113/70 mm Hg and pulse rate is 101 beats/min. Her height is 66 in (167.5 cm), and weight is 160 lb (72.6 kg) (BMI = 26 kg/m^2). She is in no apparent distress, and there are no signs of Cushing syndrome. Heart sounds are regular without murmurs, lungs are clear to auscultation, and her abdomen is soft and nontender. There is no lower-extremity edema or tremor of outstretched hands.

Laboratory test results:
- Plasma free metanephrine = 39 pg/mL (<99 pg/mL) (SI: <0.20 nmol/L [<0.50 nmol/L])
- Plasma free normetanephrine = 916 pg/mL (<165 pg/mL) (SI: 5.0 nmol/L [<0.90 nmol/L])
- Urinary metanephrine = 180 μg/24 h (<185 μg/24 h) (SI: 913 nmol/d [<938 nmol/d])
- Urinary normetanephrine = 6324 μg/24 h (<286 μg/24 h) (SI: 34,529 nmol/d [<1562 nmol/d])
- Urinary epinephrine = 4.2 μg/24 h (<21 μg/24 h) (SI: 23 nmol/d [<115 nmol/d])
- Urinary norepinephrine = 1423 μg/24 h (<80 μg/24 h) (SI: 8416 nmol/d [<473 nmol/d])

CT of the abdomen and pelvis reveals normal findings. Specifically, the adrenal glands have normal morphology and there are no abdominal masses.

Which of the following is the best next step in this patient's management?
- A. Cessation of venlafaxine for 4 to 6 weeks followed by repeated laboratory testing
- B. MRI of the abdomen and pelvis
- C. CT of the chest, mediastinum, and neck
- D. Toxicology testing for cocaine and methamphetamines
- E. No further testing; reassure the patient that symptoms are not due to a catecholamine-producing tumor

16 A previously well 19-year-old man presents to the emergency department with a 3-week history of an 11-lb (5-kg) weight loss, lethargy, palpitations, an irritating dry cough, and progressive left-sided pleuritic chest pain.

On physical examination, his blood pressure is 110/60 mm Hg and resting pulse rate is 120 beats/min and regular. He has a diffuse 30-mg goiter with an audible bruit. There is no exophthalmos or orbital inflammation. He has decreased breath sounds throughout the left hemithorax and marked bilateral 2-in (5.1 cm) gynecomastia. Testes are 2 mL bilaterally.

Laboratory test results:
- TSH = <0.03 mIU/L (0.5-5.0 mIU/L)
- Free T$_4$ = 6.3 ng/dL (0.8-1.8 ng/dL) (SI: 81.09 pmol/L [10.30-23.17 pmol/L])
- Free T$_3$ = 11.4 pg/mL (2.3-4.2 pg/mL) (SI: 17.51 pmol/L [3.53-6.45 pmol/L])
- Total testosterone = 213 ng/dL (300-900 ng/dL) (SI: 7.4 nmol/L [10.4-31.2 nmol/L])
- LH = <0.2 mIU/mL (1.0-9.0 mIU/mL) (SI: 0.2 IU/L [1.0-9.0 IU/L])
- FSH = <0.2 mIU/mL (1.0-13.0 mIU/mL) (SI: 0.7 IU/L [1.0-13.0 IU/L])
- Lactate dehydrogenase = 1374 IU/L (100-200 IU/L) (SI: 22.9 μkat/L [1.7-3.3 μkat/L])

Chest CT with intravenous contrast is shown (*see image*).

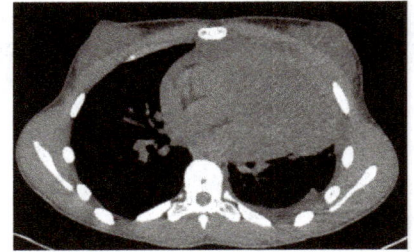

Which of the following is the most important diagnostic test to order now?
- A. β-hCG measurement
- B. TRAb assessment
- C. Nuclear medicine thyroid uptake and scan
- D. Karyotype analysis
- E. Urine androgenic steroid profile

17 A 32-year-old woman with a 5-year history of suboptimally controlled type 2 diabetes mellitus is concerned about a right lower-extremity lesion that started small and has grown over time. The lesion is solitary, not raised, and it itches but does not hurt. Her diabetes regimen includes metformin, glimepiride, and liraglutide. Additional medications are lisinopril and atorvastatin.

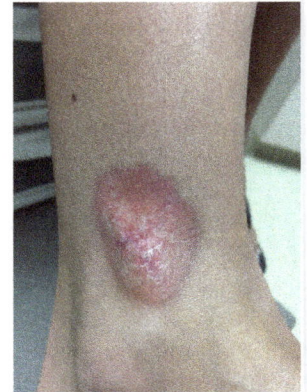

The lesion is located on the right lower extremity. It is erythematous with some yellowing in the center, with visible blood vessels within the lesion. The border is regular (*see image*). No other lesions are observed on careful skin ex amination.

Her current hemoglobin A_{1c} level is 9.4% (4.0%-5.6%) (79 mmol/mol [20-38 mmol/mol]).

Which of the following is the most likely diagnosis for the skin finding?
- A. Necrobiosis lipoidica diabeticorum
- B. Scleroderma diabeticorum
- C. Granuloma annulare
- D. Diabetic bullae
- E. Diabetic dermopathy

18 A 40-year-old woman presents for follow-up of abnormal thyroid function test results. Testing was prompted by the finding of a diffuse goiter on routine neck examination at the patient's annual visit with her gynecologist. The patient generally feels well, but she does report fatigue and hair loss. Other than 2 normal pregnancies, she has no notable medical history. She takes a progesterone-only oral contraceptive, but no other medications or supplements. Her mother has Hashimoto thyroiditis.

On physical examination, there is a diffuse goiter (25 g) without tenderness, asymmetry, or palpable nodules. Her blood pressure is 135/82 mm Hg, and pulse rate is 84 beats/min. Her height is 68 in (172.7 cm), and weight is 170 lb (77.3 kg) (BMI = 25.8 kg/m²). The rest of her examination findings are normal.

Laboratory test results:
> Six weeks ago:
>> TSH = 0.22 mIU/L (0.5-5.0 mIU/L)
> Today:
>> TSH = 0.11 mIU/L (0.5-5.0 mIU/L)
>> Free T_4 = 1.5 ng/dL (0.8-1.8 ng/dL) (SI: 19.3 pmol/L [10.30-23.17 pmol/L])
>> Total T_3 = 150 ng/dL (70-200 ng/dL) (SI: 2.3 nmol/L [1.08-3.08 nmol/L])

Which of the following is the most appropriate next step in this patient's management?
- A. Prescribe methimazole
- B. Measure TRAb
- C. Recommend radioactive iodine therapy
- D. Measure TSH and free T_4 again in 3 to 6 months
- E. Perform thyroid ultrasonography

19 A 44-year-old woman presents with a diagnosis of insulin-dependent diabetes. She would like to establish care with a new endocrinologist. She reports having been diagnosed with gestational diabetes during her first pregnancy and requiring insulin therapy to manage hyperglycemia. She continued to require insulin therapy after pregnancy. After 9 years of multiple daily insulin injections, she began insulin pump therapy. Her hemoglobin A_{1c} level has typically been around 7.0% (53 mmol/mol). She has microalbuminuria and nonproliferative retinopathy. Other than diabetes and a BMI of 31 kg/m², she has no other health issues.

The patient's mother also has insulin-dependent diabetes, managed with insulin pump therapy. The patient's daughter was diagnosed with type 2 diabetes at age 11 years. Her daughter's regimen consists of metformin, 500 mg twice daily; pioglitazone, 15 mg daily; and insulin detemir, 18 units subcutaneously at bedtime. The patient notes that her daughter has always been thin, but since starting insulin therapy 2 years ago, she has gained 15 lb (6.8 kg). Her daughter's BMI is 26 kg/m².

Which of the following would confirm the correct diagnosis?
- A. Order genetic testing for pathogenic variants in the *HNF1A* gene
- B. Order genetic testing for pathogenic variants in the *GCK* gene
- C. Measure C-peptide
- D. Assess for glutamic acid decarboxylase 65 antibodies
- E. Assess for insulin antibodies

20 A 43-year-old man with a history of depression saw an otolaryngologist for "sinus problems." CT of the head showed a sellar mass. MRI confirmed a large sellar mass with suprasellar extension and displacement of the chiasm. The patient is referred for further evaluation.

Laboratory test results:
Prolactin = 30 ng/mL (4-23 ng/mL) (SI: 1.3 nmol/L [0.17-1.00 nmol/L])
Testosterone = 262 ng/dL (300-900 ng/dL) (SI: 9.1 nmol/L [10.4-31.2 nmol/L])
Cortisol (8 AM) = 19.1 μg/dL (5-25 μg/dL) (SI: 526.9 nmol/L [137.9-689.7 nmol/L])
Serum IGF-1 = 157 ng/mL (98-261 ng/mL) (SI: 20.6 nmol/L [12.8-34.2 nmol/L])
Free T_4 = 1.3 ng/dL (0.8-1.8 ng/dL) (SI: 16.7 pmol/L [10.30-23.17 pmol/L])
TSH = 2.5 mIU/L (0.5-5.0 mIU/L)

On physical examination, his blood pressure is 130/80 mm Hg and pulse rate is 82 beats/min. His height is 72 in (182.9 cm), and weight is 192 lb (87.3 kg) (BMI = 26 kg/m²). Visual field testing shows bitemporal hemianopsia. On review of systems, he reports feeling well overall. His only medication is fluoxetine, 20 mg daily.

A nonfunctioning pituitary adenoma is diagnosed. Transsphenoidal surgery is uneventful. He is discharged on hydrocortisone, 15 mg in the morning and 5 mg in the afternoon, with a plan to measure serum cortisol 1 week after surgery. On postoperative day 6, the patient presents to your clinic because he feels unwell and has nausea and a headache. His vital signs are normal.

Which of the following is the best immediate next step?
- A. Perform a pituitary-directed MRI
- B. Administer intravenous hydrocortisone
- C. Measure sodium
- D. Measure cortisol
- E. Refer for lumbar puncture

21 A 67-year-old woman is referred for evaluation of osteoporosis. She has a history of osteoporosis documented on DXA that was performed 2 years ago. She has had no low-trauma fractures as an adult. Following the DXA scan, alendronate therapy was initiated, which she has continued to date. She reports adherence to the therapy and taking the medication correctly. She recently moved from another state and underwent another DXA scan locally within the past few weeks.

Medical history is notable for hypertension, hypothyroidism (on a stable levothyroxine dosage for the past 2 years), and osteoarthritis (bilateral hip replacement). Her medications include calcium, 600 mg twice daily; vitamin D, 800 IU daily; levothyroxine, 75 mcg daily; and hydrochlorothiazide, 25 mg daily. Family history is negative for osteoporosis or hip fracture. She does not smoke cigarettes or drink alcohol.

On physical examination, her height is 66 in (167.6 cm), which is 1 in (2.5 cm) shorter than her self-reported maximum adult height. Her examination findings are normal, including normal spinal curvature without kyphosis and a normal rib-to-pelvis distance of 2 fingerbreadths.

Laboratory test results (serum):
  Calcium = 10.4 mg/dL (8.2-10.2 mg/dL) (SI: 2.6 mmol/L [2.1-2.6 mmol/L])
  Phosphate = 3.2 mg/dL (2.3-4.7 mg/dL) (SI: 1.0 mmol/L [0.7-1.5 mmol/L])
  Creatinine = 0.9 mg/dL (0.6-1.1 mg/dL) (SI: 79.6 μmol/L [53.0-97.2 μmol/L])
  Albumin = 4.8 g/dL (3.5-5.0 g/dL) (SI: 48 g/L [35-50 g/L])
  Intact PTH = 60 pg/mL (10-65 pg/mL) (SI: 60 ng/L [10-65 ng/L])
  25-Hydroxyvitamin D = 25 ng/mL (30-80 ng/mL [optimal]) (SI: 62.4 nmol/L [74.9-199.7 nmol/L])
  TSH = 2.1 mIU/L (0.5-5.0 mIU/L)

Previous and current DXA images are shown (*see images*).

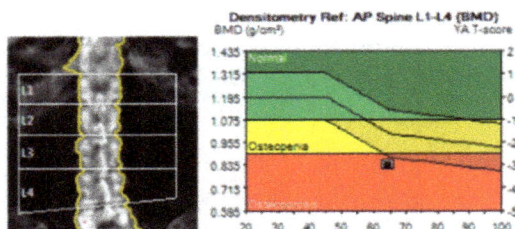

DXA scan performed with machine Brand 1 (2 years ago).

Region	BMD	Young adult		Age-matched	
	g/cm²	%	T-score	%	T-score
L1	0.767	68	−3.0	81	−1.5
L2	0.848	70	−3.0	83	−1.5
L3	0.852	71	−2.9	84	−1.4
L4	0.869	73	−2.7	86	−1.2
L1-L4	0.838	71	−2.9	84	−1.4

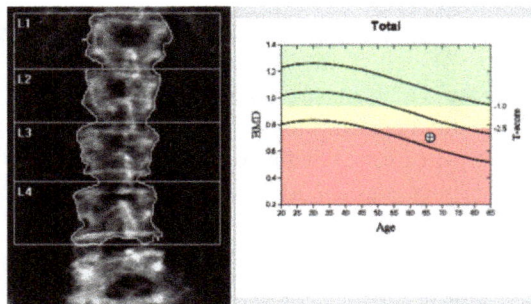

DXA scan performed with machine Brand 2 (current).

Region	BMD, g/cm²	T-score
L1	0.707	−2.6
L2	0.736	−2.7
L3	0.682	−3.7
L4	0.705	−3.2
L1-L4	0.707	−3.1

On the basis of this patient's clinical data, which of the following is the most appropriate next step in her osteoporosis management?
  A. Continue alendronate
  B. Discontinue alendronate and administer intravenous zoledronic acid
  C. Discontinue alendronate and start teriparatide
  D. Perform neck ultrasonography
  E. Start ergocalciferol, 50,000 IU once weekly

22 A 31-year-old woman is referred for evaluation of spells that started about 6 months ago. She describes these episodes as short and increasing in frequency. During the spells, she feels diaphoretic, has tremors, and is extremely weak. When asked about the timing of the episodes in relation to eating, she reports that they usually happen 2 hours after meals and that she does not experience spells when she fasts. She is worried she could have an episode while driving.

At the recommendation of a friend, she bought a glucose meter. During episodes, her point-of-care glucose concentration ranges from 40 to 60 mg/dL (2.2-3.3 mmol/L). Since learning that her symptoms are due to low glucose readings, she started eating every 2 to 3 hours. She is concerned that if she continues eating like this, she will regain the weight she lost after Roux-en-Y gastric bypass 2 years ago. She lost 100 lb (45.5 kg) after surgery, but she has gained 10 lb (4.5 kg) in the last 2 months. Her medications include a multivitamin with iron and calcium citrate.

On physical examination, her blood pressure is 120/72 mm Hg and pulse rate is 60 beats/min. Her height is 63 in (160 cm), and weight is 170 lb (77.3 kg) (BMI = 30 kg/m²). She is in no distress. Her lungs are clear to auscultation bilaterally. On cardiac examination, her heart sounds are normal, and rate and rhythm are regular. Her abdomen is soft and nontender.

Which of the following is the best next step in this patient's management?
A. Refer to a dietitian to review her current meal plan
B. Start octreotide
C. Start acarbose
D. Admit to the hospital for a 72-hour fast
E. Perform an oral glucose tolerance test

23 A 57-year-old man is found to have a new 3-cm right adrenal lesion on a whole-body surveillance CT scan. Two years ago, he underwent allogenic stem-cell transplant for acute myeloid leukemia, which was complicated by graft-vs-host disease and Epstein-Barr virus infection. He has longstanding type 2 diabetes. His current medications are amitriptyline, atorvastatin, metformin, prednisolone, ramipril, and tacrolimus.

On physical examination, his height is 71 in (180.3 cm) and weight is 202 lb (91.8 kg) (BMI = 28 kg/m²). His blood pressure is 148/92 mm Hg, and pulse rate is 76 beats/min and regular. Physical examination findings are otherwise unremarkable.

Laboratory test results:
    Serum potassium = 4.4 mEq/L (3.5-5.0 mEq/L) (SI: 4.4 mmol/L [3.5-5.0 mmol/L])
    Plasma renin activity = 3.4 ng/mL per h (0.6-4.3 ng/mL per h)
    Serum aldosterone = 6.2 ng/dL (4-21 ng/dL) (SI: 172 pmol/L [111-582.5 pmol/L])
    Cortisol following 1-mg dexamethasone-suppression test = 1.0 µg/dL (SI: 27.6 nmol/L)
    Plasma metanephrines = 82 pg/mL (<99 pg/mL) (SI: 0.42 nmol/L [<0.5 nmol/L])
    Plasma normetanephrine = 189 pg/mL (<165 pg/mL) (SI: 1.03 nmol/L [<0.90 nmol/L])
    24-Hour urinary steroid profile, within normal limits

Adrenal CT (triple phase) documents a 3.1-cm right adrenal nodule with a density of 39 Hounsfield units at baseline, 49 Hounsfield units 1 minute after contrast, and 59 Hounsfield units 10 minutes after contrast.

Whole-body PET-CT shows focal increased tracer uptake in the right adrenal nodule, but otherwise normal physiologic uptake.

Which of the following is the most likely cause of the adrenal abnormality?
A. Adrenocortical adenoma
B. Cytomegalovirus adrenalitis
C. Pheochromocytoma
D. Metastasis from unknown primary tumor
E. Secondary lymphoproliferative disease

24 A 51-year-old woman presents with swelling in the midanterior neck that has been noticeable for 3 days. This swelling is slightly tender. She had a similar episode 2 years ago that improved after antibiotic treatment. The swelling elevates with tongue protrusion or swallowing. She is otherwise healthy, and she takes no medications. Her mother has a history of hypothyroidism; the rest of the family history is unremarkable.

On physical examination, her blood pressure is 124/64 mm Hg, pulse rate is 64 beats/min, and temperature is 98.6°F (37°C). Her height is 66 in (167.6 cm), and weight is 124 lb (56.2 kg) (BMI = 20.0 kg/m²). She has a visible and palpable anterior neck mass measuring 2.0 cm, just above the hyoid bone. Her thyroid gland is not enlarged. There is no palpable cervical lymphadenopathy. Her heart rate is regular, and lungs are clear to auscultation. There is no lower-extremity edema.

Laboratory test results:
    TSH = 1.2 mIU/L (0.5-5.0 mIU/L)
    Calcium = 8.5 mg/dL (8.2-10.2 mg/dL) (SI: 2.1 mmol/L [2.1-2.6 mmol/L])

Neck ultrasonography shows a normal thyroid gland with no evidence of abnormal cervical lymphadenopathy. There is a 1.8 × 2.0 × 2.1 cm (anteroposterior × transverse × longitudinal) hypoechoic mass with posterior acoustic enhancement in the midline anterior neck with no evidence of any solid component above the thyroid gland.

Which of the following is the best next step in this patient's management?
    A. Initiate antibiotic treatment
    B. Initiate levothyroxine therapy
    C. Perform FNA biopsy of the mass
    D. Refer for excision of the mass
    E. Refer for a Sistrunk procedure

25 An 18-year-old woman is referred for a second opinion regarding hyperprolactinemia while on risperidone to treat schizophrenia. She initially sought evaluation when she developed galactorrhea and oligomenorrhea. Menarche occurred at age 13 years with normal monthly menses until the past year when her periods occurred very infrequently. Her last period was 6 months ago. Initial laboratory testing documented an elevated prolactin concentration of 47.3 ng/mL (2.1 nmol/L). Pelvic ultrasonography showed an endometrial lining of 3 mm, multifollicular appearance, and antral follicle count of 14 on the right ovary consistent with polycystic ovarian morphology. Ovarian volumes were less than 10 mL bilaterally.

After the hyperprolactinemia was first noted, oral contraceptives were prescribed, but they made her very nauseated and were discontinued. A trial of aripiprazole did not normalize her prolactin or resolve her symptoms. Her psychiatrist then tried to switch from risperidone to quetiapine. Although her prolactin normalized while on quetiapine, her psychotic symptoms worsened. She is currently back on risperidone and continues to have nipple discharge and amenorrhea, which is causing significant anxiety.

On physical examination, there is no terminal hair growth and only a few mild noninflammatory papular acne lesions on her forehead and cheeks.

Laboratory test results:
    TSH = 1.7 mIU/L (0.5-5.0 mIU/L)
    Prolactin = 50.7 ng/mL (4-30 ng/mL) (SI: 2.2 nmol/L [0.17-1.30 nmol/L])
    FSH = 5.0 mIU/mL (2.0-12.0 mIU/mL [follicular]) (SI: 5.0 IU/L [2.0-12.0 IU/L])
    Estradiol = 30 pg/mL (10-180 pg/mL [follicular]) (SI: 110.1 pmol/L [36.7-660.8 pmol/L])
    Total testosterone = 32 ng/dL (8-60 ng/dL) (SI: 1.1 nmol/L [0.3-2.1 nmol/L])
    Free testosterone = 0.33 ng/dL (0.3-1.9 ng/dL) (SI: 0.01 nmol/L [0.01-0.07 nmol/L])
    DHEA-S = 213 µg/dL (44-332 µg/dL) (SI: 5.77 µmol/L [1.19-9.00 µmol/L])

Which of the following is the best next step in this patient's management?
- A. Initiate cabergoline
- B. Refer back to her psychiatrist to consider alternative medical options
- C. Initiate progesterone for 10 days every 1 to 3 months to induce a period
- D. Order pituitary MRI
- E. Initiate metformin to induce ovulation

26 A 36-year-old man presents for follow-up 3 months after commencing medical therapy for a macroprolactinoma. Initial symptoms were headaches and a bitemporal visual field defect, and MRI of the sella revealed a pituitary macroadenoma with suprasellar extension (*see image*). He was initially commenced on cabergoline, 0.25 mg twice weekly, which has been up-titrated at monthly intervals to the current dosage of 0.75 mg twice weekly. He takes no other medications. His headache and visual symptoms resolved quickly after starting cabergoline.

On physical examination, his height is 72 in (183 cm) and weight is 198 lb (90 kg) (BMI = 27 kg/m^2). His resting pulse rate is 66 beats/min and regular, and blood pressure is 125/75 mm Hg. Visual acuity is 20/20 (6/6) in the right eye and 20/10 (6/3) in the left eye. Formal visual field assessment demonstrates full resolution of the bitemporal hemianopia.

Laboratory test results at initial presentation:
 Prolactin = 1960 ng/mL (4-30 ng/mL) (SI: 85.2 nmol/L [0.17-1.30 nmol/L])
 TSH = 1.2 mIU/L (0.5-5.0 mIU/L)
 Free T$_4$ = 1.25 ng/dL (0.8-1.8 ng/dL) (SI: 16.1 pmol/L [10.30-23.17 pmol/L])
 Cortisol (8 AM) = 15.0 µg/dL (5-25 µg/dL) (SI: 413.8 nmol/L [137.9-689.7 nmol/L])
 IGF-1 = 185 ng/mL (106-277 ng/mL) (SI: 24.2 nmol/L [13.9-36.3 nmol/L])
 FSH = 0.9 mIU/mL (1.0-13.0 mIU/mL) (SI: 0.9 IU/L [1.0-13.0 IU/L])
 LH = 1.3 mIU/mL (1.0-9.0 mIU/mL) (SI: 1.3 IU/L [1.0-9.0 IU/L])
 Total testosterone = 160 ng/dL (300-900 ng/dL) (SI: 5.6 nmol/L [10.4-31.2 nmol/L])

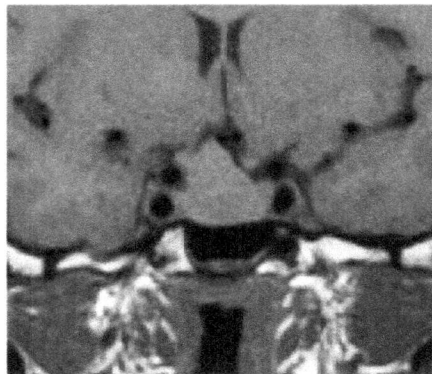

Laboratory test results after 3 months of cabergoline treatment:
 Prolactin = 10 ng/mL (4-30 ng/mL) (SI: 0.43 nmol/L [0.17-1.30 nmol/L])
 FSH = 2.1 mIU/mL (1.0-13.0 mIU/mL) (SI: 2.1 IU/L [1.0-13.0 IU/L])
 LH = 3.3 mIU/mL (1.0-9.0 mIU/mL) (SI: 3.3 IU/L [1.0-9.0 IU/L])
 Total testosterone = 480 ng/dL (300-900 ng/dL) (SI: 16.7 nmol/L [10.4-31.2 nmol/L])

MRI of the sella (T1 noncontrast) before and 3 months after commencing treatment is shown (*see images*).

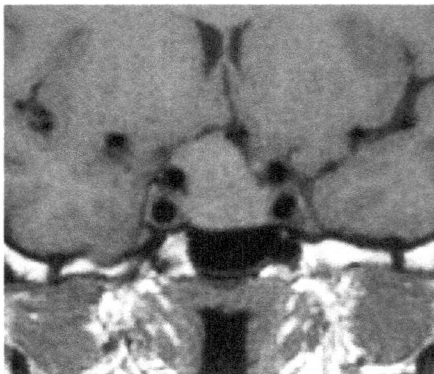

At initial presentation   After cabergoline therapy

Which of the following is the most appropriate management plan?
- A. Change cabergoline to bromocriptine
- B. Continue cabergoline at the current dosage
- C. Increase the cabergoline dosage
- D. Refer for stereotactic radiosurgery
- E. Refer for transsphenoidal surgery

27 A 31-year-old woman is referred for management of gestational diabetes mellitus. She had gestational diabetes with her first pregnancy at age 26 years and was treated with diet and glyburide. At 38 weeks' gestation, she delivered a 9 lb 12 oz (4422 g) baby by cesarean delivery. The baby had jaundice and hypoglycemia at birth. The patient has a history of obesity. She is now at 29 weeks' gestation with her second pregnancy and has again been diagnosed with gestational diabetes. She follows a diabetes meal plan and uses a glucose meter. Eight days ago, her obstetrician prescribed glyburide, 10 mg twice daily. Her mother, 2 siblings, and maternal grandfather have diabetes.

On physical examination, her height is 67.5 in (171.5 cm) and weight is 208 lb (94.5 kg) (BMI = 32 kg/m^2). Blood pressure is 128/80 mm Hg, and pulse rate is 86 beats/min. A gravid uterus is palpable. There is trace pedal edema. Reflexes are normal.

Laboratory test results:
Hemoglobin A$_{1c}$ = 5.8% (4.0%-5.6%) (40 mmol/mol [20-38 mmol/mol])
Creatinine = 0.8 mg/dL (0.6-1.1 mg/dL) (SI: 70.7 μmol/L [53.0-97.2 μmol/L])
Electrolytes, normal

Fingerstick glucose readings (point of care) are shown (*see table*).

Day	Breakfast	2-Hour postbreakfast	2-Hour postlunch	2-Hour postdinner
Tuesday	97 mg/dL (SI: 5.4 mmol/L)	117 mg/dL (SI: 6.5 mmol/L)	109 mg/dL (SI: 6.0 mmol/L)	131 mg/dL (SI: 7.3 mmol/L)
Wednesday	103 mg/dL (SI: 5.7 mmol/L)	109 mg/dL (SI: 6.0 mmol/L)	121 mg/dL (SI: 6.7 mmol/L)	135 mg/dL (SI: 7.5 mmol/L)
Thursday	102 mg/dL (SI: 5.7 mmol/L	122 mg/dL (SI: 6.8 mmol/L)	112 mg/dL (SI: 6.2 mmol/L)	127 mg/dL (SI: 7.0 mmol/L)
Friday	96 mg/dL (SI: 5.3 mmol/L)	118 mg/dL (SI: 6.5 mmol/L)	103 mg/dL (SI: 5.7 mmol/L)	121 mg/dL (SI: 6.7 mmol/L)
Saturday	105 mg/dL (SI: 5.8 mmol/L)	113 mg/dL (SI: 6.3 mmol/L)	114 mg/dL (SI: 6.3 mmol/L)	148 mg/dL (SI: 8.2 mmol/L)

After reviewing her adherence to dietary treatment, which of the following is the best next step in this patient's management?
- A. Start metformin
- B. Start insulin lispro before dinner
- C. Start NPH insulin at bedtime
- D. Double the dosage of glyburide
- E. Stop glyburide, start NPH insulin at bedtime and insulin lispro before dinner

28 A 28-year-old woman with Cushing disease undergoes surgery for a pituitary microadenoma (0.9 cm in maximal diameter).

Preoperative laboratory test results:
Urinary free cortisol = 153 μg/24 h (4-50 μg/24 h) (SI: 422.3 nmol/d [11-138 nmol/d])
ACTH = 65 pg/mL (10-60 pg/mL) (SI: 14.3 pmol/L [2.2-13.2 pmol/L])
Post-dexamethasone cortisol = 13 μg/dL (SI: 358.6 nmol/L)

Surgery is uneventful. On postoperative day 2, her morning cortisol concentration is 11 μg/dL (303.5 nmol/L) and she is discharged on no medication, feeling well. In the late evening of postoperative day 5, she presents to a local emergency department with nausea, vomiting, and fatigue. The emergency department physician calls for advice.

Which of the following is the best next step in this patient's management?
  A. Measure free T$_4$
  B. Perform a pituitary-directed MRI
  C. Measure plasma ACTH
  D. Administer hypertonic fluid
  E. Start empiric glucocorticoid therapy

29 An 18-year-old man seeks evaluation to determine his risk for type 1 diabetes mellitus. His parents accompany him to the appointment. His fraternal twin brother developed type 1 diabetes at age 16 years. There is no other family history of type 1 diabetes.

The patient's medical history includes hypothyroidism with elevated TPO antibodies and recent mononucleosis from which he has recovered. Laboratory evaluation reveals that he has elevated glutamic acid decarboxylase 65 antibodies and islet-cell antibodies. He also has a fasting blood glucose concentration of 89 mg/dL (4.9 mmol/L).

You have a discussion with the patient and his parents about the risk of developing type 1 diabetes.

Which of the following factors in this vignette confers the greatest risk that he will develop type 1 diabetes?
  A. Family history of type 1 diabetes
  B. Hashimoto disease
  C. Male sex
  D. Recent history of mononucleosis infection
  E. Autoantibody status

30 A 66-year-old man presents for management of cardiovascular risk. He had an ST-elevation myocardial infarction 2 years ago and had a coronary stent placed. He was on low-intensity atorvastatin, 10 mg daily, before his coronary event, as he had developed severe myalgias on higher atorvastatin dosages and with multiple past attempts with alternative statins, including simvastatin and rosuvastatin. Fibrate therapy was also attempted, but he again developed myalgias. His current lipid-lowering regimen includes atorvastatin, 10 mg daily, and ezetimibe, 10 mg daily. He sporadically takes an over-the-counter fish oil supplement. He has hypertension treated with lisinopril. He has a 40 pack-year history of cigarette smoking and quit 2 years ago. He drinks 2 to 4 alcoholic beverages weekly. He leads a sedentary lifestyle and has many dietary indiscretions. His father, now deceased, had coronary artery disease and underwent coronary artery bypass surgery at age 68 years. His 39-year-old son has elevated triglycerides.

On physical examination, his height is 70 in (177.5 cm) and weight is 225 lb (102.3 kg) (BMI = 32.3 kg/m^2). His blood pressure is 130/80 mm Hg. There are no skin eruptions, but abdominal adiposity is noted.

Laboratory test results (sample drawn while fasting):
   Total cholesterol = 158 mg/dL (<200 mg/dL [optimal]) (SI: 4.09 mmol/L [<5.18 mmol/L])
   Triglycerides = 225 mg/dL (<150 mg/dL [optimal]) (SI: 2.54 mmol/L [<1.70 mmol/L])
   HDL cholesterol = 36 mg/dL (>60 mg/dL [optimal]) (SI: 0.93 mmol/L [>1.55 mmol/L])
   LDL cholesterol = 77 mg/dL (<100 mg/dL [optimal]) (SI: 1.99 mmol/L [<2.59 mmol/L])
   Non-HDL cholesterol = 122 mg/dL (<130 mg/dL [optimal]) (SI: 3.16 mmol/L [<3.37 mmol/L])
   Lipoprotein (a) = 42 mg/dL (≤30 mg/dL) (SI: 1.50 μmol/L [≤1.07 μmol/L])
   Hemoglobin A$_{1c}$ = 5.9% (4.0%-5.6%) (41 mmol/mol [20-38 mmol/mol])
   Fasting glucose = 108 mg/dL (70-99 mg/dL) (SI: 5.99 mmol/L [3.9-5.5 mmol/L])
   Creatinine = 1.1 mg/dL (0.7-1.3 mg/dL) (SI: 97.2 μmol/L [61.9-114.9 μmol/L])
   TSH = 1.4 mIU/L (0.5-5.0 mIU/L)

In addition to ongoing lifestyle efforts, which of the following is the best next step in this patient's management?
- A. Switch to rosuvastatin
- B. Add extended-release niacin
- C. Add colesevelam
- D. Add purified icosapent ethyl
- E. Add dulaglutide

31 A 65-year-old woman with a longstanding history of type 2 diabetes mellitus seeks recommendations concerning her bone health. She has no history of low-trauma fractures. She has been on hemodialysis for approximately 4 years. Diabetes-related complications also include peripheral neuropathy involving her lower extremities. Her medications are insulin glargine once daily, insulin lispro before meals, atorvastatin, metoprolol, calcium acetate, and gabapentin. She does not smoke cigarettes or drink alcohol. Family history is negative for osteoporosis, including no parental history of hip fracture.

On physical examination, she is only 0.8 in (2 cm) shorter than her self-reported adult maximum height. She has a palpable thrill over her left forearm arteriovenous shunt. Her spinal curvature is normal. There is no palpable bony tenderness over the tibias. There are no ulcers or lesions on her feet. She has absent sensation to 5.07-g monofilament testing on both feet. The rest of her physical examination findings are noncontributory.

Laboratory test results (serum):
    Calcium = 9.8 mg/dL (8.2-10.2 mg/dL) (SI: 2.5 mmol/L [2.1-2.6 mmol/L])
    Phosphate = 5.5 mg/dL (2.3-4.7 mg/dL) (SI: 1.8 mmol/L [0.7-1.5 mmol/L])
    Creatinine = 8.9 mg/dL (0.6-1.1 mg/dL) (SI: 786.8 μmol/L [53.0-97.2 μmol/L])
    Serum urea nitrogen = 25 mg/dL (8-23 mg/dL) (SI: 8.9 mmol/L [2.9-8.2 mmol/L])
    Albumin = 3.6 g/dL (3.5-5.0 g/dL) (SI: 36 g/L [35-50 g/L])
    Alkaline phosphatase = 130 U/L (50-120 U/L) (SI: 2.17 μkat/L [0.84-2.00 μkat/L])
    Intact PTH = 320 pg/mL (10-65 pg/mL) (SI: 320 ng/L [10-65 ng/L])
    25-Hydroxyvitamin D = 11 ng/dL (30-80 ng/mL [optimal]) (SI: 27.5 nmol/L [74.9-199.7 nmol/L])

DXA documents the following values:
    Lumbar spine T-score = −1.2
    Right femoral neck T-score = −2.0
    Right total hip T score = −1.6
    Left proximal one-third radius T-score = −2.8

Which of the following treatments would best address the patient's underlying bone disorder?
- A. Alendronate
- B. Teriparatide
- C. Cholecalciferol
- D. Calcitriol
- E. Sevelamer hydrochloride

32 A 69-year-old man is referred by his radiation oncologist for consideration of testosterone replacement for ongoing hot flashes, fatigue, and low energy. The patient has not had low mood or depressive symptoms. He has a history of localized, intermediate-risk prostate cancer treated with definitive radiotherapy and 12 months of adjuvant androgen-deprivation therapy with a GnRH antagonist. Androgen-deprivation therapy was stopped 6 months ago, and the patient is disappointed that he does not feel any better. Other history includes a provoked pulmonary embolism 3 years ago treated with anticoagulation therapy for 6 months.

On physical examination, his height is 67 in (170.2 cm), and weight is 195 lb (88.6 kg) (BMI = 31 kg/m²). He has modest nontender gynecomastia, loss of body hair, reduced muscle bulk, and 10-mL testes bilaterally.

Laboratory test results (sample drawn at 8 AM while fasting):

   Serum total testosterone = 75 ng/dL (300-900 ng/dL) (SI: 2.6 nmol/L [10.4-31.2 nmol/L])

   LH = 3.1 mIU/mL (1.0-9.0 mIU/mL) (SI: 2.1 IU/L [1.0-9.0 IU/L])

   PSA = <0.03 ng/mL (therapeutic target, <0.03 ng/mL) (SI: <0.03 µg/L [<0.03 µg/L])

   Hemoglobin = 12.0 g/dL (13.8-17.2 g/dL) (SI: 120 g/L [138-172 g/L])

Which of the following is the best treatment to start now?

   A. Estradiol gel
   B. Long-acting intramuscular testosterone
   C. Tamoxifen
   D. Testosterone gel
   E. Venlafaxine

33 A 66-year-old white woman presents to your office for diabetes management. Type 2 diabetes mellitus was diagnosed 15 years ago. Her current treatment regimen consists of 34 units of insulin glargine at bedtime; sitagliptin, 25 mg once daily; and glipizide extended release, 5 mg once daily. She has end-stage renal disease and has been receiving hemodialysis for the past 4 years. Her diabetes has also been complicated by retinopathy and neuropathy. She reports that her last dilated eye examination was about 6 months ago at which time stable nonproliferative retinopathy was noted. She has well-controlled hypertension. She does not routinely check her blood glucose at home, but states that the few times she has checked it, values have been in the range of 100 to 200 mg/dL (5.6-11.1 mmol/L). She has not noticed any low glucose values. She reports blurry vision over the past few weeks but has no other symptoms.

On physical examination, her blood pressure is 154/86 mm Hg and pulse rate is 84 beats/min. Her height is 64 in (162.6 cm), and weight is 182 lb (82.7 kg) (BMI = 31 kg/m^2). She has stasis dermatitis in both lower extremities and +1 pitting peripheral edema. Upon auscultation, her heart has a regular rate and rhythm, with a +2/6 systolic murmur best auscultated over the right upper sternal border. Her lungs are clear to auscultation. There is no abdominal tenderness or palpable mass.

Current medications are lisinopril, amlodipine, iron sulfate, and epoetin alfa.

Laboratory test results:

   Hemoglobin A$_{1c}$ = 6.7% (4.0%-5.6%) (50 mmol/mol [20-38 mmol/mol])

   Hemoglobin = 8.9 g/dL (12.1-15.1 g/dL) (SI: 89 g/L [121-151 g/L])

   Albumin = 3.7 mg/dL (3.5-5.0 g/dL) (SI: 37 g/L [35-50 g/L])

   Electrolytes, normal

Which of the following is the best next step in this patient's management?

   A. Check for hemoglobin S variant
   B. Measure fructosamine
   C. Reduce the dosage of insulin glargine
   D. Stop glipizide
   E. Measure C-peptide

34 A 35-year-old man presents to the emergency department for evaluation of progressive substernal chest pain over the preceding 5 days and a 2-month history of palpitations, shortness of breath, diaphoresis, tremulousness, and 20-lb (9.1-kg) unintentional weight loss.

On physical examination, his blood pressure is 140/90 mm Hg and pulse rate is 120 beats/min. There is a diffuse goiter (30 g) without tenderness or palpable nodules. He has a fine tremor of his outstretched hands, his skin is warm and moist, and deep tendon reflexes are 3+. He is afebrile, and the rest of his examination findings are normal.

Electrocardiography shows sinus tachycardia without ST- or T-wave changes.

Laboratory test results:

Complete blood cell count, normal

Complete metabolic panel, normal

Troponin I = <0.05 ng/mL (<0.6 ng/mL) (SI: <0.05 μg/L [<0.6 μg/L])

TSH = <0.01 mIU/L (0.5-5.0 mIU/L)

Free T_4 = 4.2 ng/dL (0.8-1.8 ng/dL) (SI: 54.1 pmol/L [10.30-23.17 pmol/L])

Total T_3 = 510 ng/dL (70-200 ng/dL) (SI: 7.9 nmol/L [1.08-3.08 nmol/L])

Thyroid-stimulating immunoglobin = 150% of basal activity (≤120% of basal activity)

CT imaging of the chest with contrast is negative for pulmonary embolism, but reveals a solid, homogenous anterior mediastinal mass measuring 11.5 × 7.5 × 3 cm (*see image, arrow*).

The patient is admitted to the hospital and begins treatment with methimazole, 20 mg twice daily, and propranolol, 10 mg 3 times daily, with subsequent titration of propranolol and transition to an extended-release formulation. The patient's symptoms gradually improve, and his vital signs normalize over the next 2 days. He plans to pursue treatment with radioactive iodine (^{131}I) after hospital discharge.

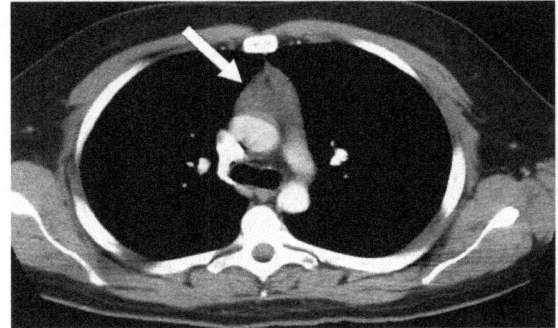

Which of the following is the most appropriate initial management of the patient's anterior mediastinal mass?

A. CT chest imaging in 6 months
B. Mediastinoscopy with biopsy
C. Measurement of serum β-hCG, α-fetoprotein, and lactate dehydrogenase
D. PET-CT scan
E. Surgical resection via median sternotomy

35 A 23-year-old transgender man with a history of depression is referred for gender dysphoria and gender-affirming hormone therapy. He reports first noticing incongruence between the sex he was assigned at birth and his gender identity at age 6 years. He recalls preferring playing with boys and dressing like male TV characters. He experienced significant distress and dysphoria at the onset of puberty, especially with menstruation and breast development. He did not tell anyone that menstruation had started for 2 years because he was too embarrassed to discuss it. During a psychology class in his junior year in high school, he had an assignment on gender dysphoria and learned the language to describe his identity. When moving to the local area 1 year ago, he shared his identity with his family and socially transitioned in the new city.

He has several goals for gender-affirming hormone therapy. The first is to stop monthly bleeding, which is emotionally difficult and triggers dysphoria and depression. He has not had any hospitalizations for depression, but he has presented to the emergency department for evaluation when bleeding was associated with suicidality. He also desires gender-affirming chest surgery, as he wears a binder. He looks forward to voice deepening and facial hair development with hormone therapy. He wants to discuss cost-effective options because he cannot afford expensive testosterone preparations. He has read about the different methods of testosterone treatment and is comfortable with possible injection therapy. He is now engaged to be married to a cisgender man, and they are interested in discussing fertility preservation.

On physical examination, his blood pressure is 124/81 mm Hg and pulse rate is 88 beats/min. His height is 66 in (167.9 cm), and weight is 199 lb (90.3 kg) (BMI = 32.1 kg/m²). There are no signs of androgen excess.

Laboratory test results:

Total testosterone = 16 ng/dL (8-60 ng/dL) (SI: 0.6 nmol/L [0.3-2.1 nmol/L])

TSH = 1.7 mIU/L (0.5-5.0 mIU/L)

DHEA-S = 127 μg/dL (44-332 μg/dL) (SI: 3.4 μmol/L [1.19-9.00 μmol/L])

Fasting glucose = 98 mg/dL (70-99 mg/dL) (SI: 5.4 mmol/L [3.9-5.5 mmol/L])

Lipid panel, normal

Day 3 FSH = 7.0 mIU/mL (2.0-12.0 mIU/mL [follicular]) (SI: 7.0 IU/L [2.0-12.0 IU/L])

Estradiol = 54 pg/mL (10-180 pg/mL [follicular]) (SI: 198.2 pmol/L [36.7-660.8 pmol/L])

Which of the following is the best next step?

A. Referral to reproductive endocrinology for controlled ovarian stimulation for embryo cryopreservation with fiancé's sperm

B. Referral to reproductive endocrinology for ovarian tissue cryopreservation now (before initiating hormone therapy)

C. Initiation of transdermal testosterone

D. Initiation of intramuscular testosterone

E. Initiation of a GnRH agonist until gender-affirming surgery when ovarian tissue cryopreservation can be performed

36 A 58-year-old man is referred for evaluation of severe hypercalcemia. He reports joint pain and mild memory loss. He has no history of fractures or kidney stones. His dietary calcium intake is approximately 600 mg daily, and he does not take any calcium or vitamin D supplements. His family history is negative for parathyroid or thyroid disease.

On physical examination, he has a palpable 5-cm, mobile, nontender, right-sided central neck mass.

Laboratory test results:

Serum calcium = 12.5 mg/dL (8.2-10.2 mg/dL) (SI: 3.1 mmol/L [2.1-2.6 mmol/L])

Serum phosphate = 2.0 mg/dL (2.3-4.7 mg/dL) (SI: 0.6 mmol/L [0.7-1.5 mmol/L])

Serum creatinine = 1.4 mg/dL (0.7-1.3 mg/dL) (SI: 123.8 μmol/L [61.9-114.9 μmol/L])

Serum intact PTH = 233 pg/mL (10-65 pg/mL) (SI: 233 ng/L [10-65 ng/L])

Serum 25-hydroxyvitamin D = 37 ng/mL (30-80 ng/mL [optimal]) (SI: 92.4 nmol/L [74.9-199.7 nmol/L])

Serum albumin = 3.5 g/dL (3.5-5.0 g/dL) (SI: 35 g/L [35-50 g/L])

Neck CT shows a 5-cm, heterogeneous, predominantly hypodense lesion in the right thyroid lobe, with mass effect on the common carotid artery and trachea, and no lymph node enlargement or distant lesions (*see image, arrow*).

He undergoes surgical removal of the neck mass and right hemithyroidectomy, and the pathology slide is shown (*see image*).

Surgical pathology reveals nests of parathyroid tumor cells entrapped within a thick, irregular capsule, with adherence to the thyroid gland, with no foci of transcapsular tumor invasion into adjacent tissues or definitive lymphovascular invasion.

Neck CT (*sagittal view*).

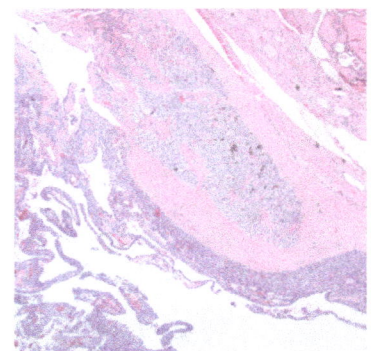

His calcium and PTH levels normalize 1 month postoperatively, and no residual mass is identified on subsequent neck CT 6 months later.

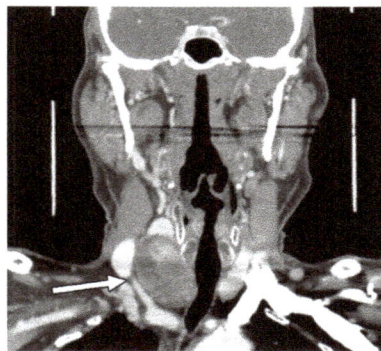

Which of the following is the best next step in this patient's management?

A. Order sestamibi scintigraphy

B. Order whole-body PET-CT

C. Repeat laboratory tests and neck imaging in 1 year

D. Refer for radiotherapy

E. Refer for chemotherapy

37 A 65-year-old man seeks consultation regarding diabetes mellitus that has been exacerbated by glucocorticoid treatment. He was admitted to the hospital 2 months ago for evaluation of headaches, fevers, and left-sided vision impairment. He was presumed to have giant-cell arteritis and was initially prescribed prednisone, 120 mg daily, which is now being tapered (current dosage 40 mg daily). The plan is to reduce the dosage by 10% weekly over the next 6 months. He has intermittent symptoms of paresthesia in his fingers and toes, but he otherwise feels well. He is up to date on screening laboratory tests and assessments, and there is no history of nephropathy.

Before the hospitalization, he was taking metformin, 1000 mg twice daily, and extended-release glipizide, 6 mg daily. On this regimen, his hemoglobin A$_{1c}$ level ranged from 6.7% to 7.0% (50-53 mmol/mol) over the preceding year (before receiving glucocorticoids). While in the hospital, his diabetes regimen was switched to insulin detemir, 30 units once daily, and insulin aspart, 12 units before meals, with supplemental insulin to be given on a correctional scale. However, he admits to often missing 1 dose of aspart daily because he forgets and expresses dissatisfaction with the current regimen. His fingerstick blood glucose measurements are noted as follows:

Fasting = 100-120 mg/dL (5.6-6.7 mmol/L)
Before lunch = 178-197 mg/dL (9.9-10.9 mmol/L)
Before dinner = 235-260 mg/dL (13.0-14.4 mmol/L)

Which of the following should be recommended to improve this patient's hyperglycemia?
  A. Continue current detemir dosage but increase the aspart dose before meals
  B. Continue current regimen but increase correctional insulin scale
  C. Continue current regimen and add liraglutide once daily
  D. Increase both detemir and aspart dosages
  E. Stop current regimen and start premixed insulin (NPH/regular) twice daily

38 A 46-year-old man with a history of multiple gastrointestinal polyps and lipomas underwent extensive abdominal surgery for his polyp burden 3 years ago and now has a colostomy bag. He was recently diagnosed with a 5-cm right thyroid nodule. He undergoes FNA biopsy of the thyroid nodule, which is documented to be Bethesda IV. Total thyroidectomy with central neck dissection is performed. The final pathology reveals an angioinvasive, well-differentiated follicular carcinoma (5 cm) with oncocytic features in the right thyroid lobe. All margins are free and 5 of 10 cervical lymph nodes are positive for metastases.

Six weeks postoperatively, he has a radioactive iodine scan while he is hypothyroid.

Laboratory test results:
  Thyroglobulin, undetectable
  Thyroglobulin antibodies = 1220 IU/mL (≤4 IU/mL) (SI: 1220 kIU/L [≤4.0 kIU/L])
  TSH = 240 mIU/L (0.5-5.0 mIU/L)

He receives 100 mCi of radioiodine treatment. His scan after therapy demonstrates an abnormal focus of increased radioiodine uptake in the midneck that was not seen on a pretherapy ^{131}I scan, corresponding to a 10 × 7-mm, soft-tissue nodule in the anterior aspect of the thyroid cartilage, consistent with a metastatic Delphian lymph node. A follow-up recombinant human TSH radioactive iodine scan is negative, with undetectable thyroglobulin but still elevated thyroglobulin antibodies of 40 IU/mL (40 kIU/L) 6 months after receiving radioiodine treatment. He has no palpable mass in his neck, dysphagia, or dysphonia. He currently takes levothyroxine, 200 mcg daily, and bupropion, 450 mg daily.

The patient is married and has a 9-year-old son with some learning difficulties. Family history is notable for colon polyps in his father and colon cancer in his paternal grandfather.

On physical examination, his blood pressure is 125/68 mm Hg and pulse rate is 70 beats/min. There is a well-healed scar at the base of his neck. There is an ileostomy stoma in the right side of his abdomen. He has no lower-extremity edema. Skin examination shows several skin-colored papules with slightly rough surfaces around his lips and in the nasolabial folds.

Laboratory test results:
    TSH = 0.92 mIU/L (0.5-5.0 mIU/L)
    Thyroglobulin = undetectable (<1.0 ng/mL) (SI: undetectable [<1.0 µg/L])
    Thyroglobulin antibodies = 10 IU/mL (≤4 IU/mL) (SI: 10 kIU/L [≤4.0 kIU/L])

In addition to increasing his levothyroxine dosage, which of the following is the most appropriate next step?
    A. Genetic testing for the *BRAF* V600E somatic variant
    B. Genetic testing for a *PTEN* germline pathogenic variant
    C. Kidney ultrasonography
    D. Neck CT
    E. Thyroid ultrasonography for the patient's son

39 A 32-year-old woman returns for management of diabetes mellitus. Monogenic diabetes was diagnosed at age 15 years. She was found to have a pathogenic variant in the gene encoding hepatic nuclear factor 1α (*HNF1A*) and was the index case for monogenic diabetes (MODY type 3) in her extended family. Her mother, 2 of 5 siblings, maternal grandmother, and several maternal great aunts and uncles have diabetes.

Initially, she was treated with glyburide and had excellent glycemic control. During a pregnancy at age 26 years, she started insulin and continued insulin therapy after delivery. She has had reasonable glycemic control during the last several years, with hemoglobin A_{1c} levels ranging from 6.4% to 7.5% (46-58 mmol/mol). She currently administers 13 units of insulin degludec at bedtime. She uses an insulin-to-carbohydrate ratio of 1 unit of insulin aspart per 14 g carbohydrate (total bolus dose of 16 units/day).

She has not had a dilated eye examination in the last 2 years. At her last exam, she was told her eyes appeared normal. She has no symptoms of neuropathy. When measured 6 months ago, her albumin-to-creatinine ratio was elevated at 88 mg/g creatinine. She has never been treated for hypertension or dyslipidemia. She does not have hypoglycemia unawareness.

On physical examination, her height is 69 in (175.3 cm), and weight is 142 lb (64.5 kg) (BMI = 21 kg/m²). Her blood pressure is 130/78 mm Hg, and pulse rate is 56 beats/min. Peripheral pulses are strong. She has normal reflexes and normal sensation for position sense and 10-g monofilament in each foot.

Laboratory test results:
    Electrolytes, normal
    Hemoglobin A_{1c} = 7.4% (4.0%-5.6%) (57 mmol/mol [20-38 mmol/mol])
    Creatinine = 0.7 mg/dL (0.6-1.1 mg/dL) (SI: 61.9 mmol/L [53.0-97.2 mmol/L])
    TSH = 1.64 mIU/L (0.5-5.0 mIU/L)
    Albumin-to-creatinine ratio = 103 mg/g creat (<30 mg/g creat)
    Urinalysis, no white or red blood cells or bacteria

Which of the following is the best next step in this patient's management?
    A. Monitor only; no therapy needed
    B. Start lisinopril
    C. Start canagliflozin
    D. Intensify insulin treatment
    E. Start a low-protein diet

40 A 33-year-old woman with hypertension is referred for assistance with weight loss. Weight gain has been a problem since she delivered her first child 3 years ago. Before her first pregnancy, her weight was 161 lb (73.2 kg). Twelve months after delivery, her weight was 187 lb (85 kg). Her current weight is 185 lb (84.1 kg). The patient has been trying to follow different diets, but she is unable to lose weight. She reports that her biggest struggle is cravings. When she sees sweets or pastries, she cannot control her cravings and ends up eating. After taking a complete history, a low-calorie meal plan and an exercise program are recommended. The patient returns 2 weeks later and has not lost any weight. She reports that despite her best efforts to follow her new meal plan, cravings are a big obstacle.

Her medications include hydrochlorothiazide, 12.5 mg daily.

On physical examination, her blood pressure is 130/85 mm Hg and pulse rate is 70 beats/min. Her height is 63.5 in (161.3 cm), and weight is 185 lb (84.1 kg) (BMI = 32 kg/m²). She is in no distress and does not look cushingoid. Her lungs are clear to auscultation, and heart sounds are regular. Findings on abdominal examination are unremarkable. She has no peripheral edema.

Her hemoglobin A_{1c} level is 5.4% (4.0%-5.6%) (36 mmol/mol [20-38 mmol/mol]).

The patient agrees to adding a weight-loss medication to her program.

Which of the following medications should be recommended for this patient?
   A. Liraglutide
   B. Naltrexone/bupropion
   C. Metformin
   D. Phentermine/topiramate
   E. Orlistat

41 A 20-year-old man with hypothyroidism due to Hashimoto thyroiditis on long-term levothyroxine therapy presents for follow-up. He also has celiac disease treated with a gluten-free diet. Interval medical history is notable for a diagnosis of focal (partial) seizures that onset 4 months ago. Today, the patient reports fatigue and a 5-lb (2.3-kg) weight gain over 3 months, but he is otherwise feeling well. Current medications are levothyroxine, 100 mcg daily, and carbamazepine, 100 mg twice daily. He has had no subsequent seizures following initiation of anticonvulsant drug therapy.

Physical examination is notable for dry skin. His blood pressure is 107/55 mm Hg, and pulse rate is 68 beats/min. His height is 69 in (175.3 cm), and weight is 150 lb (68.2 kg) (BMI = 22.1 kg/m²). The rest of his examination findings are normal.

Laboratory test results:
   TSH = 13.0 mIU/L (0.5-5.0 mIU/L)
   Free T_4 = 0.7 ng/dL (0.8-1.8 ng/dL) (SI: 9.0 pmol/L [10.30-23.17 pmol/L])
   Serum carbamazepine = 8 µg/mL (4-12 µg/mL) (SI: 33.9 µmol/L [17-51 µmol/L])

Six months ago, his serum TSH value was 2.0 mIU/L.

Which of the following is the most likely cause of the change in this patient's thyroid function tests results?
   A. Anticonvulsant drug therapy
   B. Celiac disease
   C. Nonadherence to levothyroxine therapy
   D. Nonthyroidal illness syndrome
   E. Weight gain

42 A 56-year-old woman presents with a 1-year history of worsening anxiety, palpitations, and sweating. She describes episodic anxiety with a feeling of heart racing and pounding, accompanied by drenching sweats on her upper body and face. These symptoms are not provoked by any physical or emotional triggers. The episodes occur at unpredictable times and resolve spontaneously within 15 to 60 minutes. During symptomatic episodes, her blood pressure (assessed at home) ranges from 154/80 mm Hg to 210/100 mm Hg. Pheochromocytoma is diagnosed after plasma normetanephrine levels are found to be 6-fold elevated, and abdominal CT imaging reveals an 8-cm left adrenal mass with high attenuation characteristics. On review of her family history, her father died of a metastatic gastrointestinal stromal tumor and her mother and sister have had breast cancer.

The pathogenesis of this patient's pheochromocytoma is most likely attributable to a pathogenic variant in which of the following genes?
- A. *EPAS1* (endothelial PAS domain protein 1)
- B. *SDHB* (succinate dehydrogenase subunit B)
- C. *RET* (ret proto-oncogene)
- D. *TMEM127* (transmembrane protein 127)
- E. *VHL* (von Hippel–Lindau tumor suppressor)

43 A 44-year-old woman presents for evaluation of a goiter. She first noticed enlargement of her thyroid gland 12 months ago, and she believes that it has continued to grow. She describes some pressure over her neck and difficulty swallowing. She has had no weight loss or night sweats. Hypothyroidism was diagnosed a year ago, and she takes levothyroxine, 125 mcg daily. Thyroid ultrasonography reveals hypoechoic thyroid tissue in both thyroid lobes and an ill-defined, 2.2-cm nodule in the left lobe. FNA biopsy of left thyroid nodule is nondiagnostic. A second FNA biopsy of the nodule is also nondiagnostic. She undergoes core biopsy of the left thyroid nodule, and examination shows extensive fibrosis with moderate lymphoplasmacytic infiltrate and no follicular cells. Thyroid lymphoma is ruled out.

She has no notable medical or surgical history. She has no known drug allergies, and her only medication is levothyroxine.

On physical examination, her blood pressure is 120/70 mm Hg and pulse rate is 68 beats/min. Her height is 63 in (160 cm) and weight is 130 lb (59 kg) (BMI = 23 kg/m^2). She is in no acute distress. Her thyroid gland is enlarged (3 times normal size), and the left lobe is larger than the right lobe. The gland does not move with swallowing and feels hard. There is no palpable cervical lymphadenopathy. Her heart rate is regular, and lungs are clear to auscultation. There is no lower-extremity edema. The rest of the examination findings are normal.

Laboratory test results:
TSH = 2.0 mIU/L (0.5-5.0 mIU/L)
Calcium = 8.8 mg/dL (8.2-10.2 mg/dL) (SI: 2.2 mmol/L [2.1-2.6 mmol/L])
PTH = 45 pg/mL (10-65 pg/mL) (SI:45 ng/L [10-65 ng/L])

Which of the following is the best next step in this patient's management?
- A. Perform total thyroidectomy
- B. Initiate prednisone
- C. Initiate tamoxifen
- D. Perform isthmusectomy with left lobectomy
- E. Increase the levothyroxine dosage

44 A 64-year-old woman with a 20-year history of type 2 diabetes mellitus presents for follow-up. Three months ago, her hemoglobin A$_{1c}$ level was 11.0% (97 mmol/mol). She recently retired and has been able to eat better, exercise, and take insulin more regularly. Her glycemic control has improved, and her hemoglobin A$_{1c}$ level is now 8.5% (69 mmol/mol). She also reports a 20-lb (9.1-kg) weight loss over the past year.

Her primary concern today is discomfort in her feet that is keeping her awake at night. The pain started about 4 weeks ago and is bilateral and burning in nature. Ambulation does not significantly worsen the pain.

On physical examination, her blood pressure is 134/82 mm Hg and pulse rate is 88 beats/min. Her height is 65 in (165 cm), and weight is 175.5 lb (79.8 kg) (BMI = 29 kg/m^2).

Skin examination reveals acanthosis nigricans. Strength is preserved in all extremities. She has decreased sensation to pin prick in both lower extremities up to her ankles. There is no motor dysfunction, and ankle reflexes are 1+ bilaterally. Bilateral dorsalis pedis pulses are palpable. The rest of the examination findings are normal.

Which of the following is the most likely cause of this patient's current prominent symptoms?
- A. Vascular insufficiency
- B. Diabetic polyneuropathy
- C. Radiculopathy
- D. Treatment-induced neuropathy of diabetes
- E. Diabetic neuropathic cachexia

45 A 32-year-old woman is referred because of recently diagnosed acromegaly due to a 1.9-cm pituitary macroadenoma. She developed symptoms of enlarging hands, sweating, carpal tunnel syndrome, facial feature changes, and snoring that started about 9 years ago. Her father is 64 years old and healthy. She has a paternal cousin with acromegaly, another paternal cousin (from different uncle) with a prolactinoma, and a paternal uncle (now deceased) whom she remembers had very large hands. She produces a picture of this uncle, who looks frankly acromegalic. There is no family history of recurrent kidney stones, hypercalcemia, pancreatic tumors, or cardiac problems. Her mother is alive and well. No pituitary adenomas are present in her mother's side of the family. The patient has 2 children (9-year-old boy and 7-year-old girl), and she asks whether they are at risk for pituitary adenomas.

A pathogenic variant in which of the following genes is the most likely culprit underlying this syndrome?
- A. *MEN1* (menin 1)
- B. *RET* (ret proto-oncogene)
- C. *AIP* (aryl hydrocarbon receptor interacting protein)
- D. *PRKAR1A* (protein kinase cAMP-dependent type I regulatory subunit alpha)
- E. *GNAS* (GNAS complex locus)

46 A 67-year-old man presents for ongoing cardiovascular risk management and genetic dyslipidemia. He has known cardiovascular disease and had a myocardial infarction and 3-vessel coronary artery bypass grafting at age 47 years. Since then, he has required 2 more percutaneous coronary interventions, the most recent being 8 months ago, while on therapy. He has treated hypertension, as well as type 2 diabetes treated with metformin. Mixed-pattern dyslipidemia has been treated for many years with rosuvastatin, 40 mg daily; ezetimibe, 10 mg daily; and fenofibrate, 145 mg daily. As he is at very high cardiovascular risk, therapy is initiated with evolocumab, a PCSK9 inhibitor. Ezetimibe is stopped after initiation of injectable therapy. He returns for a follow-up visit, and he has no concerns and feels well.

On physical examination, his height is 68 in (173 cm), and weight is 182.5 lb (83 kg) (BMI = 27.7 kg/m²). His blood pressure is 118/64 mm Hg.

Laboratory test results are presented in the table.

Measurement	Previous (on rosuvastatin, 40 mg daily, ezetimibe, 10 mg daily, and fenofibrate 145 mg daily)	Present (on rosuvastatin, 40 mg daily, fenofibrate, 145 mg daily, and evolocumab, 140 mg every 2 weeks)	Reference ranges
Total cholesterol	169 mg/dL (SI: 4.38 mmol/L)	59 mg/dL (SI: 1.53 mmol/L)	<200 mg/dL (optimal) (SI: 5.18 mmol/L)
Triglycerides	395 mg/dL (SI: 4.46 mmol/L)	114 mg/dL (SI: 1.29 mmol/L)	<150 mg/dL (optimal) (SI: <1.70 mmol/L)
HDL cholesterol	26 mg/dL (SI: 0.67 mmol/L)	33 mg/dL (SI: 0.85 mmol/L)	>60 mg/dL (optimal) (>1.55 mmol/L)
LDL cholesterol	64 mg/dL (SI: 1.66 mmol/L)	3 mg/dL (SI: 0.78 mmol/L)	<100 mg/dL (optimal) (SI: 2.59 mmol/L)
Non-HDL cholesterol	143 mg/dL (SI: 3.70 mmol/L)	26 mg/dL (SI: 0.67 mmol/L)	<130 mg/dL (optimal) (SI: 3.37 mmol/L)
Hemoglobin A₁c	6.2% (44 mmol/mol)	6.4% (46 mmol/mol)	4.0%-5.6% (20-38 mmol/mol)
Fasting plasma glucose	113 mg/dL (SI: 6.27 mmol/L)	109 mg/dL (SI: 6.05 mmol/L)	70-99 mg/dL (SI: 3.9-5.5 mmol/L)
Creatinine	1.14 mg/dL (SI: 100.8 µmol/L)	1.18 mg/dL (SI: 104.3 µmol/L)	0.7-1.3 mg/dL (SI: 61.9-114.9 µmol/L)

Which of the following is the best next step in this patient's ongoing management?
- A. Stop evolocumab
- B. Stop rosuvastatin
- C. Stop fenofibrate
- D. Add semaglutide
- E. Recommend no change at this time

47 A 50-year-man is referred for evaluation of newly identified hypercalcemia after presenting to his primary care physician with symptoms of fatigue and polyuria over the last 6 months. He is otherwise healthy and has no history of notable medical problems. Specifically, he has no history of fractures, nephrolithiasis, or craniocervical radiation. He does not take medications or over-the-counter supplements. Family history is negative for osteoporosis, nephrolithiasis, endocrine tumors, or head and neck malignancies.

On physical examination, he appears well. Vital signs are unremarkable, including a BMI of 27 kg/m². Findings on examination of the eyes, ears, nose, and throat (including oral exam) are normal. There is a fullness appreciated over the right lower anterior neck without associated precervical or supraclavicular adenopathy. The rest of the examination findings are normal.

Laboratory test results (serum):
Calcium = 12.9 mg/dL (8.2-10.2 mg/dL) (SI: 3.2 mmol/L [2.1-2.6 mmol/L])
Phosphate = 3.0 mg/dL (2.3-4.7 mg/dL) (SI: 1.0 mmol/L [0.7-1.5 mmol/L])
Creatinine = 0.8 mg/dL (0.7-1.3 mg/dL) (SI: 70.7 μmol/L [61.9-114.9 μmol/L])
Albumin = 4.2 g/dL (3.5-5.0 g/dL) (SI: 42 g/L [35-50 g/L])
Alkaline phosphatase = 125 U/L (50-120 U/L) (SI: 2.09 μkat/L [0.84-2.00 μkat/L])
Intact PTH = 350 pg/mL (10-65 pg/mL) (SI: 350 ng/L [10-65 ng/L])
25-Hydroxyvitamin D = 15 ng/dL (30-80 ng/mL [optimal]) (SI: 37.4 nmol/L [74.9-199.7 nmol/L])

Technetium ^{99}Tc parathyroid scan shows delayed uptake in the right lower neck.

Which of the following is the best next step in this patient's management?
- A. Refer to endocrine surgery for minimally invasive parathyroidectomy
- B. Start cholecalciferol and measure intact PTH again in 6 weeks
- C. Start cinacalcet
- D. Perform neck ultrasonography
- E. Perform renal ultrasonography

48 A 35-year-old man presents for evaluation of suspected hypogonadism. He requested that his primary care physician measure his testosterone because he did not react with anger when his girlfriend broke up with him, which his family thought was unusual.

Laboratory test results:
Serum total testosterone (sample drawn at 4 PM) = 181 ng/dL (300-900 ng/dL) (SI: 6.3 nmol/L [10.4-31.2 nmol/L])
Repeat total testosterone (sample drawn at 8 AM while fasting) = 268 ng/dL (300-900 ng/dL) (SI: 9.3 nmol/L [10.4-31.2 nmol/L])
LH = 4.0 mIU/mL (1.0-9.0 mIU/mL) (SI: 4.0 IU/L [1.0-9.0 IU/L])

He underwent normal puberty at age 12 years and denies sexual dysfunction. He plays badminton on a regular basis and has not noticed recent fatigue or muscle loss. He is currently not in a relationship and is not planning a family.

On physical examination, his height is 68 in (173 cm) and weight is 207 lb (94 kg) (BMI = 32 kg/m²). His blood pressure is 134/91 mm Hg, and resting pulse rate is 67 beats/min. His waist circumference is 40 in (101.6 cm). Neck inspection reveals acanthosis nigricans. There is no clinical visual field defect, and he has full range of eye movements. He has mildly enlarged breasts but no palpable breast tissue. Muscle bulk appears normal, and testes are 25 mL bilaterally.

Which of the following is the best test to order now to further evaluate his gonadal axis?

- A. SHBG measurement and free testosterone estimation
- B. Pituitary-directed MRI
- C. Prolactin measurement
- D. Iron studies
- E. Estradiol measurement

49 A 26-year-old woman presents with a 3-month history of intermittent headaches. Her neurologist thinks she most likely has a variant of migraine but arranges for brain MRI to exclude an underlying structural cause. This reveals a possible pituitary abnormality that is confirmed on further dedicated imaging. MRI of the sella is shown (T1 contrast) (*see image*). The patient is referred to endocrinology.

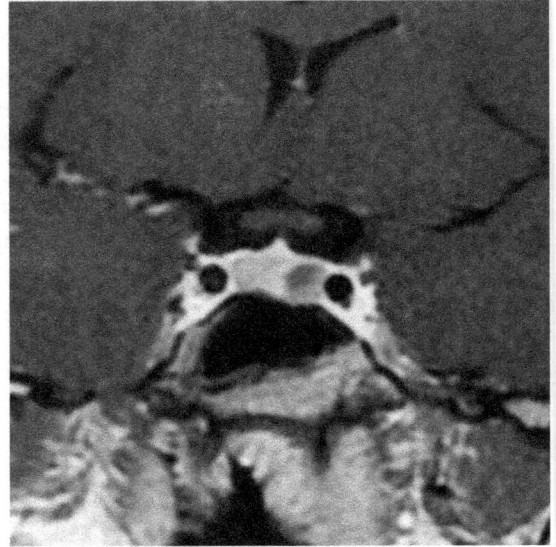

On questioning, she has no features of pituitary dysfunction. In childhood, she was diagnosed with attention-deficit/hyperactivity disorder and had recurrent middle ear infections. She has no other relevant medical history and is not taking any medications.

On physical examination, her height is 65 in (165 cm) and weight is 159 lb (72 kg) (BMI = 26 kg/m^2). Her resting pulse rate is 88 beats/min and regular, and blood pressure is 105/75 mm Hg. She has a symmetric, smooth goiter (30 g). Visual acuity is 20/20 (6/6) in both eyes and visual fields are full to confrontation. The rest of the physical examination findings are normal.

Initial laboratory test results:
    TSH = 2.4 mIU/L (0.5-5.0 mIU/L)
    Free T$_4$ = 2.5 ng/dL (0.8-1.8 ng/dL) (SI: 32.18 pmol/L [10.30-23.17 pmol/L])
    Free T$_3$ = 5.9 pg/mL (2.3-4.2 pg/mL) (SI: 9.06 pmol/L [3.53-6.45 pmol/L])
    Cortisol (8 AM) = 14.0 µg/dL (5-25 µg/dL) (SI: 386.2 nmol/L [137.9-689.7 nmol/L])
    Prolactin = 28 ng/mL (4-30 ng/mL) (SI: 1.22 nmol/L [0.17-1.30 nmol/L])
    IGF-1 = 160 ng/mL (117-321 ng/mL) (SI: 21.0 nmol/L [14.8-38.9 nmol/L])
    FSH = 6.2 mIU/mL (2.0-12.0 mIU/mL [follicular]) (SI: 6.2 IU/L [2.0-12.0 IU/L])
    LH = 5.0 mIU/mL (1.0-18.0 mIU/mL [follicular]) (SI: 5.0 IU/L [1.0-18.0 (IU/L])
    Estradiol = 60 pg/mL (10-180 pg/mL [follicular]) (SI: 220.3 pmol/L [36.7-660.8 pmol/L])

Follow-up laboratory test results:
    TSH = 2.5 mIU/L (0.5-5.0 mIU/L)
    Free T$_4$ = 2.4 ng/dL (0.8-1.8 ng/dL) (SI: 30.89 pmol/L [10.30-23.17 pmol/L])
    Free T$_3$ = 5.7 pg/mL (2.3-4.2 pg/mL) (SI: 8.76 pmol/L [3.53-6.45 pmol/L])
    TRAb = 0.1 IU/L (≤1.75 IU/L)
    SHBG = 6.9 µg/mL (2.2-14.6 µg/mL) (SI: 61.4 nmol/L [20-130 nmol/L])
    α-Subunit of pituitary glycoprotein hormones = 0.6 ng/mL (<1.2 ng/mL) (SI: 0.6 µg/L [<1.2 µg/L])

There is no evidence of laboratory assay interference in the free thyroid hormone and TSH assays.

Which of the following is the most appropriate next step in this patient's management?

A. Arrange for another pituitary MRI in 3 months
B. Initiate methimazole
C. Initiate octreotide LAR
D. Refer for genetic testing
E. Refer for transsphenoidal surgery

50 A 54-year-old woman presents with nausea, a few episodes of emesis, fatigue, and general malaise over the past few days. She has a 5-year history of type 2 diabetes mellitus that is currently managed with metformin, 500 mg twice daily; canagliflozin, 100 mg daily; insulin aspart, 10 units at each meal; and insulin degludec, 42 units daily at bedtime. This regimen has been stable for the past 6 months.

After a brief trial of oral therapy at the time of diagnosis 8 years ago (hemoglobin A_{1c} = 8.6% [70 mmol/mol]), insulin was initiated to control glycemia. Her most recent hemoglobin A_{1c} measurement is 7.2% (55 mmol/mol). She checks her blood glucose before each meal and at bedtime. She reports that her blood glucose values have been in the usual range of 80 to 150 mg/dL (4.4-8.3 mmol/L) with occasional higher readings (180-250 mg/dL [10.0-13.9 mmol/L]).

She contacted her primary care physician earlier this week, and she was given a prescription for ondansetron, 4 mg oral dissolving tablet, to help with the nausea, which was presumed to be secondary to gastroenteritis. Although ondansetron has ameliorated her nausea, she still does not feel better overall. She reports that she has increased her fluid intake over the past few weeks but has not noticed any increase in the frequency of urination.

Which of the following is the best step in this patient's management?

A. Order a basic metabolic panel and measure serum ketones
B. Perform urine analysis
C. Perform a gastric-emptying study
D. Perform esophagogastroduodenoscopy
E. Stop metformin

51 A 51-year-old woman with ischemic congestive heart failure, hypertension, obstructive sleep apnea, seizure disorder, depression, glaucoma, and Crohn disease is referred for assistance with weight loss. The patient reports that weight gain has been a problem since she was in elementary school. Her weight gain has been gradual; however, every time she initiates steroids for Crohn disease, she gains more weight than usual. She has followed commercial weight-loss programs but has been unable to keep the weight off. The patient eats 3 meals a day and describes her portions as large. She snacks on cookies, chips, cake, and ice cream. She cannot currently exercise because of deconditioning.

Her home medications include duloxetine, metoprolol, eluxadoline, fluticasone/salmeterol, aspirin, potassium chloride, levetiracetam, and esomeprazole.

On physical examination, her height is 66 in (168 cm) and weight is 278 lb (126.4 kg) (BMI = 45 kg/m^2). Her blood pressure is 121/80 mm Hg, and pulse rate is 78 beats/min. Findings on pulmonary and cardiovascular examination are normal.

Bariatric surgery is not an option given her history of Crohn disease. A low-calorie meal plan (1500 calories daily) is recommended. Six weeks after starting her new plan, she has lost 6 lb (2.7 kg). However, she is struggling with hunger. The patient believes hunger is a barrier that will impair further weight loss. Starting a weight-loss medication is discussed.

Which of the following medications should be recommended for this patient?

A. Naltrexone/bupropion
B. Liraglutide
C. Orlistat
D. Phentermine
E. Phentermine/topiramate

52 A 25-year-old man with a 15-year history of type 1 diabetes mellitus presents for routine follow-up. He has microvascular complications, including background retinopathy and microalbuminuria. His treatment consists of a basal-bolus insulin regimen (insulin aspart, 4 to 6 units with meals; insulin detemir, 6 units in the morning with 4 units at bedtime) and ramipril, 5 mg daily. He has recently been feeling more tired than usual, which he attributes to waking up at night with an increased frequency of nocturnal hypoglycemic episodes.

On physical examination, his height is 72 in (182.9 cm) and weight is 160 lb (72.7 kg) (BMI = 22 kg/m²). His blood pressure is 110/70 mm Hg, and pulse rate 88 beats/min and regular. The rest of the examination findings are normal.

Laboratory test results:
Hemoglobin A_{1c} = 6.1% (4.0%-5.6%) (43.2 mmol/mol [20-38 mmol/mol])
Serum sodium = 133 mEq/L (136-142 mEq/L) (SI: 133 mmol/L [136-142 mmol/L])
Serum potassium = 5.3 mEq/L (3.5-5.0 mEq/L) (SI: 5.3 mmol/L [3.5-5.0 mmol/L])
Serum creatinine = 1.3 mg/dL (0.7-1.3 mg/dL) (SI: 114.9 mmol/L [61.9-114.9 mmol/L])
Serum urea nitrogen = 24.3 mg/dL (8-23 mg/dL) (SI: 8.7 mmol/L [2.9-8.2 mmol/L])

Which of the following is the most appropriate next step in management?
A. Reduce the insulin detemir dosage
B. Reduce the insulin-to-carbohydrate ratio
C. Measure serum tissue transglutaminase antibodies
D. Measure serum TSH
E. Perform a 250-mcg cosyntropin-stimulation test

53 A 65-year-old woman presents for evaluation of a nodule in the thyroid isthmus that was detected on examination at her annual preventative visit with her primary care provider. The patient has no symptoms and has no personal history of head or neck radiation and no family history of thyroid cancer.

On physical examination, her blood pressure is 120/82 mm Hg and pulse rate is 80 beats/min. Her height is 65 in (165.1 cm), and weight is 160 lb (72.7 kg) (BMI = 26.6 kg/m²). Examination is notable for a soft, mobile, 1.5-cm nodule in the thyroid isthmus. The rest of the findings, including palpation of the right and left thyroid lobes and cervical lymph nodes, are normal.

The TSH concentration is 3.0 mIU/L (0.5-5.0 mIU/L).

Neck ultrasonography demonstrates a 1.8 × 1.4 × 1.0-cm nodule in the thyroid isthmus (*see image, arrow*). No abnormal cervical lymph nodes or additional thyroid nodules are observed.

Which of the following is the most appropriate diagnostic test to perform next?
A. Neck ultrasonography in 24 months
B. Neck CT
C. Radioactive iodine uptake and scan
D. Serum calcitonin measurement
E. Ultrasound-guided FNA biopsy

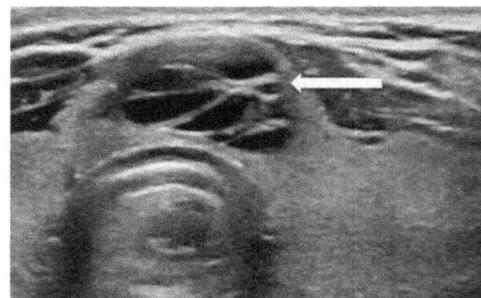

54 A 52-year-old man seeks consultation regarding type 2 diabetes mellitus. Diabetes was diagnosed 6 years ago on the basis of routine laboratory tests that documented a hemoglobin A_{1c} value of 8.2% (66 mmol/mol). His current regimen consists of metformin, 500 mg twice daily, and glimepiride, 4 mg once daily. He has no acute concerns today, and there is no history of hypoglycemia.

On physical examination, his blood pressure is 168/102 mm Hg and pulse rate is 78 beats/min. His height is 71 in (180.3 cm), and weight is 202 lb (91.8 kg) (BMI = 28.2 kg/m²). On foot examination, he has normal pulses and there are no wounds. On neurologic examination, both vibratory sensation and 10-g microfilament testing are normal.

Review of records indicates that blood pressure was similarly elevated at a previous primary care visit.

Laboratory test results:

Serum urea nitrogen = 16 mg/dL (8-23 mg/dL) (SI: 5.7 mmol/L [2.9-8.2 mmol/L])
Creatinine = 0.9 mg/dL (0.7-1.3 mg/dL) (SI: 79.6 μmol/L [61.9-114.9 μmol/L])
Hemoglobin A_{1c} = 6.9% (4.0%-5.6%) (52 mmol/mol [20-38 mmol/mol])
Urine albumin-to-creatinine ratio = 14 mg/g (<30 mg/g creat)

In addition to lifestyle management, which of the following options for pharmacologic management is the best next step for this patient?

A. Lisinopril
B. Amlodipine
C. Lisinopril and valsartan
D. Amlodipine and chlorthalidone
E. Amlodipine and metoprolol

55 A 48-year-old woman is referred for management of hyperthyroidism. Four months ago, she saw her primary care physician because of palpitations and a 10-lb (4.5-kg) weight loss. At that time, laboratory testing revealed suppressed TSH and elevated free T_4. Her primary care physician diagnosed thyroiditis and prescribed atenolol, 100 mg daily. However, she continues to experience palpitations and has developed diarrhea and tremors. She also has irregular menses and mild left lower abdominal pain. She has no known drug allergies and takes a daily multivitamin. Her family history is remarkable for hypothyroidism in her mother.

On physical examination, her blood pressure is 110/60 mm Hg and pulse rate is 90 beats/min. Her height is 64 in (162.6 cm), and weight is 136 lb (61.8 kg) (BMI = 23.3 kg/m²). Her thyroid gland is not palpable. She has no neck pain. Her heart rate is regular, and lungs are clear to auscultation. There is no lower-extremity edema. Her abdomen is tender in the left lower quadrant without a palpable mass. The rest of the examination findings are normal.

Laboratory test results:

Basic metabolic panel, normal
Complete blood cell count, normal
TSH = <0.01 mIU/L (0.5-5.5 mIU/L)
Free T_4 = 3.2 ng/dL (0.8-1.8 ng/dL) (SI: 41.2 pmol/L [10.30-23.17 pmol/L])
Thyroglobulin = 56 ng/mL (3-42 ng/mL) (SI: 56 μg/L [3-42 μg/L])
Pregnancy test, negative

She also undergoes a pinhole thyroid scan, which demonstrates decreased tracer uptake in both thyroid lobes.

Which of the following is the best next step in this patient's management?

A. Order thyroid ultrasonography
B. Initiate methimazole
C. Measure thyroid-stimulating immunoglobulin
D. Order ¹²³I whole-body scan with SPECT-CT
E. Initiate prednisone

56 A 23-year-old woman presents with irregular and heavy menses. Menarche was at age 12 years, adrenarche occurred at age 10 years, and thelarche occurred about a year later. The interval between her menstrual periods is typically 45 to 60 days.

On physical examination, her blood pressure is 110/74 mm Hg. Her height is 65 in (165.1 cm), and weight is 140 lb (63.5 kg) (BMI = 23.3 kg/m²). She has no terminal hair growth or acanthosis. Sexual development is Tanner stage 5.

Laboratory test results on cycle day 3:

    TSH = 3.1 mIU/L (0.5-5.0 mIU/L)

    Prolactin = 13 ng/mL (4-30 ng/mL [nonlactating female]) (SI: 0.56 nmol/L [0.17-1.30 nmol/L])

    LH = 15.5 mIU/mL (1.0-18.0 mIU/mL [follicular]) (SI: 3.5 IU/L [1.0-18.0 IU/L])

    FSH = 5.6 mIU/mL (2.0-12.0 mIU/mL [follicular]) (SI: 5.6 IU/L [2.0-12.0 IU/L])

    Estradiol = 35 pg/mL (10-180 pg/mL [follicular]) (SI: 128.5 pmol/L [367.1-660.8 pmol/L])

    Total testosterone = 68 ng/dL (8-60 ng/dL) (SI: 2.4 nmol/L [0.3-2.1 nmol/L])

    Free testosterone = 0.43 ng/dL (0.3-1.9 ng/dL) (SI: 0.01 nmol/L [0.01-0.07 nmol/L])

    DHEA-S = 257 μg/dL (44-332 μg/dL) (SI: 6.96 μmol/L [1.19-9.00 μmol/L])

    Androstenedione = 137 ng/dL (30-200 ng/dL) (SI: 4.78 nmol/L [1.05-6.98 nmol/L])

    17-Hydroxyprogesterone = 45 ng/dL (<80 ng/dL [follicular]) (SI: 1.36 nmol/L [<2.42 nmol/L])

    Hemoglobin A$_{1c}$ = 5.1% (4.0%-4.6%) (32 mmol/mol [20-38 mmol/mol])

Which of the following is the best next step in this patient's evaluation?

    A. Pelvic ultrasonography

    B. Measurement of antimullerian hormone

    C. Measurement of day 21 progesterone

    D. Cosyntropin-stimulation test with measurement of cortisol and 17-hydroxyprogesterone

    E. 2-Hour 75-g oral glucose tolerance test

57 A 31-year-old pregnant woman at 28 weeks' gestation seeks evaluation of hypercalcemia. She was found to be mildly hypercalcemic on routine blood work performed during her prenatal care. She has a history of Hodgkin lymphoma treated with chemotherapy at age 21 years. She is taking a prenatal multivitamin daily but no other supplements. She reports no nausea, vomiting, or changes in her bowel movements. She has no fractures or kidney stones. She has no known family history of calcium or parathyroid disease.

On physical examination, her weight is 149 lb (67.7 kg) and she has a gravid abdomen. Findings are otherwise unremarkable.

Laboratory test results:

    Serum calcium = 10.6 mg/dL (8.2-10.2 mg/dL) (SI: 2.7 mmol/L [2.1-2.6 mmol/L])

    Serum phosphate = 2.6 mg/dL (2.3-4.7 mg/dL) (SI: 0.8 mmol/L [0.7-1.5 mmol/L])

    Serum creatinine = 0.6 mg/dL (0.6-1.1 mg/dL) (SI: 53.0 μmol/L [53.0-97.2 μmol/L])

    Serum intact PTH = 35 pg/mL (10-65 pg/mL) (SI: 35 ng/L [10-65 ng/L])

    Serum 25-hydroxyvitamin D = 30 ng/mL (30-80 ng/mL [optimal]) (SI: 74.9 nmol/L [74.9-199.7 nmol/L]

    Serum 1,25-dihydroxyvitamin D = 117 pg/mL (16-65 pg/mL) (SI: 304.2 pmol/L [41.6-169.0 pmol/L])

    Serum albumin = 3.8 g/dL (3.5-5.0 g/dL) (SI: 38 g/L [35-50 g/L])

    Urinary calcium = 338 mg/24 h (100-300 mg/24 h) (SI: 8.5 mmol/d [2.5-7.5 mmol/d])

Which of the following is the most appropriate next step in the management of this patient's hypercalcemia?

    A. Initiate cinacalcet therapy

    B. Treat with intravenous pamidronate

    C. Refer for parathyroid surgery

    D. Refer to oncology for evaluation of possible lymphoma recurrence

    E. Monitor laboratory values for the remainder of her pregnancy

58 A 30-year-old woman presents for ongoing management of polycystic ovary syndrome after recently moving to the area. She was diagnosed at age 17 years when she developed irregular menses and increased terminal hair growth on her face, chin, and below the umbilicus. Menses have been irregular for several years. She is not sexually active. Her parents are alive and well in their 60s, and there is no family history of premature cardiovascular disease.

On physical examination, her height is 63.5 in (161 cm) and weight is 200 lb (91 kg) (BMI = 34.9 kg/m²). Her blood pressure is 104/70 mm Hg. She has evidence of tweezed hairs on her chin. Central adiposity is present, but she has no purple striae or bruising. Examination findings are otherwise unremarkable.

Laboratory studies confirm mild hyperandrogenism without evidence of Cushing syndrome or other hyperandrogenic states. Additional laboratory test results:

Total cholesterol = 257 mg/dL (<200 mg/dL [optimal]) (SI: 6.66 mmol/L [<5.18 mmol/L])

Triglycerides = 236 mg/dL (<150 mg/dL [optimal]) (SI: 2.67 mmol/L [<1.70 mmol/L])

HDL cholesterol = 49 mg/dL (>60 mg/dL [optimal]) (SI: 1.27 mmol/L [>1.55 mmol/L])

LDL cholesterol = 161 mg/dL (<100 mg/dL [optimal]) (SI: 4.17 mmol/L [<2.59 mmol/L])

Non-HDL cholesterol = 208 mg/dL (<130 mg/dL [optimal]) (SI: 5.39 mmol/L [<3.37 mmol/L])

Apolipoprotein B = 175 mg/dL (50-110 mg/dL) (SI: 1.8 g/L [0.5-1.1 g/L])

Fasting plasma glucose = 99 mg/dL (70-99 mg/dL) (SI: 5.5 mmol/L [3.9-5.5 mmol/L])

Hemoglobin A_{1c} = 5.6% (4.0%-5.6%) (38 mmol/mol [20-38 mmol/mol])

TSH = 2.7 mIU/L (0.5-5.0 mIU/L)

AST = 59 U/L (20-48 U/L) (SI: 0.99 μkat/L [0.33-0.80 μkat/L])

ALT = 66 U/L (10-40 U/L) (SI: 1.10 μkat/L [0.17-0.67 μkat/L])

Creatinine = 0.6 mg/dL (0.6-1.1 mg/dL) (SI: 53.0 μmol/L [53.0-97.2 μmol/L])

Which of the following is the best next step in the management of this patient's lipids?
A. Refer to a dietitian for lifestyle modification
B. Start a statin
C. Start fibrate
D. Start omega-3 fish oil
E. Start metformin

59 A 59-year-old man is admitted to the hospital with severe hypoglycemia. His wife called paramedics after finding him unconscious. The initial point-of-care glucose value was 34 mg/dL (1.9 mmol/L). He was treated with glucagon and 2 ampules of D50 and transported to the emergency department. The initial plasma glucose value at the hospital was 54 mg/dL (3.0 mmol/L). He was treated again with glucagon and started on a D5 infusion.

He is now alert and able to answer questions. He last ate food about 18 hours ago. He reports that he vomited twice in the last day. He has stage 4 chronic kidney disease due to hypertension. Medications include losartan, diltiazem, doxazosin, furosemide, clopidogrel, and a statin. He started metoprolol 4 weeks ago. Ciprofloxacin was initiated 4 days ago for treatment of a urinary tract infection. He has no history of diabetes.

In the last 4 years, he has gone through treatment twice for alcohol dependency. He stopped drinking alcohol for 14 months, but he relapsed and has been drinking daily for the last 2 months (sometimes up to three-quarters of a liter of vodka per day). He does not smoke cigarettes.

On physical examination, his height is 70 in (177.8 cm), and weight is 146 lb (66.4 kg) (BMI = 21 kg/m²). His blood pressure is 158/83 mm Hg, and pulse rate is 82 beats/min. He does not appear inebriated. The epigastric area is slightly tender. The liver edge is palpable and nontender. There is +1 pedal edema. Distal pulses are good.

Initial laboratory test results:

Hemoglobin A_{1c} = 4.9% (4.0%-5.6%) (30 mmol/mol [20-38 mmol/mol])

Creatinine = 2.4 mg/dL (0.7-1.3 mg/dL) (SI: 212.2 μmol/L [61.9-114.9 μmol/L])

Serum urea nitrogen = 36 mg/dL (8-23 mg/dL) (SI: 12.8 mmol/L [2.9-8.2 mmol/L])

Plasma glucose = 79 mg/dL (70-99 mg/dL) (SI: 4.4 mmol/L [3.9-5.5 mmol/L])

Ethanol level = 204 mg/dL

The D5 infusion is stopped and his glucose concentration is monitored. Ninety minutes later, his point-of-care glucose value is 48 mg/dL (2.7 mmol/L).

Laboratory test results (sample collected at the time of hypoglycemia):
    Plasma glucose = 51 mg/dL (70-99 mg/dL) (SI: 2.8 mmol/L [3.9-5.5 mmol/L])
    Insulin = 3.0 μIU/mL (1.4-14.0 μIU/mL) (SI: 20.8 pmol/L [9.7-97.2 pmol/L])
    C-peptide = 1.0 ng/mL (0.9-4.3 ng/mL) (SI: 0.33 nmol/L [0.30-1.42 nmol/L])
    Proinsulin = 42.3 pg/mL (26.5-176.4 pg/mL) (SI: 4.8 nmol/L [3.0-20.0 nmol/L])
    Sulfonylurea/hypoglycemia agent screen, negative

Which of the following is the most likely etiology of this patient's hypoglycemia?
    A. Insulin-secreting neuroendocrine tumor
    B. Ethanol
    C. Stage 4 chronic kidney disease
    D. Metoprolol
    E. Ciprofloxacin

60 A 20-year-old woman presents for follow-up of papillary thyroid carcinoma, which was diagnosed after thyroid nodules were detected on neck examination 2 months ago. Neck ultrasonography revealed a well-circumscribed, 2.1-cm, isoechoic, mixed cystic and solid nodule in the right thyroid lobe. A similar-appearing, 2.5-cm nodule was also observed in the left lobe. There were no abnormal lymph nodes. The patient underwent ultrasound-guided FNA biopsy of both nodules 1 week ago. The left thyroid nodule was benign, but the right nodule demonstrated findings consistent with the cribriform-morular variant of papillary thyroid cancer. A photograph of the cytopathology smear is shown (*see image*).

The patient presents to discuss the next management steps. She reports chronic diarrhea and intermittent rectal bleeding over the past year, but no other symptoms. Family history is notable for both thyroid and colon cancer in her father. Her paternal grandfather died of metastatic colon cancer. Her 25-year-old brother has a history of multiple adenomatous colon polyps and underwent resection of an abdominal desmoid tumor earlier this year. Her mother and younger sister are healthy.

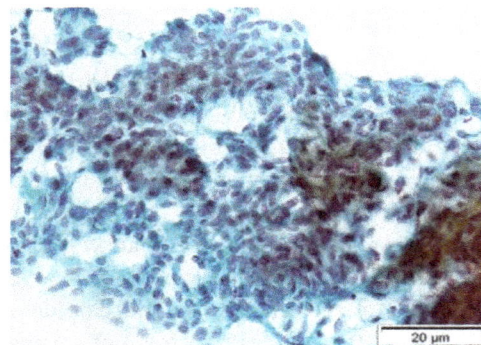

On physical examination, her blood pressure is 110/70 mm Hg and pulse rate is 72 beats/min. Her height is 66 in (167.6 cm), and weight is 145 lb (65.9 kg) (BMI = 23 kg/m²). She has bilateral thyroid nodules and no cervical lymphadenopathy. Examination of the skin is notable for multiple epidermoid cysts on her arms and trunk, but no other cutaneous findings. The rest of the findings are normal.

The TSH concentration is 1.2 mIU/L (0.5-5.0 mIU/L).

Which of the following is this patient's most likely diagnosis?
    A. Carney complex
    B. *PTEN* hamartoma tumor syndrome (Cowden syndrome)
    C. Familial adenomatous polyposis
    D. Hereditary nonpolyposis colorectal cancer (Lynch syndrome)
    E. Multiple endocrine neoplasia type 2B

61 A 40-year-old man presents with new-onset hot flashes, sweats, worsening fatigue, and low libido. He first noted these symptoms about 4 weeks ago.

Laboratory test results:
    Serum testosterone 2 weeks ago (sample drawn at 8 AM while fasting) = 66 ng/dL (300-900 ng/dL)
        (SI: 2.3 nmol/L [10.4-31.2 nmol/L])
    Serum testosterone 6 months ago = 400 ng/dL (SI: 13.9 nmol/L)

He has stage IV adrenocortical carcinoma. Four months ago, he commenced combination immune checkpoint inhibitor therapy with ipilimumab plus nivolumab for progressive disease. Two months ago, he was hospitalized (very unwell) with grade 4 immune-related hepatitis treated with high-dosage glucocorticoid therapy and mycophenolate mofetil. He also sustained an above-knee deep venous thrombosis. At that time, endocrine testing was consistent with immune-related thyroiditis and adrenalitis. Immunotherapy was stopped, but remarkably, a current fluorodeoxyglucose-PET scan shows no evidence of disease activity. He also has a microprolactinoma treated with cabergoline. Current medications include mycophenolate mofetil, 500 mg twice daily; prednisolone, 25 mg daily (weaning dose); fludrocortisone, 150 mcg daily; methadone, 10 mg twice daily; cabergoline, 0.25 mg twice weekly; a proton-pump inhibitor; and a non–vitamin K antagonist oral anticoagulant.

On physical examination, his height is 70 in (178 cm) and weight is 209 lb (95 kg) (BMI = 30 kg/m²). His blood pressure is 134/89 mm Hg without a postural drop. He has a mildly cushingoid appearance and mild proximal myopathy. There is no goiter. He has normal body hair. There is no gynecomastia. Testes are 15 mL bilaterally and soft, without palpable masses.

Current laboratory test results (sample drawn at 8 AM while fasting):
    Total testosterone = 55 ng/dL (300-900 ng/dL) (SI: 1.9 nmol/L [10.4-31.2 nmol/L])
    LH = 73.0 mIU/mL (1.0-9.0 mIU/mL) (SI: 73.0 IU/L [1.0-9.0 IU/L])
    FSH = 71.6 mIU/mL (1.0-13.0 mIU/mL) (SI: 71.6 IU/L [1.0-13.0 IU/L])
    Hemoglobin = 12.6 g/dL (13.8-17.2 g/dL) (SI: 126 g/L [138-172 g/L])
    Prolactin = 52 ng/mL (4-23 ng/mL) (SI: 2.26 nmol/L [0.17-1.00 nmol/L])
    TSH = 2.9 mIU/L (0.5-5.0 mIU/L)
    Free T$_4$ = 1.1 ng/dL (0.8-1.8 ng/dL) (SI: 14.16 pmol/L [10.30-23.17 pmol/L])
    Free T$_3$ = 2.5 pg/mL (2.3-4.2 pg/mL) (SI: 3.84 pmol/L [3.53-6.45 pmol/L])

Which of the following is the most likely explanation for his low testosterone?
    A. Treatment with glucocorticoids
    B. Immune checkpoint inhibitor therapy–associated orchitis
    C. Inadequately treated prolactinoma
    D. Thyroiditis-related changes in SHBG
    E. Recovery phase from severe illness

62 A 58-year-old woman returns for consultation regarding type 2 diabetes mellitus. She wants to know if there is a diet that could help her avoid increasing her medication burden. Diabetes was diagnosed 7 years ago based on routine screening blood tests that documented a hemoglobin A$_{1c}$ level of 7.8% (62 mmol/mol). She was prescribed metformin and engaged in lifestyle modification that mostly involved increasing her physical activity. Initially, she had a good response, with hemoglobin A$_{1c}$ values in the range of 6.7% to 7.0% (50-53 mmol/mol). However, over the last year, her hemoglobin A$_{1c}$ has increased to 7.6% (60 mmol/mol). Current medications include metformin, 1000 mg twice daily, and sitagliptin, 100 mg daily. She has no microvascular complications of diabetes.

On physical examination, her blood pressure is 132/78 mm Hg and pulse rate is 78 beats/min. Her height is 64 in (162.5 cm), and weight is 158.5 lb (72 kg) (BMI = 27.2 kg/m²). There is no evidence of peripheral neuropathy. The rest of the examination findings are unremarkable.

Laboratory test results, including a basic metabolic panel, hepatic function panel, and urine albumin excretion, are normal.

Regarding diet, which of the following eating patterns should be recommended for this patient to improve her glycemic control?
    A. Low-carbohydrate (less than 40% of calories from carbohydrates)
    B. Paleo
    C. Low-fat (less than 30% of calories from fat)
    D. DASH (Dietary Approaches to Stop Hypertension)
    E. Intermittent fasting

63 A 53-year-old man is referred for management of hypogonadism. Five years ago, he noticed reduced libido and laboratory test results at that time documented the following:

Serum testosterone = 92 ng/dL (300-900 ng/dL) (SI: 3.2 nmol/L [10.4-31.2 nmol/L])
FSH = 2.3 mIU/mL (1.0-13.0 mIU/mL) (SI: 2.3 IU/L [1.0-13.0 IU/L])
LH = 4.5 mIU/mL (1.0-9.0 mIU/mL) (SI: 4.5 IU/L [1.0-9.0 IU/L])
Prolactin = 10.0 ng/mL (4-23 ng/mL) (SI: 0.43 nmol/L [0.17-1.00 nmol/L])

Pituitary MRI revealed a pituitary macroadenoma, and he underwent surgical removal. Current MRI shows an enlarged, mostly empty sella. There is no evidence of residual adenoma.

He is already using a testosterone gel. He feels overall well and has no concerns except for constipation and fatigue. Physical examination findings are normal, with the exception of small testes (approximately 6-8 mL in volume).

Current laboratory test results:
Testosterone = 425 ng/dL (300-900 ng/dL) (SI: 14.7 nmol/L [10.4-31.2 nmol/L])
Free T$_4$ = 0.6 ng/dL (0.8-1.8 ng/dL) (SI: 7.7 pmol/L [10.30-23.17 pmol/L])
TSH = 2.9 mIU/L (0.5-5.0 mIU/L)
Cortisol (8 AM) = 18.5 μg/dL (5-25 μg/dL) (SI: 510.4 nmol/L [137.9-689.7 nmol/L])
IGF-1 = 120 ng/mL (84-233 ng/mL) (SI: 15.7 nmol/L [11.0-30.5 nmol/L])

Which of the following best describes the chance that he has GH deficiency?
A. Very low, as his IGF-1 level is normal
B. Very high, as he has other impaired pituitary axes
C. Very high, as he has an empty sella on imaging
D. Very low, as he has no symptoms
E. Irrelevant, as he is an adult

64 A 67-year-old woman with osteoporosis presents for evaluation of hyperparathyroidism. She has a history of an L1 vertebral compression fracture and was on bisphosphonate therapy but stopped this 12 months ago because she sustained a right atypical femur fracture. Recent DXA scan reveals declining bone mineral density in the forearm compared with 2 years prior, with a T-score of −2.4 in the spine, −3.0 in the left femoral neck, and −3.2 in the left one-third radius. She is on calcium and vitamin D supplementation.

Laboratory test results:
Serum calcium = 10.1 mg/dL (8.2-10.2 mg/dL) (SI: 2.5 mmol/L [2.1-2.6 mmol/L])
Serum phosphate = 3.0 mg/dL (2.3-4.7 mg/dL) (SI: 1.0 mmol/L [0.7-1.5 mmol/L])
Serum creatinine = 0.6 mg/dL (0.6-1.1 mg/dL) (SI: 53.0 μmol/L [53.0-97.2 μmol/L])
Glomerular filtration rate (estimated) = >90 mL/min per 1.73 m^2 (>60 mL/min per 1.73 m^2)
Serum intact PTH = 103 pg/mL (10-65 pg/mL) (SI: 103 ng/L [10-65 ng/L])
Serum 25-hydroxyvitamin D = 32 ng/mL (30-80 ng/mL [optimal]) (SI: 79.9 nmol/L [74.9-199.7 nmol/L])
Serum albumin = 4.6 g/dL (3.5-5.0 g/dL) (SI: 46 g/L [35-50 g/L])
Serum magnesium = 1.9 mg/dL (1.5-2.3 mg/dL) (SI: 0.8 mmol/L [0.6-0.9 mmol/L])
Urinary calcium = 180 mg/24 h (100-300 mg/24 h) (SI: 4.5 mmol/d [2.5-7.5 mmol/d])
Urinary creatinine = 0.7 g/24 h (1.0-2.0 g/24 h) (SI: 6.2 mmol/d [8.8-17.7 mmol/d])
Fractional excretion of calcium = 0.015

Which of the following is the most likely diagnosis?
A. Normocalcemic primary hyperparathyroidism
B. Secondary hyperparathyroidism
C. Tertiary hyperparathyroidism
D. Familial hypocalciuric hypercalcemia
E. Pseudohypoparathyroidism type 1a

65 A 67-year-old woman was diagnosed with dermatomyositis 1 year ago. As part of surveillance for dermatomyositis-associated malignancies, abdominal CT was performed, which revealed a unilateral adrenal mass. Noncontrast CT of the abdomen 1 month later showed a 1.6 × 1.5-cm left adrenal mass that was round and had an unenhanced attenuation value of –2 Hounsfield units. She now presents for further evaluation 1 year after her last CT.

On physical examination, her blood pressure is 121/78 mm Hg and pulse rate is 66 beats/min. Her height is 64 in (162.6 cm), and weight is 140 lb (63.6 kg) (BMI = 24 kg/m²). She does not have moon facies, dorsocervical or supraclavicular fat pads, hirsutism, acne, acanthosis nigricans, hyperpigmentation, or striae.

Results of a basic metabolic panel show normal electrolytes and kidney function. Her morning serum cortisol concentration following overnight 1-mg dexamethasone is 1.4 µg/dL (SI: 38.6 nmol/L).

Which of the following is the best next step in this patient's management?
A. Measurement of aldosterone and renin
B. Measurement of DHEA-S
C. Measurement of plasma metanephrines
D. Abdominal CT now (1 year after the last CT)
E. Reassurance and no further testing

66 A 32-year-old woman presents for follow-up of papillary thyroid carcinoma. She has a history of stage I (T2N1bM0) papillary thyroid carcinoma that was diagnosed 6 months ago. She underwent near-total thyroidectomy and central and right lateral neck dissections. Pathologic examination demonstrated a 2.5-cm primary tumor in the right thyroid lobe and no vascular invasion or extrathyroidal extension. The surgical margins were negative. A total of 13 of 40 lymph nodes were positive for metastasis. Seven days ago, she was treated with radioactive iodine therapy (75 mCi ¹³¹I) with recombinant human TSH. Her posttherapy whole-body scan shows uptake in the thyroid bed and physiologic uptake in the salivary glands, but no evidence of metastasis.

Today, the patient reports that for the past week she has been experiencing mild discomfort, fullness, and intermittent swelling in the right and left upper neck just inferior to the lower jaw. The swelling is usually associated with eating. She has no other symptoms. She is taking levothyroxine daily and no other medications.

On physical examination, her blood pressure is 95/50 mm Hg, pulse rate is 55 beats/min, and temperature is 98.2°F (36.8°C). Her height is 62 in (157.5 cm), and weight is 120 lb (54.5 kg) (BMI = 22 kg/m²). Examination is notable for a palpable mass in right zone 1B, which correlates with the patient's area of clinical concern, and it is mildly tender to the touch. The rest of her examination findings are normal.

Laboratory test results:
    1 month after surgery (before radioactive iodine therapy):
        TSH = 0.5 mIU/L
        Thyroglobulin = 0.8 ng/mL (SI: 0.8 µg/L)
        Thyroglobulin antibodies = <4 IU/mL (SI: <4 kIU/L)
    7 days ago (at the time of radioactive iodine therapy):
        TSH = 65 mIU/L
        Stimulated thyroglobulin = 0.8 ng/mL (SI: 0.8 µg/L)
        Thyroglobulin antibodies = <4 IU/mL (SI: <4 kIU/L)

Which of the following is the most appropriate initial treatment of the patient's right neck mass?
A. Initiate amoxicillin-clavulanate twice daily
B. Increase the levothyroxine dosage to achieve a serum TSH value <0.1 mIU/L
C. Recommend massage, warm compresses, oral hydration, and nonsteroidal antiinflammatory drugs as needed for pain
D. Perform FNA biopsy
E. Administer radioactive iodine therapy again with a higher administered activity of ¹³¹I

67 A 47-year-old man presents to your office with questions regarding a recent diagnosis of prediabetes. His most recent hemoglobin A_{1c} values were 5.9% (41 mmol/mol) and 6.2% (44 mmol/mol). He also reports that his fasting blood glucose values have been in the range of 100 to 115 mg/dL (5.6-6.4 mmol/L) over the last year.

He has obstructive sleep apnea but states he cannot tolerate continuous positive airway pressure (CPAP). He has not used CPAP for the past few years. He experiences fatigue that affects his quality of life. He has smoked 1 pack of cigarettes daily for the past 30 years. He has been employed in the rubber manufacturing industry for the past 25 years. Secondary hypogonadism was recently diagnosed, most likely due to obesity. Two recent serum total testosterone measurements were 255 and 228 ng/dL (8.8 and 7.9 nmol/L) (both drawn between 8 and 10 AM). He has not yet initiated testosterone therapy, but he is interested in exploring this option.

He has had difficulty maintaining a healthy weight most of his adult life. While he continues to try to exercise and reduce caloric intake, he always relapses to his old dietary and sedentary habits. He is concerned about developing type 2 diabetes and asks about starting a therapy to reduce his risk.

On physical examination, his blood pressure is 122/76 mm Hg and pulse rate is 88 beats/min. His height is 70 in (177.8 cm), and weight is 225 lb (102.3 kg) (BMI = 32 kg/m²). He has +1 pitting edema in both lower extremities. The rest of the examination findings are normal.

Laboratory test results:
  Creatinine = 1.1 mg/dL (0.7-1.3 mg/dL) (SI: 97.2 µmol/L [61.9-114.9 µmol/L])
  Hematocrit = 54% (41%-50%) (SI: 0.54 [0.41-0.50])

Which of the following interventions is the best choice to reduce this patient's risk of progression to type 2 diabetes?
  A. Vitamin D_3
  B. Pioglitazone
  C. Testosterone therapy
  D. Liraglutide
  E. Angiotensin-receptor blocker

68 A 61-year-old woman with a history of hypertension, type 2 diabetes mellitus, and hyperlipidemia is diagnosed with a 3.6-cm right thyroid nodule. She reports that an FNA biopsy of this nodule 8 months ago had benign results. Recent follow-up thyroid ultrasonography shows an increase in the nodule's size with a more heterogeneous appearance and microcalcifications. A second FNA biopsy documents follicular neoplasm. She undergoes total thyroidectomy, which confirms the diagnosis of differentiated widely invasive follicular thyroid carcinoma. She then develops hematuria 4 weeks later. Abdominal CT demonstrates a 2.6-cm, heterogeneous right adrenal mass. The unenhanced CT attenuation is 20 Hounsfield units, and 10 minutes after contrast injection the absolute contrast medium washout is only 30%. No kidney stone is visualized. An evaluation for pheochromocytoma, primary aldosteronism, and Cushing syndrome is negative.

Her family history is notable for type 2 diabetes, hypertension, and kidney stones. Current medications are atorvastatin, losartan, and NPH insulin/regular insulin 70/30.

On physical examination, her blood pressure is 120/80 mm Hg and pulse rate is 74 beats/min. There is a well-healed scar at the base of her neck. There is no cervical adenopathy. Her lungs are clear to auscultation bilaterally. Her abdomen is soft and nontender. She has no lower-extremity edema.

In addition to measuring serum thyroglobulin, which of the following is the best next step in this patient's management?
  A. FNA biopsy of the right adrenal mass
  B. Neck ultrasonography
  C. ^{131}I whole-body scan with SPECT-CT
  D. Right adrenalectomy
  E. Chest CT

69   A 22-year-old woman seeks a second opinion regarding the diagnosis of polycystic ovary syndrome. At age 16 years, she was told she most likely had polycystic ovary syndrome because she had not yet started her period and had significant cystic acne requiring isotretinoin. Oral contraceptives were initiated to start her period and for the purpose of contraception while on isotretinoin. She did not have any laboratory tests done. Adrenarche occurred at age 11 years and breast development began around the same time. She continued oral contraceptives through college and only recently stopped taking them to see if she would have her period spontaneously. She has not had her period for the past 6 months, and her cystic acne has recurred. Before starting isotretinoin and oral contraceptives again, she would like to reassess her diagnosis of polycystic ovary syndrome.

On physical examination, her blood pressure is 110/74 mm Hg. Her height is 61 in (154.9 cm), and weight is 110 lb (49.9 kg) (BMI = 21 kg/m^2). On her face, she has multiple inflammatory papules and a few deeper nodules, especially along the jaw line. She has terminal hair growth on her upper lip and abdomen. She has had this hair growth for a few years and notes that it is similar to her sister's. The rest of the examination findings are normal.

Laboratory test results:
TSH = 2.9 mIU/L (0.5-5.0 mIU/L)
Prolactin = 9 ng/mL (4-30 ng/mL [nonlactating female]) (SI: 0.39 nmol/L [0.17-1.30 nmol/L])
LH = 4.5 mIU/mL (1.0-18.0 mIU/mL [follicular]) (SI: 4.5 IU/L [1.0-18.0 IU/L])
FSH = 2.6 mIU/mL (2.0-12.0 mIU/mL [follicular]) (SI: 2.6 IU/L [2.0-12.0 IU/L])
Estradiol = 32 pg/mL (10-180 pg/mL [follicular]) (SI: 117.5 pmol/L [36.7-660.8 pmol/L])
Total testosterone = 33 ng/dL (8-60 ng/dL) (SI: 1.1 nmol/L [0.3-2.1 nmol/L])
DHEA-S = 157 μg/dL (44-332 μg/dL) (SI: 4.25 μmol/L [1.19-9.00 μmol/L])

Which of the following is the best next step in this patient's management?
A. Androstenedione and free testosterone measurement
B. Pituitary MRI
C. Progesterone test for withdrawal bleed
D. Antimullerian hormone measurement
E. 17-Hydroxyprogesterone measurement

70   A 23-year-old white woman is referred for evaluation of hypercalcemia. She initially presented to her primary care physician with bilateral hip pain. Clinical and radiographic investigations have been unrevealing. Laboratory studies documented mildly elevated creatinine and calcium, which prompted referral to your clinic. She takes no medications and does not take calcium or vitamin D supplements. She does not smoke cigarettes or drink alcohol. Her family history is notable for hypertension and history of nephrolithiasis and osteoporosis in her father. Review of systems is negative for fevers, weight loss, cough, back pain, or hematuria.

On physical examination, she appears well. Her blood pressure is 125/80 mm Hg, and pulse rate is 82 beats/min. Her height is 65 in (165 cm), and weight is 125 lb (56.8 kg) (BMI = 21 kg/m^2). There are no palpable thyroid or other neck masses. There is no flank tenderness to percussion. Spinal examination shows normal curvature without vertebral tenderness to palpation. The rest of her examination findings are normal.

Current laboratory test results:
Serum calcium = 10.9 mg/dL (8.2-10.2 mg/dL) (SI: 2.7 mmol/L [2.1-2.6 mmol/L])
Serum phosphate = 3.8 mg/dL (2.3-4.7 mg/dL) (SI: 1.2 mmol/L [0.7-1.5 mmol/L])
Serum creatinine = 1.3 mg/dL (0.6-1.1 mg/dL) (SI: 114.9 μmol/L [53.0-97.2 μmol/L])
Serum albumin = 4.0 g/dL (3.5-5.0 g/dL) (SI: 40 g/L [35-50 g/L])
Serum total protein = 6.8 g/dL (6.0-8.3 g/dL) (SI: 68 g/L [60-83 g/L])
Serum intact PTH = 15 pg/mL (10-65 pg/mL) (SI: 15 ng/L [10-65 ng/L])
Serum 25-hydroxyvitamin D = 25 ng/mL (30-80 ng/mL [optimal]) (SI: 62.4 nmol/L [74.9-199.7 nmol/L])
Serum 1,25-dihydroxyvitamin D = 105 pg/mL (16-65 pg/mL) (SI: 273 pmol/L [41.6-169.0 pmol/L])
Urinary calcium = 340 mg/24 h (100-300 mg/24 h) (SI: 8.5 mmol/d [2.5-7.5 mmol/d])
Urinary creatinine = 0.6 g/24 h (1.0-2.0 g/24 h) (SI: 5.3 mmol/d [8.8-17.7 mmol/d])

Findings on chest x-ray are normal. Renal ultrasonography shows no evidence of frank nephrolithiasis, but it does show increased echogenicity of the renal medullae bilaterally, consistent with nephrocalcinosis.

Which of the following is the best next step in this patient's management?
- A. Measure serum angiotensin-converting enzyme
- B. Perform serum protein electrophoresis
- C. Measure serum vitamin A
- D. Measure serum 24,25-dihydroxyvitamin D
- E. Perform purified protein derivative testing for tuberculosis

71 A 32-year-old woman is referred for management of diabetes mellitus. The patient recently presented with symptoms of polydipsia, polyuria, nocturia, and 14-lb (6.4-kg) weight loss that developed over 4 weeks. She was evaluated in the emergency department and documented to have the following laboratory test results:

Plasma glucose = 378 mg/dL (70-99 mg/dL) (SI: 21.0 mmol/L [3.9-5.5 mmol/L])
Bicarbonate = 20 mEq/L (21-28 mEq/L) (SI: 20 mmol/L [21-28 mmol/L])
β-Hydroxybutyrate = 3.6 mg/dL (<3.0 mg/dL) (SI: 345.8 μmol/L [<288.8 μmol/L])
Hemoglobin A$_{1c}$ = 9.6% (4.0%-5.6%) (81 mmol/mol [20-38 mmol/mol])

She was treated with intravenous fluids and was given 10 units of regular insulin subcutaneously. Three hours later, the plasma glucose concentration was 204 mg/dL (11.3 mmol/L). She was discharged and told to administer 10 units of insulin glargine at bedtime.

She has seen a dietician, modified her diet, and has been doing home glucose monitoring. She now administers 13 units of insulin glargine at bedtime. She had gestational diabetes with her most recent pregnancy 8 months ago. She was treated with insulin detemir and insulin aspart given twice daily during the last 10 weeks of pregnancy. The insulin was stopped when she went into labor and was never restarted. She delivered vaginally, and the baby's birth weight was 8 lb, 11 oz (3941 g). The baby had no complications at birth. The patient did not return for a scheduled oral glucose tolerance test 6 weeks after delivery.

She gained 38 lb (17.3 kg) during her pregnancy and lost 31 lb (14.1 kg) in the first 6 months after delivery. She has a history of primary hypothyroidism and is treated with levothyroxine, 112 mcg daily. She has no history of hypertension, dyslipidemia, or coronary heart disease. She does not smoke cigarettes and has 1 serving of alcohol 2 to 3 times per week. Her maternal grandmother, maternal aunt, and maternal uncle have diabetes. Her mother has hypothyroidism.

On physical examination, her height is 66 in (167.6 cm) and weight is 157 lb (71.4 kg) (BMI = 25 kg/m^2). Her blood pressure is 122/74 mm Hg, and pulse rate is 76 beats/min. Peripheral pulses are strong. Findings on neurologic examination are unremarkable.

Laboratory test results:
Plasma glucose (3 hours postprandial) = 178 mg/dL (70-99 mg/dL) (SI: 9.9 mmol/L [3.9-5.5 mmol/L])
Bicarbonate = 26 mEq/L (21-28 mEq/L) (SI: 26 mmol/L [21-28 mmol/L])
Creatinine = 0.78 mg/dL (0.6-1.1 mg/dL) (SI: 69.0 μmol/L [53.0-97.2 μmol/L])
TSH = 2.1 mIU/L (0.5-5.0 mIU/L)
C-peptide = 1.0 mg/dL (0.9-4.3 ng/mL) (SI: 0.3 nmol/L [0.30-1.42 nmol/L])

Results of point-of-care fingerstick glucose readings are shown (*see table*).

Day	Breakfast	Prelunch	Predinner	Bedtime
Friday	137 mg/dL (SI: 7.6 mmol/L)	135 mg/dL (SI: 7.5 mmol/L)	...	131 mg/dL (SI: 7.3 mmol/L)
Saturday	119 mg/dL (SI: 6.6 mmol/L)	...	121 mg/dL (SI: 6.7 mmol/L)	107 mg/dL (SI: 5.9 mmol/L)
Sunday	128 mg/dL (SI: 7.1 mmol/L)	109 mg/dL (SI: 6.0 mmol/L)	99 mg/dL (SI: 5.5 mmol/L)	...
Monday	...	118 mg/dL (SI: 6.5 mmol/L)	133 mg/dL (SI: 7.4 mmol/L)	...
Tuesday	117 mg/dL (SI: 6.5 mmol/L)	96 mg/dL (SI: 5.3 mmol/L)	114 mg/dL (SI: 6.3 mmol/L)	128 mg/dL (SI: 7.1 mmol/L)

Which of the following is the most likely etiology of this patient's diabetes?
- A. Type 1 diabetes mellitus
- B. Latent autoimmune diabetes in adults
- C. Type 2 diabetes mellitus
- D. Maturity-onset diabetes of the young
- E. Insufficient data to make a diagnosis

72 An 18-year-old man is evaluated for cervical lymphadenopathy. Biopsy confirms a diagnosis of classic Hodgkin lymphoma. He undergoes 12 cycles of chemotherapy with doxorubicin, bleomycin, vinblastine, and dacarbazine. Subsequent imaging shows resolution of the cervical lymphadenopathy. A staging PET scan demonstrates a new 1.6 × 1.2-cm, intensely fluorodeoxyglucose-avid left adrenal mass without evidence of extra-adrenal involvement or new lymphadenopathy. On CT, the unenhanced attenuation value of the left adrenal mass is 35 Hounsfield units. He has no hyperadrenergic symptoms such as palpitations, sweating, tremulousness, or headache.

On physical examination, his blood pressure is 115/65 mm Hg and pulse rate is 64 beats/min. His height is 69 in (175.3 cm), and weight is 143 lb (65 kg) (BMI = 21.1 kg/m²). The patient is in no apparent distress. There are no overt signs of Cushing syndrome such as moon facies, lipodystrophy or lipoatrophy, striae, or proximal muscle weakness.

Which of the following is the best next step in this patient's management?
- A. Core-needle biopsy of the left adrenal mass
- B. FNA of the left adrenal mass
- C. Measurement of plasma metanephrines
- D. Resumption of lymphoma-directed chemotherapy
- E. Surgical resection of the left adrenal mass

73 A 37-year-old man is referred from the liver transplant clinic for evaluation of very high lipid levels. He has a history of Crohn disease and primary sclerosing cholangitis with progressive liver failure. He is being considered as a candidate for liver transplant. He takes ursodiol, mesalamine, sertraline, and hydroxyzine. He does not smoke cigarettes and does not drink alcohol or use controlled substances. His family history is remarkable for liver disease and cirrhosis in his brother, but there is no cardiovascular disease.

On physical examination, he is a chronically ill-appearing, cachectic man. His height is 68.5 in (176.5 cm), and weight is 152 lb (69.1 kg) (BMI = 22.1 kg/m²). His blood pressure is 102/72 mm Hg. Icteric conjunctivae are observed. There are no eruptive or tendon xanthomas, corneal arcus, or xanthelasma. His skin is dry and scaly. The abdomen is mildly distended and nontender.

Laboratory test results (nonfasting):
    Total cholesterol = 1484 mg/dL (<200 mg/dL [optimal]) (SI: 38.44 mmol/L [<5.18 mmol/L])
    Triglycerides = 538 mg/dL (<150 mg/dL [optimal]) (SI: 6.08 mmol/L [<1.70 mmol/L])
    HDL cholesterol = 31 mg/dL (>60 mg/dL [optimal]) (SI: 0.80 mmol/L [>1.55 mmol/L])
    LDL cholesterol = 1345 mg/dL (<100 mg/dL [optimal]) (SI: 34.84 mmol/L [<2.59 mmol/L])
    Creatinine = 0.6 mg/dL (0.7-1.3 mg/dL) (SI: 53.0 µmol/L [61.9-114.9 µmol/L])
    AST = 87 U/L (20-48 U/L) (SI: 1.45 µkat/L [0.33-0.80 µkat/L])
    ALT = 55 U/L (10-40 U/L) (SI: 0.92 µkat/L [0.17-0.67 µkat/L])
    Alkaline phosphatase = 1094 U/L (50-120 U/L) (SI: 18.27 µkat/L [0.84-2.00 µkat/L])
    Total bilirubin = 7.0 mg/dL (0.3-1.2 mg/dL) (SI: 119.7 µmol/L [5.1-20.5 µmol/L])
    Direct bilirubin = 5.0 mg/dL (0-0.3 mg/dL)

Which of the following is the most likely explanation for this patient's very high lipid levels?
- A. Homozygous familial hypercholesterolemia
- B. Familial form of hypertriglyceridemia
- C. Hepatic lipase deficiency
- D. Ursodiol therapy
- E. Cholestatic liver disease

74 A 36-year-old woman presents with a 1-month history of odynophagia, weight loss, and subacute mental status decline. She was previously healthy. She is found to be lymphopenic with an absolute neutrophil count of 800/mm³. HIV/AIDS is diagnosed. She is presumed to have *Pneumocystis jirovecii* pneumonia based on x-ray findings. Endocrinology is consulted because of hypoglycemia that develops in the late mornings of hospital days 5 and 6, in the nonfasting state. Plasma glucose levels are documented to be 45 and 49 mg/dL (2.5 and 2.7 mmol/L). Notably, plasma glucose values on the first day of admission ranged between 65 and 89 mg/dL (3.6-4.9 mmol/L).

On physical examination, the patient is agitated. Her blood pressure is 117/88 mm Hg, pulse rate is 100 beats/min, respiratory rate is 16 breaths/min, and oxygen saturation is normal. Examination findings are nonfocal; however, the patient is unable to answer questions.

Current medications are ciprofloxacin eye drops; fluconazole, 200 mg intravenously every 24 hours; iron sucrose, 200 mg intravenously daily; lidocaine transdermal patch; miconazole topical; quetiapine, 50 mg nightly; trimethoprim-sulfamethoxazole, 600 mg intravenously every 24 hours; and thiamine, 300 mg intravenously daily.

Laboratory test results:
  White blood cell count = 1100/µL (4500-11,000/µL) (SI: 1.1 × 10⁹/L [4.5-11.0 × 10⁹/L])
  Hemoglobin = 7.7 g/dL (12.1-15.1 g/dL) (SI: 77 g/L [121-151 g/L])
  Platelet count = 326 × 10³/µL (150-450 × 10³/µL) (SI: 326 × 10⁹/L [150-450 × 10⁹/L])
  Sodium = 143 mEq/L (136-142 mEq/L) (SI: 143 mmol/L [136-142 mmol/L])
  Potassium = 4.3 mEq/L (3.5-5.0 mEq/L) (SI: 4.3 mmol/L [3.5-5.0 mmol/L])
  Chloride = 113 mEq/L (96-106 mEq/L) (SI: 113 mmol/L [96-106 mmol/L])
  Bicarbonate = 17 mEq/L (21-28 mEq/L) (SI: 17 mmol/L [21-28 mmol/L])
  Serum urea nitrogen = 7 mg/dL (8-23 mg/dL) (SI: 2.5 mmol/L [2.9-8.2 mmol/L])
  Creatinine = 0.3 mg/dL (0.6-1.1 mg/dL) (SI: 26.5 µmol/L [53.0-97.2 µmol/L])
  Protein = 4.9 g/dL (6.0-8.0 g/dL) (SI: 49 g/L [60-80 g/L])
  Albumin = 2.0 g/dL (3.5-5.0 g/dL) (SI: 20 g/L [35-50 g/L])

Which of the following is the most likely cause of this patient's hypoglycemia?
- A. Iron
- B. Fluconazole
- C. Malnutrition
- D. Trimethoprim-sulfamethoxazole
- E. Primary adrenal insufficiency

75 A 69-year-old man with hepatitis C liver cirrhosis is referred for evaluation and management of osteoporosis, which was diagnosed based on a screening bone density test done 6 months ago (lowest T-score of –4.2 at the left total hip, Z-score –3.2). He sustained a Colles fracture of his right wrist after falling 1 year ago. He has no history of thyroid disease or parathyroid disease. He has limited dietary calcium intake and was recently started on calcium and vitamin D supplements.

On physical examination, he has an intact gait and no spine tenderness to palpation.

Laboratory test results:
   Serum calcium = 9.6 mg/dL (8.2-10.2 mg/dL) (SI: 2.4 mmol/L [2.1-2.6 mmol/L])
   Serum phosphate = 4.0 mg/dL (2.3-4.7 mg/dL) (SI: 1.3 mmol/L [0.7-1.5 mmol/L])
   Serum creatinine = 0.9 mg/dL (0.7-1.3 mg/dL) (SI: 79.6 μmol/L [61.9-114.9 μmol/L])
   Serum intact PTH = 29 pg/mL (10-65 pg/mL) (SI: 29 ng/L [10-65 ng/L])
   Serum 25-hydroxyvitamin D = 26 ng/mL (30-80 ng/mL [optimal]) (SI: 64.9 nmol/L [74.9-199.7 nmol/L])
   Serum albumin = 3.5 g/dL (3.5-5.0 g/dL) (SI: 35 g/L [35-50 g/L])
   Serum total alkaline phosphatase = 90 U/L (50-120 U/L) (SI: 1.50 μkat/L [0.84-2.00 μkat/L])
   Serum bone-specific alkaline phosphatase = 35.0 μg/L (≤25.1 μg/L)
   TSH, normal
   Morning testosterone, normal

In addition to dietary counseling and adequate calcium and vitamin D supplementation, which of the following is the best next step?
   A. Perform serum protein electrophoresis
   B. Measure 24-hour urinary calcium excretion
   C. Perform whole-body bone scan
   D. Start alendronate
   E. Start teriparatide

76 A 41-year-old woman is referred for evaluation of possible Cushing syndrome. Hypertension was diagnosed 2 years ago and type 2 diabetes mellitus was diagnosed last year. She has gained 25 lb (11.4 kg) over 2 years, mostly in her midsection.

Laboratory test results (ordered by her internist):
   Urinary free cortisol = 45 μg/24 h (4-50 μg/24 h) (SI: 124.2 nmol/d [11-138 nmol/d])
   Serum cortisol after 1-mg overnight dexamethasone-suppression test = 3.2 μg/dL (SI: 88.3 nmol/L)
   Dexamethasone = 234 ng/dL (180-550 ng/dL [suppressive level])

Her current medications are losartan, 100 mg daily; metformin, 500 mg twice daily; oral contraceptive pill; and cetirizine, 10 mg daily.

   On physical examination, her blood pressure is 140/90 mm Hg and pulse rate is 76 beats/min. Her height is 66.5 in (169 cm), and weight is 202.5 lb (92 kg) (BMI = 32 kg/m²). She has some facial rounding and an obese abdomen with no striae.

Which of the following is the best next step in this patient's management?
   A. Obtain 2 bedtime salivary cortisol measurements
   B. Measure plasma ACTH
   C. Perform pituitary-directed MRI
   D. Perform another dexamethasone-suppression test (2 mg)
   E. Measure 24-hour urinary free cortisol after stopping the oral contraceptive

77 A 58-year-old woman who has had type 1 diabetes mellitus since she was 4 years old presents for regular follow-up. She has no known complications, but she does have suboptimal glycemic control, and her hemoglobin A$_{1c}$ level is 8.3% (67 mmol/mol) at the current visit.

   Some mornings, she exercises for 1 hour. She eats her first meal of the day around 9 AM. The timing of lunch and dinner is inconsistent. She uses an insulin pump with the following rates:

Basal

Midnight: 0.6 units/h
6:00 AM: 0.9 units/h
9:00 AM: 0.6 units/h
11:00AM: 0.6 units/h
1:00 PM: 0.7 units/h
Total basal insulin = 16.4 units

Bolus insulin

Midnight-11:00 AM: 1 unit per 14 g carbohydrate; sensitivity factor: 1 unit per 85 mg/dL (4.7 mmol/L)
11:00 AM-midnight: 1 unit per 11 g carbohydrate; sensitivity factor: 1 unit per 65 mg/dL (3.6 mmol/L)

Her glucose target is 150 mg/dL (8.3 mmol/L) around the clock. She provides a 90-day tracing from her continuous glucose monitor for review (*see image*).

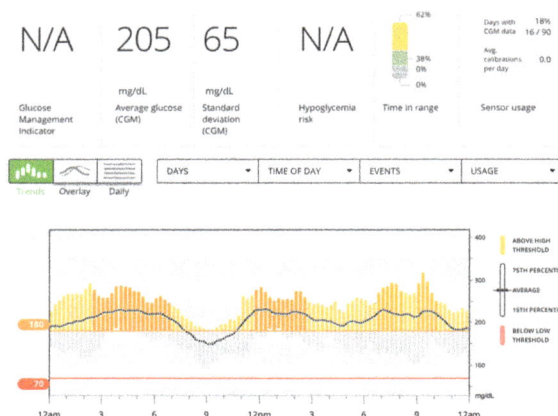

In addition to counseling her about eating meals at regular times, which of following is the best next step?

A. Reassess continuous glucose monitoring data over a different interval before making recommendations
B. Increase overnight basal insulin to 0.8 units per hour from midnight to 6 AM
C. Increase each basal rate by 10%
D. Increase the insulin-to-carbohydrate ratio with breakfast
E. Recommend that she change from insulin pump therapy to multiple daily injections

78 A 46-year-old woman presents for follow-up of stage I (T2N0M0) papillary thyroid carcinoma that was initially diagnosed and treated with a near-total thyroidectomy 9 months ago. Surgical pathology demonstrated a 2.2-cm classic papillary thyroid carcinoma with no evidence of extrathyroidal extension or lymphatic or vascular invasion. The surgical margins were negative.

Six weeks after surgery, the patient's thyroglobulin concentration was noted to be elevated at 11.2 ng/mL (11.2 μg/L) with negative thyroglobulin antibodies and a serum TSH value of 0.8 mIU/L. Postoperative neck ultrasonography and diagnostic radioactive iodine (^{123}I) whole-body scan were performed, and both were negative for evidence of metastasis. The patient was treated with radioactive iodine (100 mCi ^{131}I), and her posttreatment whole-body scan demonstrated uptake in the thyroid bed, but was again negative for metastasis. Since treatment with ^{131}I, the patient has continued to have elevated serum thyroglobulin measurements. CT of the neck and chest was subsequently performed, but no suspicious findings were observed.

On physical examination, her blood pressure is 130/80 mm Hg and pulse rate is 88 beats/min. Her height is 65 in (165.1 cm), and weight is 170 lb (77.3 kg) (BMI = 28.3 kg/m²). The rest of the examination findings are normal.

Laboratory test results:
  Six months ago (at the time of radioactive iodine therapy):
    TSH = 52 mIU/L
    Stimulated thyroglobulin = 9.9 ng/mL (SI: 9.9 μg/L)
    Thyroglobulin antibodies = <4 IU/mL (SI: <4 kIU/L)
  Two months ago:
    TSH = 0.4 mIU/L
    Thyroglobulin = 10.4 ng/mL (SI: 10.4 μg/L)
    Thyroglobulin antibodies = <4 IU/mL (SI: <4 kIU/L)

Which of the following is the most appropriate diagnostic test to recommend next?

A. Bone scintigraphy
B. Diagnostic radioactive iodine (^{123}I) whole-body scan
C. Exploratory central neck dissection
D. Thyroglobulin measurement by radioimmunoassay
E. PET-CT whole-body imaging

79 A 42-year-old man returns for continued management of type 1 diabetes mellitus, which was diagnosed at age 22 years. Glycemic control has been variable, and recent hemoglobin A_{1c} measurements have been in the range of 6.7% to 8.2% (50-66 mmol/mol). Two years ago, he started insulin pump therapy and began using a continuous glucose sensor because of hypoglycemia unawareness. The last time he required assistance to treat severe hypoglycemia was 2.5 years ago. He can now recognize hypoglycemia when his glucose concentration is in the range of 60 to 70 mg/dL (3.3-3.9 mmol/L).

He uses insulin lispro in the pump. The total daily insulin dose is 48 units, 45% of which is basal insulin. He changes his pump site every 3 days and his glucose sensor every 7 days. He does not have lipohypertrophy.

The basal insulin rates are as follows:
  Midnight to 3 AM: 0.8 units per h
  3 AM to 7 AM: 1.2 units per h
  7 AM to 1 PM: 0.9 units per h
  1 PM to 6 PM: 0.7 units per h
  6 PM to 12 PM: 0.9 units per h

He uses a ratio of 1 unit of insulin aspart per 10 g carbohydrate (insulin-to-carbohydrate ratio) as a bolus before meals. He boluses the insulin 10 to 15 minutes before eating. His meals are eaten at 7:30 AM, 12:30 PM, and 6:30 PM.

Diabetes-related complications include nonproliferative retinopathy and mild distal polyneuropathy. He walks for 45 minutes 4 days per week and does not adjust the basal rate for activity.

Laboratory test results:
  Hemoglobin A_{1c} = 8.0% (4.0%-5.6%) (64 mmol/mol [20-38 mmol/mol])
  Creatinine = 1.1 mg/dL (0.7-1.3 mg/dL) (SI: 97.2 μmol/L [61.9-114.9 μmol/L])
  TSH = 1.87 mIU/L (0.5-5.0 mIU/L)
  Electrolytes, normal

The downloaded 2-week continuous glucose sensor data are shown (*see image, black arrows indicate mealtimes*).

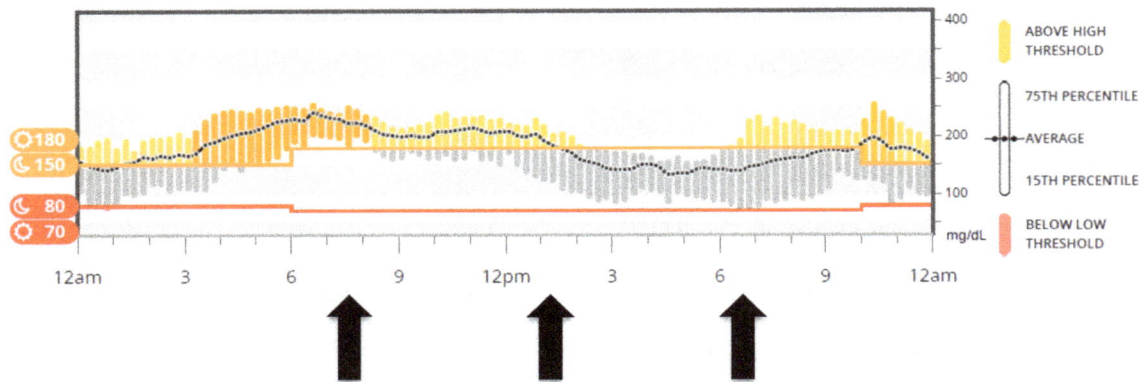

In addition to increasing the basal rate at 3 AM, which of the following is the best option to improve this patient's glycemic control?
A. Increase the basal rate at 7 AM
B. Increase the basal rate at 7 AM, 1 PM, and 6 PM
C. Increase the basal rate at 7 AM and change the insulin-to-carbohydrate ratio to 1 to 8 at 6:30 PM
D. Change the insulin-to-carbohydrate ratio to 1 to 8 at 7:30 AM
E. Change the insulin-to-carbohydrate ratio to 1 to 8 at 7:30 AM and 6:30 PM

80 A 57-year-old man with hypertension, osteoarthritis, and mixed hyperlipidemia seeks assistance with weight loss. He would like to lose weight before his upcoming high school reunion. He reports always feeling tired and says he could take a nap at any time during the day. He hopes weight loss will help with this as well. He eats out for most of his meals and often stops at fast-food restaurants. He has not been exercising because of fatigue. He has no shortness of breath or chest pain on exertion. His wife complains about his snoring at night.

On physical examination, his blood pressure is 140/85 mm Hg and pulse rate is 90 beats/min. His height is 69 in (173.3cm), and weight is 258 lb (117.3 kg) (BMI = 38 kg/m^2). His neck circumference is 18 in (45.7 cm), and waist circumference is 51.5 in (131 cm). He is in no distress and does not have moon facies. There is no goiter. His lungs are clear to auscultation bilaterally, heart sounds are regular, and no murmur is detected. His abdomen is soft, and he has white stretch marks but no purple striae. He has no peripheral edema. He has normal proximal muscle strength in both upper and lower extremities.

Laboratory test results (ordered by his primary care physician 2 weeks ago):
TSH = 2.4 mIU/L (0.5-5.0 mIU/L)
Hemoglobin A$_{1c}$ = 6.2% (4.0%-5.6%) (44 mmol/mol [20-38 mmol/mol])

In addition to recommending a meal and exercise plan, which of the following should be suggested for this patient?
A. IGF-1 measurement
B. Fasting insulin measurement
C. 24-Hour urine collection for cortisol
D. Referral to sleep medicine
E. Echocardiography

81 A 63-year-old man is referred for further assessment of hypertension, which has proved increasingly difficult to control in recent months. He also reports swelling of both ankles and is now getting up several times each night to pass urine. His current medications are atorvastatin, amlodipine, doxazosin, indapamide, and ramipril. He has never smoked cigarettes and does not consume alcohol or licorice. Review of his case records reveals that his blood pressure was normal until age 55 years, when he first commenced antihypertensive therapy.

On physical examination, his height is 69 in (175.3 cm) and weight is 192 lb (87.3 kg) (BMI = 28 kg/m^2). His blood pressure is 182/105 mm Hg, and pulse rate is 72 beats/min and regular. There is bilateral pitting edema to the mid-calf, but no other abnormalities on cardiorespiratory examination.

Laboratory test results:
Serum sodium = 143 mEq/L (136-142 mEq/L) (SI: 143 mmol/L [136-142 mmol/L])
Serum potassium = 2.1 mEq/L (3.5-5.0 mEq/L) (SI: 2.1 mmol/L [3.5-5.0 mmol/L])
Serum creatinine = 1.0 mg/dL (0.7-1.3 mg/dL) (SI: 88.4 µmol/L [61.9-114.9 µmol/L])
Plasma renin activity = 0.3 ng/mL per h (0.6-4.3 ng/mL per h)
Plasma aldosterone concentration = <2.5 ng/dL (4-21 ng/dL) (SI <69.4 pmol/L [111-582.5 pmol/L])
Urinary free cortisol = 38 µg/24 h (4-50 µg/24 h) (SI: 104.9 nmol/d [11-138 nmol/d])

Which of the following is the most likely cause of this patient's presentation?
A. Bilateral renal artery stenosis
B. Deoxycorticosterone-producing adrenal tumor
C. Glucocorticoid-remediable (suppressible) aldosteronism
D. Liddle syndrome
E. Syndrome of apparent mineralocorticoid excess

82 At 20 week's gestation, a 29-year-old woman (G2P1) presents for evaluation of a left-sided neck lump. She has a history of hypothyroidism and takes levothyroxine, 125 mcg daily. She has no history of radiation therapy to her head and neck and no family history of thyroid cancer. She takes a daily prenatal vitamin.

On physical examination, her blood pressure is 124/64 mm Hg and pulse rate is 72 beats/min. Her height is 64 in (162.6 cm) and weight is 135 lb (61.4 kg) (BMI = 23.2 kg/m^2). Her thyroid gland is 40 g with a palpable, 1.5-cm left thyroid nodule. There is no palpable cervical lymphadenopathy. Her abdomen is gravid and soft. The rest of the examination findings are normal.

Laboratory test results:
TSH = 1.2 mIU/L (0.5-5.0 mIU/L)
Total T$_4$ = 15 µg/dL (5.5-12.5 µg/dL) (SI: 193.1 nmol/L [94.02-213.68 nmol/L])
Calcium = 8.9 mg/dL (8.2-10.2 mg/dL) (SI: 2.2 mmol/L [2.1-2.6 mmol/L])

Thyroid ultrasonography shows a nodule in the left lobe (*see image, sagittal view*) and this nodule measures 1.0 × 1.0 × 1.5 cm (anteroposterior × transverse × longitudinal).

Which of the following is the best next step in this patient's management?
A. Refer her to a surgeon for thyroidectomy
B. Increase her levothyroxine dosage to suppress her TSH
C. Perform a thyroid scan
D. Perform FNA biopsy of the left thyroid nodule
E. Perform thyroid ultrasonography again after delivery

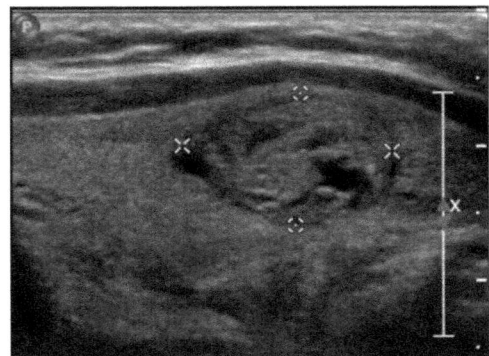

83 A 29-year-old woman seeks advice regarding difficulty conceiving. Her medical history is notable for polycystic ovary syndrome diagnosed at age 16 years. She was treated with oral contraceptive pills for several years. However, after stopping oral contraceptive pills, she and her partner have been unable to conceive for the last 2 years despite unprotected intercourse. Her primary care physician prescribed metformin for the last 6 months, but this has been unsuccessful. In the 10 years preceding treatment with metformin, she gained 40 lb (18.1 kg). Since starting metformin, her weight has been stable. Metformin was recently discontinued in favor of clomiphene citrate. Menstrual cycles are normal. Family history is notable for recently diagnosed type 2 diabetes in her mother.

Findings on physical examination are unremarkable. Her height is 68 in (172.7 cm), and weight is 205 lb (93.2 kg) (BMI = 31 kg/m^2). There is no acanthosis nigricans.

Her hemoglobin A_{1c} value is 7.9% (4.0%-5.6%) (63 mmol/mol [20-38 mmol/mol]).

You repeat the hemoglobin A_{1c} measurement and obtain a similar value. Which of the following is the best next step?
  A. Continue clomiphene and prescribe insulin
  B. Discontinue clomiphene and prescribe insulin
  C. Discontinue clomiphene and start GLP-1 receptor agonist
  D. Continue clomiphene and prescribe glimepiride
  E. Discontinue clomiphene and prescribe glimepiride

84 A 72-year-old woman is referred for recommendations regarding osteoporosis treatment. She has no history of low-trauma fractures. Her mother had vertebral and hip fractures. Current medications include omeprazole; atorvastatin; meloxicam; calcium, 600 mg twice daily; and cholecalciferol, 400 IU twice daily. Review of systems is negative for fevers, weight loss, abdominal pain, diarrhea, or hematuria.

On physical examination, her blood pressure is 125/70 mm Hg and pulse rate is 88 beats/min. Her height is 64 in (162.6 cm) (1 in [2.5 cm] shorter than her self-reported maximum adult height), and weight is 110 lb (50 kg) (BMI = 18.9 kg/m^2). The thyroid gland is not palpable. There is no appreciable adenopathy. Findings on abdominal examination are normal. Spinal curvature is normal without kyphosis or vertebral tenderness.

Laboratory test results:
  Serum calcium = 10.0 mg/dL (8.2-10.2 mg/dL) (SI: 2.5 mmol/L [2.1-2.6 mmol/L])
  Serum phosphate = 3.2 mg/dL (2.3-4.7 mg/dL) (SI: 1.0 mmol/L [0.7-1.5 mmol/L])
  Serum creatinine = 0.8 mg/dL (0.6-1.1 mg/dL) (SI: 70.7 μmol/L [53.0-97.2 μmol/L])
  Serum albumin = 3.6 g/dL (3.5-5.0 g/dL) (SI: 36 g/L [35-50 g/L])
  Serum intact PTH = 55 pg/mL (10-65 pg/mL) (SI: 55 ng/L [10-65 ng/L])
  Serum 25-hydroxyvitamin D = 32 ng/mL (30-80 ng/mL [optimal]) (SI: 79.9 nmol/L [74.9-199.7 nmol/L])
  Urinary calcium = 250 mg/24 h (100-300 mg/24 h) (SI: 6.3 mmol/d [2.5-7.5 mmol/d])
  Urinary creatinine = 0.8 g/24 h (1.0-2.0 g/24 h) (SI: 7.1 mmol/d [8.8-17.7 mmol/d])
  Fractional excretion of calcium = 0.025

DXA documents the following values:
  Lumbar spine T-score = −2.5
  Right femoral neck T-score = −2.4
  Right total hip T-score = −2.1
  Left proximal one-third radius T-score = −3.5

FRAX 10-year fracture risk:
  Hip = 9.9%
  Major = 21%

On the basis of her clinical history and high fracture risk, you recommend initiating teriparatide. After 3 weeks of treatment, she returns with concerns of fatigue and nocturia. Her serum calcium concentration is 11.2 mg/dL (2.8 mmol/L).

On the basis of this patient's clinical history, which of the following is the most likely underlying disorder that explains her current hypercalcemia?
- A. Sarcoidosis
- B. Familial hypocalciuric hypercalcemia
- C. Primary hyperparathyroidism
- D. Multiple myeloma
- E. Renal cell carcinoma

85 A 67-year-old man is hospitalized after low-trauma fracture of the femoral neck sustained 1 week ago. The fracture has been treated with total hip arthroplasty. Clinical risk factors for osteoporosis include regular alcohol intake (3 standard drinks per day) and a low BMI. His only regular mediations are a vitamin D supplement, thiamine, and pantoprazole. On review of symptoms, the patient reports longstanding low libido, low mood, and fatigue. His postoperative pain is controlled on opioids.

On physical examination, his height is 67 in (170.2 cm) and weight is 121 lb (55 kg) (BMI = 18.9 kg/m²). Visual fields are normal to confrontation, and eye movements are full. He has low muscle bulk, scattered spider nevi, and palmar erythema. His liver is palpable 2 cm below the costal margin. There is no ascites. Testes are 15 mL bilaterally.

Laboratory test results (performed on postoperative day 2 (sample drawn at 8 AM while fasting):
    ALT = 55 U/L (10-40 U/L) (SI: 0.92 µkat/L [0.17-0.67 µkat/L])
    AST = 77 U/L (20-48 U/L) (SI: 1.29 µkat/L [0.33-0.80 µkat/L])
    γ-Glutamyltransferase = 89 U/L (2-30 U/L) (SI: 1.49 µkat/L [0.03-0.50 µkat/L])
    Total testosterone = 55 ng/dL (300-900 ng/dL) (SI: 1.9 nmol/L [10.4-31.2 nmol/L])
    LH = 1.0 mIU/mL (1.0-9.0 mIU/mL) (SI: 1.0 IU/L [1.0-9.0 IU/L])
    FSH = 0.7 mIU/mL (1.0-13.0 mIU/mL) (SI: 0.7 IU/L [1.0-13.0 IU/L])
    Prolactin = 28 ng/mL (4-23 ng/mL) (SI: 1.22 nmol/L [0.17-1.00 nmol/L])
    25-Hydroxyvitamin D = 28 ng/mL (30-80 ng/mL [optimal]) (SI: 69.9 nmol/L [74.9-199.7 nmol/L])
    Serum electrolytes, normal
    Serum creatinine, normal
    Serum phosphate, normal
    Serum magnesium, normal

A repeated total testosterone measurement on postoperative day 4 (sample drawn at 8 AM while fasting) is 66 ng/dL (SI: 2.3 nmol/L).

Which of the following is the most appropriate next step in this patient's management?
- A. Administer zoledronic acid infusion
- B. Initiate testosterone replacement
- C. Initiate anastrozole
- D. Administer zoledronic acid infusion and initiate testosterone replacement
- E. Hold treatment, perform pituitary-directed MRI first

86 A 43-year-old woman presents for follow-up of hypocalcemia due to hypoparathyroidism that occurred as a result of thyroidectomy for thyroid lymphoma 3 years ago. Despite adherence to treatment with 4 g of elemental calcium daily in divided doses and calcitriol, 1 mcg daily, she continued to have intermittent mild-to-moderate symptoms of hypocalcemia. She tried hydrochlorothiazide in the past, but this resulted in significant hypokalemia despite potassium supplementation, with minimal benefit in terms of her calcium level, so she was started on recombinant human PTH (rhPTH) (1-84) injections once daily. She had been doing well on a dosage of 75 mcg daily with a significant reduction in her calcium supplement and calcitriol requirements (down to 2 g daily of calcium and 0.5 mcg daily of calcitriol). However, she states that she has been unable to take her rhPTH (1-84) since yesterday because of a medication recall. She now reports recurrence of the hypocalcemia symptoms that she had before starting this therapy.

On physical examination, she has a positive Chvostek sign. Neck examination reveals a surgically absent thyroid gland with an intact scar. Her examination findings are otherwise normal.

Laboratory test results:
Serum calcium = 7.3 mg/dL (8.2-10.2 mg/dL) (SI: 1.8 mmol/L [2.1-2.6 mmol/L])
Serum phosphate = 5.5 mg/dL (2.3-4.7 mg/dL) (SI: 1.8 mmol/L [0.7-1.5 mmol/L])
Serum creatinine = 0.7 mg/dL (0.6-1.1 mg/dL) (SI: 61.9 μmol/L [53.0-97.2 μmol/L])
Serum intact PTH = 4 pg/mL (10-65 pg/mL) (SI: 4 ng/L [10-65 ng/L])
Serum 25-hydroxyvitamin D = 43 ng/mL (30-80 ng/mL [optimal]) (SI: 107.3 nmol/L [74.9-199.7 nmol/L])
Serum albumin = 3.9 g/dL (3.5-5.0 g/dL) (SI: 39 g/L [35-50 g/L])
Serum magnesium = 1.9 mg/dL (1.5-2.3 mg/dL) (SI: 0.8 mmol/L [0.6-0.9 mmol/L])

Which of the following is the most appropriate next step in managing this patient's hypocalcemia?
A. Recommend no changes to her current medications
B. Increase the calcium dosage to 4 g daily
C. Increase the calcitriol dosage to 1 mcg daily
D. Increase the dosages of calcium to 4 g daily and calcitriol to 2 mcg daily
E. Start once-daily teriparatide injections

87 A 65-year-old woman with a 30-year history of type 2 diabetes mellitus seeks help for an ulcer on her left foot. She has significant peripheral neuropathy, including left Charcot foot. She has had ulcers in the past and was admitted to the hospital 6 months ago with a foot ulcer that required antibiotics and ultimately resulted in amputation of the second digit of the left foot. She has a history of methicillin-resistant *Staphylococcus aureus* infection in a foot ulcer.

She previously had suboptimal glycemic control, with hemoglobin A_{1c} values around 9.0% (75 mmol/mol). However, her hemoglobin A_{1c} level is currently 6.7% (50 mmol/mol). In addition to neuropathy, she has diabetic nephropathy with microalbuminuria and moderate proliferative diabetic retinopathy. Her diabetes regimen includes metformin, insulin glargine, and insulin aspart.

On physical examination, her temperature is 98.9°F (37.2°C), blood pressure is 131/71 mm Hg, pulse rate is 84 beats/min, and respiratory rate is 20 breaths/min. Her height is 68 in (173 cm), and weight is 207.5 lb (94.3 kg) (BMI = 32 kg/m²). The ulcer is quarter-sized and is located on the plantar surface over the first metatarsal head. There is purulent drainage and erythema extending less than 2 cm around the wound, with streaking up her leg. There is no evidence of gangrene or necrosis. The probe does not extend to the bone. Amputation of the second digit of the left foot is noted. On the right foot, the dorsalis pedis pulse and posterior tibial pulse are 1+. On the left side, dorsalis pedis pulse is nonpalpable and the posterior tibial pulse is 1+.

On laboratory testing, the white blood cell count is noted to be 10,100/μL (4500-11,000/μL) (SI: 10.1 × 10⁹/L [4.5-11.0 × 10⁹/L]).

On plain film, no gas is noted.

In addition to debridement and offloading, which of the following therapeutic options is most appropriate?
A. Cephalexin
B. Clindamycin
C. Topical antimicrobial agent
D. Hyperbaric oxygen therapy
E. No additional treatment

88 A 32-year-old man is referred for assistance with weight loss. Ten years ago, he was in a motor vehicle accident and he has since struggled with weight gain. Five years ago, he began following a meal replacement plan (1 meal each day), and he successfully lost 20 lb (9.1 kg). However, when he stopped adhering to the meal replacement plan, he regained the weight. He has not tried any weight-loss medications. In a typical day, he eats 2 sausage biscuits for breakfast, skips lunch, and consumes double portions for dinner (usually a meat and a carbohydrate). The patient usually logs 6000 to 7000 steps per day.

On physical examination, his blood pressure is 134/90 mm Hg and pulse rate is 87 beats/min. His height is 72.5 in (184.2 cm), and weight is 286 lb (130 kg) (BMI = 38 kg/m^2). His waist circumference is 51 in (129.5 cm). He is in no distress, has normal work of breathing, has no kyphosis, and has a normal gait. He has no rash or skin lesions. On neurologic examination, he is alert, and findings on cranial nerve examination are normal.

Which of the following adipokines is most likely decreased in this patient?
  A. Leptin
  B. Tumor necrosis factor α
  C. Resistin
  D. Plasminogen activator inhibitor-1
  E. Adiponectin

89 A 36-year-old man seeks evaluation for a 2-month history of increasing tiredness, excessive thirst, and polyuria. He has also noticed intermittent back pain and some shortness of breath when exercising. He has no relevant medical history. He drinks 10 units of alcohol per week and has a 20 pack-year cigarette smoking history.

On physical examination, his height is 74 in (188 cm) and weight is 190 lb (86.4 kg) (BMI = 24 kg/m^2). His resting pulse rate is 68 beats/min and regular, and blood pressure is 125/80 mm Hg. He has no clinical stigmata of endocrine dysfunction. There is mild tenderness over the midthoracic vertebrae, but the rest of the physical examination findings are normal.

Laboratory test results:
  Fasting plasma glucose = 75 mg/dL (70-99 mg/dL) (SI: 4.2 mmol/L [3.9-5.5 mmol/L])
  Serum calcium = 8.8 mg/dL (8.2-10.2 mg/dL) (SI: 2.2 mmol/L [2.1-2.6 mmol/L])
  Serum sodium = 142 mEq/L (136-142 mEq/L) (SI: 142 mmol/L [136-142 mmol/L])
  Serum potassium = 3.9 mEq/L (3.5-5.0 mEq/L) (SI: 3.9 mmol/L [3.5-5.0 mmol/L])
  Serum creatinine = 1.2 mg/dL (0.7-1.3 mg/dL) (SI: 106.1 μmol/L [61.9-114.9 μmol/L])
  TSH = 0.9 mIU/L (0.5-5.0 mIU/L)
  Free T$_4$ = 1.2 ng/dL (0.8-1.8 ng/dL) (SI: 15.44 pmol/L [10.30-23.17 pmol/L])
  Cortisol (8 AM) = 13.5 μg/dL (5-25 μg/dL) (SI: 372.4 nmol/L [137.9-689.7 nmol/L])
  Prolactin = 34 ng/mL (4-30 ng/mL) (SI: 1.48 nmol/L [0.17-1.30 nmol/L])
  FSH = 2.7 mIU/mL (1.0-13.0 mIU/mL) (SI: 2.7 IU/L [1.0-13.0 IU/L])
  LH = 2.5 mIU/mL (1.0-9.0 mIU/mL) (SI: 2.5 IU/L [1.0-9.0 IU/L])
  Total testosterone = 330 ng/dL (300-900 ng/dL) (SI: 11.5 nmol/L [10.4-31.2 nmol/L])

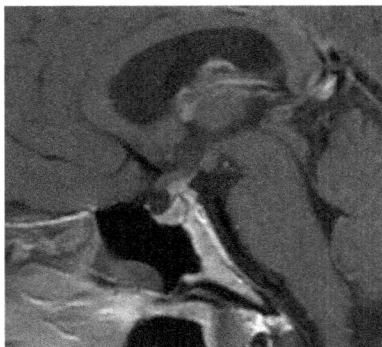

Water-deprivation test:

Time	Urine osmolality
0 h	123 mOsm/kg
8 h	147 mOsm/kg
After desmopressin (2 mcg intramuscular)	685 mOsm/kg

MRI of the sella (sagittal T1 contrast) is shown (*see image*).

CT of the chest shows bilateral upper and middle zone micronodular and cystic infiltrates. Radionuclide bone scan shows increased focal tracer uptake in several vertebrae.

Which of the following is the most likely unifying diagnosis?
  A. Hodgkin lymphoma
  B. Langerhans cell histiocytosis
  C. Lymphangitis carcinomatosis
  D. Sarcoidosis
  E. Tuberculosis

90 A 56-year-old man returns for continued management of diabetes mellitus. Type 2 diabetes was diagnosed 12 years ago. He was initially treated with oral antihyperglycemic agents, but after sustaining a non-ST segment myocardial infarction 8 months ago, his regimen was changed to basal plus bolus insulin, as well as metformin. Glycemic control has been fair to suboptimal, with hemoglobin A_{1c} values ranging from 7.2% to 8.8% (55-73 mmol/mol) over the last 14 months.

He currently takes metformin, 1000 mg twice daily, and administers 14 units of insulin lispro before breakfast and 18 units before the evening meal (he does not eat lunch). He administers 38 units of insulin glargine at bedtime.

He has a history of microalbuminuria, and the albumin level has increased over time. He is being treated with fosinopril, 40 mg daily. He also takes clopidogrel, metoprolol, and hydrochlorothiazide. He has dyslipidemia treated with rosuvastatin. At the time of the myocardial infarction, he was found to have a left ventricular ejection fraction of 45% by echocardiography. He leads a sedentary lifestyle. He does not smoke cigarettes, and he consumes 2 beers 3 days per week. There is a strong family history of type 2 diabetes, hypertension, and coronary heart disease.

On physical examination, his height is 72 in (182.9 cm) and weight is 247 lb (112.3 kg) (BMI = 34 kg/m^2). His blood pressure is 138/86 mm Hg, and pulse rate is 84 beats/min. On cardiac examination, he has a grade I/VI systolic ejection murmur heard over the base and aortic interspaces and an S_4. The distal pulses are good. There is +1 pedal edema. Findings on neurologic examination are unremarkable.

Laboratory test results:
  Electrolytes, normal
  Creatinine = 1.4 mg/dL (0.7-1.3 mg/dL) (SI: 123.8 μmol/L [61.9-114.9 μmol/L])
  Estimated glomerular filtration rate = >60 mL/min per 1.73 m^2 (>60 mL/min per 1.73 m^2)
  TSH = 2.54 mIU/L (0.5-5.0 mIU/L)
  Hemoglobin A_{1c} = 8.3% (4.0%-5.6%) (67 mmol/mol [20-38 mmol/mol])
  Albumin-to-creatinine ratio = 313 mg/g creat (<30 mg/g creat)

Which of the following is the best next step in the treatment of this patient's diabetes?
  A. Start extended-release exenatide
  B. Increase all insulin doses by 10%
  C. Start lixisenatide
  D. Start canagliflozin
  E. Start pioglitazone

91 A 28-year-old woman with a history of primary hypothyroidism due to Hashimoto thyroiditis, Sjogren syndrome, and abnormal pap smears with high-risk human papillomavirus presents for evaluation of a new neck mass. Hypothyroidism was diagnosed 5 years ago, and she has since been on a stable levothyroxine dosage. Today, she reports a new area of swelling in the right neck that she first noticed 4 weeks ago. It is mildly tender to the touch, but there is no associated dyspnea, dysphagia, or change in voice. She reports chronic dry eyes and dry mouth, which are unchanged from baseline. She has no personal history of head or neck radiation or family history of thyroid or hematologic malignancy. Her current medications are levothyroxine, 112 mcg daily, and lubricant eye drops.

On physical examination, her blood pressure is 110/60 mm Hg and pulse rate is 90 beats/min. Her height is 64 in (162.6 cm), and weight is 130 lb (59.1 kg) (BMI = 22.3 kg/m²). There is asymmetric enlargement of the right thyroid lobe with a firm texture but no discrete palpable nodule. Her mucous membranes are dry. The rest of the examination findings are normal.

Laboratory test results:
   TSH = 0.7 mIU/L (0.5-5.0 mIU/L)
   Free T₄ = 1.3 ng/dL (0.8-1.8 ng/dL) (SI: 16.7 pmol/L
      [10.30-23.17 pmol/L])

Neck ultrasonography demonstrates hyperemia of the entire thyroid gland with heterogeneous echotexture and diffuse microcalcifications in the right thyroid lobe as shown (*see images*). Several small but abnormal-appearing lymph nodes containing calcifications are observed in the right lateral neck.

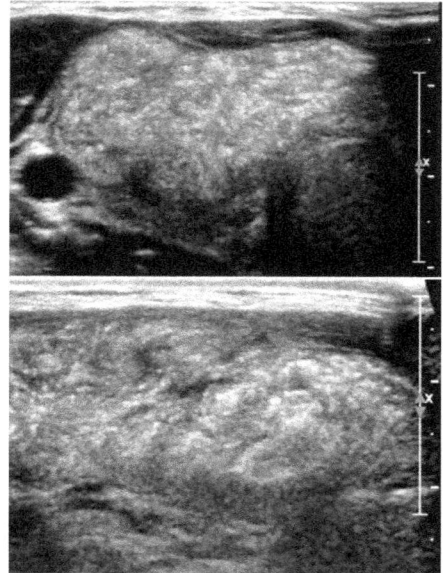

Which of the following is the most likely diagnosis?
   A. Classic papillary thyroid carcinoma
   B. Diffuse sclerosing variant of papillary thyroid carcinoma
   C. Metastatic squamous-cell carcinoma of the cervix
   D. Subacute thyroiditis
   E. Thyroid lymphoma

92 A 28-year-old woman seeks evaluation after an elevated serum prolactin concentration was documented during the workup of longstanding irregular periods and infertility (96 ng/mL [4-30 ng/mL] [SI: 4.2 nmol/L (0.17-1.30 nmol/L)]). A repeated prolactin measurement was again elevated at 91 ng/mL (4.0 nmol/L). She takes sertraline, 50 mg daily.
   On physical examination, her blood pressure is 125/80 mm Hg and pulse rate is 88 beats/min. Her height is 66.5 in (169 cm), and weight is 167.2 lb (76 kg) (BMI = 27 kg/m²). Examination findings are normal.

Laboratory test results:
   Prolactin = 91 ng/mL (4-30 ng/mL) (SI: 4.0 nmol/L [0.17-1.30 nmol/L])
   IGF-1 = 294 ng/mL (117-321 ng/mL) (SI: 38.5 nmol/L [15.3-42.1 nmol/L])
   TSH = 3.2 mIU/L (0.5-5.0 mIU/L)
   Pregnancy test, negative

Which of the following is the best next step in this patient's management?
   A. Perform pituitary-directed MRI
   B. Measure a random serum GH value
   C. Measure macroprolactin
   D. Measure free T₄
   E. Measure prolactin again after stopping sertraline

93 A 31-year-old woman seeks evaluation for nonclassic congenital adrenal hyperplasia. Her neonatal history was unremarkable; she was healthy at birth, without genital abnormalities or salt wasting. Growth, development, and puberty were unremarkable, and menarche occurred at age 12 years followed by regular periods initially. At age 14, she had irregular periods and at age 18 she developed oligomenorrhea and facial hirsutism. Results of a 1-hour 250-mcg cosyntropin-stimulation test at age 18 documented the following values:

Measurement	Baseline	1 Hour
17-Hydroxyprogesterone	1000 ng/dL (SI: 30.3 nmol/L)	3712 ng/dL (SI: 112.5 nmol/L)
Cortisol	19 µg/dL (SI: 524.2 nmol/L)	29 µg/dL (SI: 800.1 nmol/L)

Genetic testing revealed pathogenic variants in the *CYP21A2* gene. Nonclassic 21-hydroxylase deficiency was diagnosed.

She was treated with nocturnal dexamethasone, 0.25 to 0.5 mg nightly for nearly 10 years. This treatment resolved her hirsutism and initially normalized her menses. However, she was also on an estradiol-containing oral contraceptive for much of this time. She experienced weight gain of 10 to 15 lb (6.8 kg) during treatment and wanted to stop dexamethasone. Over the next 2 years, she gradually tapered her dexamethasone dosage after she learned of potential adverse effects. She has now been off dexamethasone for 2 years.

Her only current medication is an estradiol-containing oral contraceptive. She has no concerns. Menses are regular on the oral contraceptive. She is not interested in pregnancy now, but she would like to consider it in 3 to 4 years. She does have mild hirsutism that is bothersome, but she is able to manage it with various hair-removal strategies.

On physical examination, she appears healthy and athletic. Her blood pressure is 111/76 mm Hg, and pulse rate is 80 beats/min. Her height is 65 in (165.1 cm), and weight is 140 lb (63.6 kg) (BMI = 23 kg/m²). There is evidence of removed terminal hairs on the upper lip and chin. She has no acne or androgenic alopecia.

Laboratory test results (sample drawn at 8 AM):
   Urine hCG, negative
   17-Hydroxyprogesterone = 367 ng/dL (<80 ng/dL [follicular]; <285 ng/dL [luteal]) (SI: 11.1 nmol/L
      [<2.42 nmol/L (follicular); <5.64 nmol/L (luteal)])
   Androstenedione = 92 ng/dL (30-200 ng/dL) (SI: 3.2 nmol/L [1.0-7.0 nmol/L])
   DHEA-S = 43 µg/dL (31-228 µg/dL) (SI: 1.17 µmol/L [0.84-6.18 µmol/L])
   Total testosterone = 24 ng/dL (8-60 ng/dL) (SI: 0.8 nmol/L [0.3-2.1 nmol/L])
   SHBG = 40.6 µg/mL (2.2-14.6 µg/mL) (SI: 361 nmol/L [20-130 nmol/L])
   ACTH = 26 pg/mL (10-60 pg/mL) (SI: 5.7 pmol/L [2.2-13.2 pmol/L])
   Cortisol = 27.4 µg/dL (5-25 µg/dL) (SI: 755.9 nmol/L [137.9-689.7 nmol/L])
   Plasma renin activity = 1.2 ng/mL per h (0.6-4.3 ng/mL per h)
   Aldosterone = 18 ng/dL (4-21 ng/dL) (SI: 499.3 pmol/L [111.0-582.5 pmol/L])

Which of the following is the best next step in this patient's management?
A. Initiate low-dosage nocturnal prednisone
B. Initiate low-dosage prednisone in the morning
C. Initiate low-dosage dexamethasone in the morning
D. Resume low-dosage nocturnal dexamethasone therapy
E. Provide reassurance and do not change current therapy

94 A 26-year-old woman with a history of hypothyroidism since age 14 years has just learned she is pregnant (home pregnancy test). This is her first pregnancy. She currently takes levothyroxine, 100 mcg daily. Her blood is drawn for laboratory tests and she comes for a clinic visit.

Laboratory test results:
   TSH = 2.0 mIU/L (0.5-5.0 mIU/L)
   Free T₄ = 1.3 ng/dL (0.8-1.8 ng/dL) (SI: 16.7 pmol/L [10.30-23.17 pmol/L])
   β-hCG = 902 mIU/mL (<3.0 mIU/mL) (SI: 902 IU/L [<3.0 IU/L])

Her mother has Hashimoto thyroiditis and her father has celiac disease.

On physical examination, her blood pressure is 106/72 mm Hg and pulse rate is 68 beats/min. Her height is 66 in (167.6 cm), and weight is 124 lb (56.2 kg) (BMI = 20 kg/m²). She has a slightly enlarged thyroid gland that is firm and nontender. She has a regular heart rate and rhythm. There is no lower-extremity edema and no tremor in her hands.

In addition to starting a daily prenatal vitamin, which of the following is the most appropriate next step?
- A. Continue levothyroxine at the current dosage of 100 mcg daily
- B. Increase the levothyroxine dosage to 125 mcg daily
- C. Increase the levothyroxine dosage to 150 mcg daily
- D. Continue levothyroxine at the current dosage of 100 mcg daily and add liothyronine, 25 mcg daily
- E. Increase the levothyroxine dosage to 125 mcg daily and add liothyronine, 25 mcg daily

95

A 29-year-old woman seeks a second opinion regarding a diagnosis of polycystic ovary syndrome. The diagnosis was mentioned a year ago when she presented with hirsutism. She is most bothered by hair growth on her face and abdomen.

Menarche was at age 13 years and menses occurred monthly until age 15 when she started oral contraceptives to suppress ovarian cysts that ruptured. She discontinued oral contraceptives at age 21 and conceived without difficulty. Between ages 23 and 25, she experienced 2 first-trimester miscarriages. She conceived spontaneously again at age 27, and during that pregnancy she noticed terminal hair growth on her face and abdomen. For the past several years, she has noted darkening and thicker hairs and the need to shave her face and wax her abdomen more frequently. She is also seeing new hair growth.

She describes experiencing a 20-lb (9.1-kg) weight gain during the last pregnancy and difficulty losing that weight. Weight loss has been encouraged because a fasting glucose concentration of 111 mg/dL (6.2 mmol/L) was recently documented and because she had gestational diabetes in her most recent pregnancy. Her father, paternal grandmother, and grandfather have diabetes, and her mother has prediabetes. Her father's side of the family is of American Indian ancestry.

Her most recent pelvic ultrasonography demonstrates right ovarian volume of 11 mL with a dominant cyst of 13 mm and left ovarian volume of 7.8 mL. The report does not describe the exact number of follicles, but states that she does not meet criteria for polycystic ovarian morphology.

On physical examination, she has no signs of facial plethora, rounding, thinning of the skin, or striae. Her blood pressure is 139/92 mm Hg, and pulse rate is 94 beats/min. Her height is 62 in (157.5 cm), and weight is 210 lb (95.5 kg) (BMI = 38 kg/m^2).

Examination of her skin reveals terminal hair growth with the following modified Ferriman-Gallwey scores:
Chin = 3
Abdomen = 3
Lower abdomen = 1
Inner thigh = 3

Her overall modified Ferriman-Gallwey score is elevated at 10. She has acanthosis nigricans. There are no visible acne lesions.

Laboratory test results:
TSH = 1.7 mIU/L (0.5-5.0 mIU/L)
Total testosterone = 25 ng/dL (8-60 ng/dL) (SI: 0.9 nmol/L [0.3-2.1 nmol/L])
Free testosterone = 0.33 ng/dL (0.3-1.9 ng/dL) (SI: 0.01 nmol/L [0.01-0.07 nmol/L])
DHEA-S = 250 µg/dL (44-332 µg/dL) (SI: 6.78 µmol/L [1.19-9.00 µmol/L])
17-Hydroxyprogesterone = 45 ng/dL (<80 ng/dL [follicular]) (SI: 1.4 nmol/L [<2.42 nmol/L])
Fasting glucose = 120 mg/dL (70-99 mg/dL) (SI: 6.7 mmol/L [3.9-5.5 mmol/L])
Total cholesterol = 138 mg/dL (<200 mg/dL [optimal]) (SI: 3.57 mmol/L [<5.18 mmol/L])
HDL cholesterol = 38 mg/dL (>60 mg/dL [optimal]) (SI: 0.98 mmol/L [>1.55 mmol/L])
LDL cholesterol = 67 mg/dL (<100 mg/dL [optimal]) (SI: 1.73 mmol/L [<2.59 mmol/L])
Triglycerides = 230 mg/dL (<150 mg/dL [optimal]) (SI: 2.60 mmol/L [<1.70 mmol/L])

Which of the following is the most likely explanation for her hirsutism?
- A. Polycystic ovary syndrome
- B. An adrenal adenoma
- C. Idiopathic hirsutism
- D. Luteoma of pregnancy
- E. Ovarian hyperthecosis

96 A 69-year-old man is referred by his primary care physician for evaluation of very low HDL cholesterol. He reports no major health issues on detailed health history except for mild fatigue and has had no weight loss, anorexia, or gastrointestinal or cardiac symptoms. He has treated hypertension. He does not smoke cigarettes, and he drinks 4 alcoholic beverages a week. He exercises 3 to 4 times a week. His medications are lisinopril; aspirin, 81 mg daily; and a multivitamin. He takes no supplements. There is no family history of cardiovascular disease.

On physical examination, his blood pressure is 132/84 mm Hg and pulse rate is 85 beats/min. His height is 71 in (180.3 cm), and weight is 165 lb (75 kg) (BMI = 23 kg/m^2). He is lean with minimal abdominal adiposity. The rest of the examination findings are unremarkable.

Laboratory test results (sample drawn while fasting):

Measurements	2 years ago	Current
Total cholesterol	156 mg/dL (SI: 4.04 mmol/L)	144 mg/dL (SI: 3.73 mmol/L)
Triglycerides	80 mg/dL (SI: 0.90 mmol/L)	79 mg/dL (SI: 0.89 mmol/L)
HDL cholesterol	41 mg/dL (SI: 1.06 mmol/L)	5 mg/dL (SI: 0.13 mmol/L)
LDL cholesterol	99 mg/dL (SI: 2.56 mmol/L)	123 mg/dL (SI: 3.19 mmol/L)
Non-HDL cholesterol	115 mg/dL (SI: 2.98 mmol/L)	139 mg/dL (SI: 3.60 mmol/L)

Complete blood cell count reveals mild anemia.

Hemoglobin A$_{1c}$ = 5.3% (4.0%-5.6%) (34 mmol/mol [20-38 mmol/mol])
Creatinine = 1.1 mg/dL (0.7-1.3 mg/dL) (SI: 97.2 μmol/L [61.9-114.9 μmol/L])
TSH = 1.4 mIU/L (0.5-5.0 mIU/L)
AST = 14 U/L (20-48 U/L) (SI: 0.23 μkat/L [0.33-0.80 μkat/L])
ALT = 22 U/L (10-40 U/L) (SI: 0.37 μkat/L [0.17-0.67 μkat/L])
Albumin = 3.5 g/dL (3.5-5.0 g/dL) (SI: 35 g/L [35-50 g/L])

A repeated lipid panel is obtained, and the results remain unchanged.

Which of the following is the best next step in this patient's management?
- A. Measure apolipoprotein A-1
- B. Perform serum protein electrophoresis
- C. Measure serum testosterone
- D. Determine HDL-cholesterol efflux capacity
- E. Measure lipoprotein(a)

97 A 52-year-old woman is referred for evaluation of a "calcium disorder" based on an abnormal shoulder x-ray. She recently presented to her primary care physician with increasing right shoulder pain for the past 3 months. She describes right lateral shoulder pain that is worse at night and when she raises her arm above her shoulder. She reports no history of antecedent injury. Her medical history is notable for 2 metatarsal fractures that occurred in her early 40s when she was hiking. The fractures healed over 6 to 9 months with an equalizer boot. She is not physically active. Family history is notable for femur fracture in her mother while on bisphosphonate treatment in her 50s. The patient's only medication is acetaminophen for pain. She does not smoke cigarettes or drink alcohol.

On physical examination, she is in moderate discomfort. Her blood pressure is 120/75 mm Hg, and pulse rate is 85 beats/min. She is afebrile. She has moderate focal tenderness over the right lateral shoulder at the insertion of the deltoid muscle. There is mild warmth and erythema. The rest of the examination findings are normal.

Laboratory test results:
    Hemoglobin = 13.5 g/dL (12.1-15.1 g/dL) (SI: 135 g/L [121-151 g/L])
    White blood cell count = 6500/μL (4500-11,000/μL) (SI: 6.5 × 10⁹/L [4.5-11.0 × 10⁹/L])
    Serum calcium = 10.2 mg/dL (8.2-10.2 mg/dL) (SI: 2.6 mmol/L [2.1-2.6 mmol/L])
    Serum phosphate = 3.5 mg/dL (2.3-4.7 mg/dL) (SI: 1.1 mmol/L [0.7-1.5 mmol/L])
    Serum creatinine = 1.0 mg/dL (0.6-1.1 mg/dL) (SI: 88.4 μmol/L [53.0-97.2 μmol/L])
    Serum albumin = 4.4 g/dL (3.5-5.0 g/dL) (SI: 44 g/L [35-50 g/L])
    Serum intact PTH = 45 pg/mL (10-65 pg/mL) (SI: 45 ng/L [10-65 ng/L])
    Serum 25-hydroxyvitamin D = 30 ng/mL (30-80 ng/mL [optimal]) (SI: 74.9 nmol/L [74.9-199.7 nmol/L])
    Serum AST = 35 U/L (20-48 U/L) (SI: 0.58 μkat/L [0.33-0.80 μkat/L])
    Serum ALT = 30 U/L (10-40 U/L) (SI: 0.50 μkat/L [0.17-0.67 μkat/L])
    Serum alkaline phosphatase = 25 U/L (50-120 U/L) (SI: 0.42 μkat/L [0.84-2.00 μkat/L])
    Serum bilirubin (total) = 1.0 mg/dL (0.3-1.2 mg/dL) (SI: 17.1 μmol/L [5.1-20.5 μmol/L])

DXA images (obtained from another facility and technically valid) are reviewed and provide the following results:
    Lumbar spine T-score = −1.2
    Right femoral neck T-score = −2.4
    Right total hip T-score = −1.8

Anteroposterior and lateral plain radiographs of the left shoulder show curvilinear calcification superior-lateral to the right glenohumeral joint consistent with calcific periarthritis.

Which of the following is the most likely cause of this patient's shoulder pain?
    A. Tumoral calcinosis
    B. Hypophosphatasia
    C. Hyperparathyroidism
    D. Tumor-induced osteomalacia
    E. Infectious arthritis

98 A 34-year-old woman (G1P0) with a recent diagnosis of Graves hyperthyroidism is currently 21 weeks pregnant. Hyperthyroidism was diagnosed 4 weeks ago when thyroid function testing was performed by the patient's obstetrician to evaluate for recent-onset palpitations and dyspnea, as well as a 10-lb (4.5-kg) weight loss. The patient was prescribed methimazole, 5 mg daily, which she has been taking regularly with no perceived adverse effects. She reports today that her palpitations and dyspnea have significantly improved since starting treatment, and she has gained 6 lb (2.7 kg). She has no eye pain, diplopia, or vision changes.

On physical examination, her blood pressure is 110/60 mm Hg and pulse rate is 80 beats/min. Her height is 68 in (172.7 cm), and weight is 155 lb (70.5 kg) (BMI = 24 kg/m²). She has mild, symmetric enlargement of the thyroid gland without nodules and a gravid uterus. The rest of her examination findings are normal.

Laboratory test results:
    17 weeks' gestation:
        TSH = <0.01 mIU/L (0.5-5.0 mIU/L)
        Total T₄ = 21 μg/dL (5.5-12.5 μg/dL) (SI: 270.3 nmol/L [94.02-213.67 nmol/L])
        Total T₃ = 340 ng/dL (70-200 ng/dL) (SI: 5.2 nmol/L [1.08-3.08 nmol/L])
        Thyroid-stimulating immunoglobulin = 140% of basal activity (≤120% of basal activity)
        Complete blood cell count, normal
        Complete metabolic panel, normal

Today:

    TSH = <0.01 mIU/L

    Total T$_4$ = 17 µg/dL (SI: 218.8 nmol/L)

    Total T$_3$ = 290 ng/dL (SI: 4.5 nmol/L)

In addition to repeating the patient's thyroid function tests in 4 weeks, which of the following is the best next step in her care?

A. Continue methimazole at the current dosage

B. Increase the methimazole dosage

C. Discontinue methimazole and monitor thyroid function

D. Discontinue methimazole, start propylthiouracil

E. Refer for thyroidectomy

99 A 56-year-old woman presents for management of type 2 diabetes mellitus complicated by nonproliferative retinopathy and microalbuminuria. She has hypertension and hyperlipidemia controlled with lisinopril/hydrochlorothiazide, 20 mg/12.5 mg once daily, and atorvastatin, 20 mg daily. Diabetes was diagnosed 8 years ago. She currently takes metformin, 850 mg twice daily, and insulin glargine, 60 units once daily at bedtime. Her most recent hemoglobin A$_{1c}$ measurement is 7.7% (61 mmol/mol). She reports that her blood glucose values usually range from 100 to 130 mg/dL (5.6-7.2 mmol/L) in the morning. She has not had hypoglycemia on a regular basis over the past year. However, 2 years ago she had a very low glucose value while sleeping, and this scared her and her husband. She often takes only half of her insulin glargine dose at night if her bedtime glucose measurement is below 150 mg/dL (<8.3 mmol/L) because of fear of hypoglycemia while sleeping. She notes that her blood glucose concentration at bedtime is usually much higher than morning values.

On physical examination, her blood pressure is 136/78 mm Hg and pulse rate is 78 beats/min. Her height is 63 in (160 cm), and weight is 176 lb (80 kg) (BMI = 31 kg/m^2).

Her serum creatinine concentration is 1.1 mg/dL (97.2 µmol/L) and estimated glomerular filtration rate is 65 mL/min per 1.73 m^2.

A log of her blood glucose measurements is shown (*see table*).

Day	Prebreakfast	Prelunch	Predinner	Bedtime
1	106 mg/dL (SI: 5.8 mmol/L)	144 mg/dL (SI: 8.0 mmol/L)	178 mg/dL (SI: 9.9 mmol/L)	240 mg/dL (SI: 13.3 mmol/L)
2	119 mg/dL (SI: 6.6 mmol/L)	139 mg/dL (SI: 7.7 mmol/L)	164 mg/dL (SI: 9.1 mmol/L)	222 mg/dL (SI: 12.3 mmol/L)
3	92 mg/dL (SI: 5.1 mmol/L)	166 mg/dL (SI: 9.2 mmol/L)	172 mg/dL (SI: 9.5 mmol/L)	137 mg/dL (SI: 7.6 mmol/L)
4	122 mg/dL (SI: 6.8 mmol/L)	135 mg/dL (SI: 7.5 mmol/L)	157 mg/dL (SI: 8.7 mmol/L)	190 mg/dL (SI: 10.5 mmol/L)
5	128 mg/dL (SI: 7.1 mmol/L)	...	...	...

Which of the following is the best next step in this patient's management?

A. Move the timing of the insulin glargine dose to the morning

B. Add glipizide extended release, 5 mg once daily

C. Increase the metformin dosage to 1000 mg twice daily

D. Add a dose of prandial insulin at the evening meal

E. Add an SGLT-2 inhibitor and reduce her basal insulin dosage

100 A 32-year-old man with panhypopituitarism following resection of a nonfunctioning pituitary macroadenoma at age 25 years would like to have a child. He has a 12-year-old child from a previous relationship. Since his pituitary surgery, he has been on testosterone replacement. A recent pituitary-directed MRI shows no residual pituitary tumor. He is otherwise healthy. His 25-year-old wife has regular ovulatory cycles. His current medications include intramuscular testosterone, levothyroxine, and hydrocortisone.

On physical examination, his blood pressure is 122/76 mm Hg and pulse rate is 64 beats/min. His height is 70.5 in (179 cm), and weight is 176 lb (80 kg) (BMI = 25 kg/m^2). He is well androgenized and testes are 10 mL bilaterally.

Recent laboratory test results:
Total testosterone = 440 ng/dL (300-900 ng/dL) (SI: 15.3 nmol/L [10.4-31.2 nmol/L])
Free T$_4$ = 1.3 ng/dL (0.8-1.8 ng/dL) (SI: 16.73 pmol/L [10.30-23.17 pmol/L])

Semen analysis shows azoospermia.

Apart from stopping testosterone replacement, which of the following is the best initial treatment to stimulate spermatogenesis?
A. Clomiphene
B. Recombinant FSH
C. hCG
D. GnRH
E. Human menopausal gonadotropin

101 An 18-year-old woman is transitioning to adult endocrinology for management of congenital adrenal hyperplasia. She presented with precocious puberty at age 6 years with the development of pubic hair and adult body odor. Bone age was 8 years and 10 months at the chronologic age of 6 years and 2 months. There is no history of ambiguous genitalia, adrenal crisis at birth, or need for genital surgery. However, the mother was told that her daughter would always need to be on "steroids."

Laboratory test results at diagnosis at age 6 years (samples drawn at 8 AM):
17-Hydroxyprogesterone = 4040 ng/dL (<100 ng/dL) (SI: 122.4 nmol/L [<3.0 nmol/L])
Repeated 17-hydroxyprogesterone = 1880 ng/dL (<100 ng/dL) (SI: 57.0 nmol/L [<3.0 nmol/L])
ACTH = 28 pg/mL (10-60 pg/mL) (SI: 6.2 pmol/L [2.2-13.2 pmol/L])
Cortisol = 8.4 µg/dL (5-25 µg/dL) (SI: 231.7 nmol/L [137.9-689.7 nmol/L])

Hydrocortisone was initiated, 5 mg in the morning and 10 mg at bedtime. Menarche occurred spontaneously at age 10 years with regular monthly menses.

She is still on the same treatment regimen and knows to take stress-dose corticosteroids during illness. She is concerned about new facial hair growth and increased hair on her lower back, abdomen, and thighs. Her primary concern is difficulty losing weight.

On physical examination, her blood pressure is 110/74 mm Hg. Her height is 63 in (160 cm), and weight is 205 lb (93.2 kg) (BMI = 36 kg/m^2). She has terminal hair growth on her chin, neck, lower back, abdomen, and thighs with an elevated modified Ferriman-Gallwey score of 12. The rest of her examination findings are unremarkable.

Laboratory test results:
TSH = 2.9 mIU/L (0.5-5.0 mIU/L)
Prolactin = 9 ng/mL (4-30 ng/mL [nonlactating female]) (SI: 0.39 nmol/L [0.17-1.30 nmol/L])
LH = 4.5 mIU/mL (1.0-18.0 mIU/mL [follicular]) (SI: 4.5 IU/L [1.0-18.0 IU/L])
FSH = 2.6 mIU/mL (2.0-12.0 mIU/mL [follicular]) (SI: 2.6 IU/L [2.0-12.0 IU/L])
Estradiol = 32 pg/mL (10-180 pg/mL [follicular]) (SI: 117.5 pmol/L [36.7-660.8 pmol/L])
Total testosterone = 68 ng/dL (8-60 ng/dL) (SI: 2.4 nmol/L [0.3-2.1 nmol/L])
DHEA-S = 257 µg/dL (15-200 µg/dL) (SI: 6.96 µmol/L [0.41-5.42 µmol/L])
Androstenedione = 137 ng/dL (80-240 ng/dL) (SI: 4.78 nmol/L [2.79-8.38 nmol/L])
Fasting glucose = 105 mg/dL (70-99 mg/dL) (SI: 5.8 mmol/L [3.9-5.5 mmol/L])

Results are shown from a standard 250-mcg cosyntropin-stimulation test 24 hours after holding hydrocortisone (*see table*).

Measurement	Baseline	8:30 AM	9:00 AM
ACTH	26 pg/mL (SI: 5.7 pmol/L)	...	...
Cortisol	12.7 µg/dL (SI: 350.4 nmol/L)	13.0 µg/dL (SI: 358.6 nmol/L)	26.0 µg/dL (SI: 717.3 nmol/L)
17-Hydroxyprogesterone	673 ng/dL (SI: 20.4 nmol/L)	1343 ng/dL (SI: 40.7 nmol/L)	4750 ng/dL (SI: 143.9 nmol/L)

Which of the following is the best next step in this patient's management?
A. Initiate an oral contraceptive
B. Initiate metformin
C. Switch from hydrocortisone to dexamethasone
D. Taper off hydrocortisone and initiate an oral contraceptive
E. Adjust the hydrocortisone regimen to 10 mg in the morning and 5 mg at bedtime

102 A 54-year-old woman is referred for evaluation of low bone density, which was diagnosed based on a screening axial bone density test done 2 months ago (lowest T-score of −2.1 at the left femoral neck). The FRAX calculator reveals 10-year probabilities for major fracture and hip fracture of 15% and 2.7%, respectively. She had surgical menopause at age 40 years and has been on long-term prednisone therapy for rheumatoid arthritis; her current dosage is 10 mg daily. She does not smoke cigarettes and has no personal history of fractures. She has a history of esophageal stricture. She has good dietary calcium intake and is on adequate calcium and vitamin D supplementation. She has no family history of osteoporosis or fractures.

Physical examination findings are remarkable for arthritis deformities in her hands.

Her laboratory test results, including a 25-hydroxyvitamin D level, are normal.

Which of the following is the most appropriate next step in the management of this patient's low bone density?
A. Measure fasting C-telopeptide
B. Order bone density test of the one-third distal radius
C. Start alendronate
D. Start teriparatide
E. Recommend no therapy at this time

103 A 24-year-old man is referred for further investigation of recurrent unexplained episodes of hyponatremia. His medical history includes depression treated with citalopram and well-controlled asthma treated with beclometasone and salbutamol inhalers. He is a lifelong nonsmoker and drinks fewer than 10 units of alcohol each week.

On physical examination, his height is 73 in (185.4 cm) and weight is 195 lb (88.6 kg) (BMI = 26 kg/m²). His blood pressure is 130/80 mm Hg, and pulse rate is 66 beats/min and regular. He is clinically euvolemic. The rest of the physical examination findings are unremarkable.

Laboratory test results:
Serum sodium = 126 mEq/L (136-142 mEq/L) (SI: 126 mmol/L [136-142 mmol/L])
Serum potassium = 4.0 mEq/L (3.5-5.0 mEq/L) (SI: 4.0 mmol/L [3.5-5.0 mmol/L])
Serum creatinine = 0.85 mg/dL (0.7-1.3 mg/dL) (SI: 75.1 µmol/L [61.9-114.9 µmol/L])
Serum urea nitrogen = 8.3 mg/dL (8-23 mg/dL) (SI 3.0 mmol/L [2.9-8.2 mmol/L])
Plasma glucose = 75 mg/dL (70-99 mg/dL) (SI: 4.2 mmol/L [3.9-5.5 mmol/L])
Serum osmolality = 268 mOsm/kg (275-295 mOsm/kg) (SI: 268 mmol/kg [275-295 mmol/kg])
Serum copeptin = <1.3 pmol/L (<13.1 pmol/L)
Urine osmolality = 810 mOsm/kg (150-1150 mOsm/kg) (SI: 810 mmol/kg [150-1150 mmol/kg])
Spot urine sodium = 118 mEq/L (SI: 118 mmol/L)
Cortisol (8 AM) = 13.6 µg/dL (5-25 µg/dL) (SI: 375.2 nmol/L [137.9-689.7 nmol/L])
TSH = 1.2 mIU/L (0.5-5.0 mIU/L)
Free T₄ = 1.25 ng/dL (0.8-1.8 ng/dL) (SI: 16.09 pmol/L [10.30-23.17 pmol/L])

Which of the following is the most likely cause of his recurrent hyponatremia?
- A. Citalopram therapy
- B. Hypoadrenalism
- C. Nephrogenic syndrome of inappropriate antidiuresis
- D. Porphyria
- E. Pulmonary neuroendocrine tumor

104 A 49-year-old woman seeks consultation regarding management of diabetes mellitus. Type 2 diabetes was diagnosed 9 years ago. For the first 4 years after her diagnosis, her treatment consisted of diet and exercise and her hemoglobin A_{1c} level was maintained around 6.7% (50 mmol/mol). However, over the last 4 years she has gained 25 lb (11.4 kg). She is concerned that it is "all in her belly." Her mother has commented that her face and abdomen "look fat." Her hemoglobin A_{1c} level has risen to 10.6% (92 mmol/mol), and she was recently hospitalized for severe hyperglycemia. Insulin therapy was started at that time. Her medical history is also notable for hypertriglyceridemia. She has had no fractures, easy bruising, increased hair growth, change in hat/shoe/ring size, snoring, or sweating. She notes recent joint discomfort, particularly in her hands, and a scaly rash on her elbows and knees.

Her family history is notable for diabetes in her father, diagnosed in his early 50s, and hypertriglyceridemia in a paternal uncle.

Current medications are insulin degludec, 80 units once daily; insulin aspart, 30 units 3 times daily with meals + correctional scale (she reports using >200 units daily); pioglitazone; levothyroxine; omega-3 acid ethyl esters; and venlafaxine.

On physical examination, she is a well-appearing woman in no acute distress. Her height is 69 in (175.3 cm), and weight is 164 lb (74.5 kg) (BMI = 24 kg/m²). Her blood pressure is 122/78 mm Hg, and pulse rate is 88 beats/min. There is mild facial plethora. She has supraclavicular fullness but no dorsocervical fat pad fullness and no preauricular fullness. There is central fat accumulation. Superficial veins are not prominent, but her thighs appear quite muscular. Skin is notable for a scaly, mildly erythematous rash on the extensor surfaces of her elbows and fingers. Pertinent negatives include the absence of lipemia retinalis, eruptive xanthoma, acanthosis nigricans (back of the neck, axillae), wide pigmented striae, and evidence of spontaneous bruising.

Laboratory test results:
- Hemoglobin A_{1c} = 8.7% (4.0%-5.6%) (72 mmol/mol [20-38 mmol/mol])
- Total cholesterol = 300 mg/dL (<200 mg/dL [optimal]) (SI: 7.8 mmol/L [<5.18 mmol/L])
- Triglycerides = 920 mg/dL (<150 mg/dL [optimal]) (SI: 10.40 mmol/L [<1.70 mmol/L])
- HDL cholesterol = 31 mg/dL (>60 mg/dL) (SI: 0.80 mmol/L [>1.55 mmol/L])
- Glucose = 277 mg/dL (70-99 mg/dL) (SI: 15.4 mmol/L [3.9-5.5 mmol/L])
- C-peptide = 2.73 ng/mL (0.9-4.3 ng/mL) (SI: 0.90 nmol/L [0.30-1.42 nmol/L])
- Metabolic panel, normal
- Liver function, normal

Which of the following is this patient's most likely diagnosis?
- A. Type B insulin resistance (mediated by antibodies to the insulin receptor)
- B. Type A insulin resistance (mediated by genetic defects in insulin signaling)
- C. Partial lipodystrophy
- D. Cushing syndrome
- E. Acromegaly

105 A 61-year-old man with type 2 diabetes mellitus, hypertension, hypercholesterolemia, and gout presents for a follow-up appointment. He initially came to clinic 4 weeks ago when he was referred for assistance with weight loss. During the initial visit, a low-calorie meal plan (1800 calories daily) was recommended. He was also referred to an exercise physiologist, so he could obtain recommendations for an exercise program. The patient has made several dietary changes: he is eating smaller portions and avoiding meals at restaurants. He is unsure which type of oil he should use for cooking, as he has read conflicting information on the Internet. He would like to use an oil that is good for his heart. His brother recently had a myocardial infarction, and he is worried he will have one too.

His medications include metformin, liraglutide, losartan, and atorvastatin.

On physical examination, his blood pressure is 125/85 mm Hg and pulse rate is 76 beats/min. His height is 69 in (175.3 cm), and weight is 216 lb (98.2 kg) (BMI = 32 kg/m²). He is in no distress, his lungs are clear to auscultation bilaterally, and his heart sounds are regular. Findings on thyroid examination are normal, and his abdomen is soft and nontender.

Which of the following should this patient start using in his cooking?
- A. Soybean oil
- B. Coconut oil
- C. Olive oil
- D. Palm kernel oil
- E. Butter

106 A 62-year-old woman is referred for recommendations on management of osteopenia in the context of ongoing medical therapy for breast cancer. Her pertinent history is notable for breast cancer diagnosed 2 years ago, treated with lumpectomy and external beam radiotherapy. Her oncologist prescribed anastrozole 18 months ago, with plans to continue for at least 5 years. She has no history of fragility fractures. Her medical history is otherwise notable for rheumatoid arthritis, which is presently well managed with infliximab. She is not on glucocorticoid therapy. Family history is negative for osteoporosis, including no parental history of hip fracture. Her current medications include calcium, 600 mg twice daily; cholecalciferol, 400 IU twice daily; meloxicam; atorvastatin; and infliximab every 6 weeks.

On physical examination, her height is 64 in (162.6 cm) (only 1 inch shorter than her self-reported maximal height) and weight is 143 lb (65 kg) (BMI = 25 kg/m²). She has obvious rheumatoid changes involving her hands and wrists. The oropharynx appears normal without overt lesions. The thyroid gland is not palpable. Findings on spinal examination are normal without significant kyphosis or vertebral tenderness.

Laboratory test results (serum):
    Calcium = 9.5 mg/dL (8.2-10.2 mg/dL) (SI: 2.4 mmol/L [2.1-2.6 mmol/L])
    Phosphate = 3.5 mg/dL (2.3-4.7 mg/dL) (SI: 1.1 mmol/L [0.7-1.5 mmol/L])
    Creatinine = 1.0 mg/dL (0.6-1.1 mg/dL) (SI: 88.4 μmol/L [53.0-97.2 μmol/L])
    Albumin = 4.0 mg/dL (3.5-5.0 g/dL) (SI: 40 g/L [35-50 g/L])
    25-Hydroxyvitamin D = 27 ng/dL (30-80 ng/mL [optimal]) (SI: 67.4 nmol/L [74.9-199.7 nmol/L])
    TSH = 2.5 mIU/L (0.5-5.0 mIU/L)

Baseline and technically valid DXA results:
    Lumbar spine T-score = −2.8
    Right femoral neck T-score = −3.0
    Right total hip T-score = −2.6

FRAX 10-year fracture risk:
    Hip = 6.1%
    Major = 20%

Which of following is the most appropriate therapy for this patient's skeletal management?
   A. Raloxifene
   B. Zoledronic acid
   C. Alendronate
   D. Denosumab
   E. Teriparatide

107 A 63-year-old man seeks evaluation for persistent tiredness and fatigue. He is no longer able to work because of poor concentration. He underwent transsphenoidal surgery for acromegaly due to a pituitary macroadenoma 18 months ago. He is currently treated with octreotide LAR, 30 mg every 4 weeks; testosterone undecanoate, 1000 mg every 12 weeks; levothyroxine, 125 mcg daily; metformin, 850 mg twice daily; ramipril, 10 mg daily; and atorvastatin, 40 mg daily.

On physical examination, his height is 70 in (177.8 cm) and weight is 262 lb (119.1 kg) (BMI = 38 kg/m²). His resting pulse rate is 70 beats/min and regular, and blood pressure is 155/90 mm Hg. He has mild residual features of acromegaly.

Laboratory test results:
   TSH = 1.9 mIU/L (0.5-5.0 mIU/L)
   Free T$_4$ = 1.6 ng/dL (0.8-1.8 ng/dL) (SI: 20.59 pmol/L [10.30-23.17 pmol/L])
   Free T$_3$ = 4.0 pg/mL (2.3-4.2 pg/mL) (SI: 6.14 pmol/L [3.53-6.45 pmol/L])
   Cortisol (8 AM) = 17.0 μg/dL (5-25 μg/dL) (SI: 469.0 nmol/L [137.9-689.7 nmol/L])
   IGF-1 = 180 ng/mL (72-207 ng/mL) (SI: 23.6 nmol/L [9.4-27.1 nmol/L])
   Hemoglobin A$_{1c}$ = 7.4% (4.0%-5.6%) (57 mmol/mol [20-38 mmol/mol])

Laboratory test results at the time of his most recent testosterone injection:
   Total testosterone (trough level) = 235 ng/dL (300-900 ng/dL) (SI: 8.2 nmol/L [10.4-31.2 nmol/L])
   Hemoglobin = 16.8 g/dL (13.8-17.2 g/dL) (SI: 168 g/L [138-172 g/L])
   Hematocrit = 50% (41%-51%) (SI: 0.50 [0.41-0.51])
   Serum creatinine = 1.0 mg/dL (0.7-1.3 mg/dL) (SI: 88.4 μmol/L [61.9-114.9 μmol/L])
   Serum ALT = 85 U/L (10-40 U/L) (SI: 1.42 μkat/L [0.17-0.67 μkat/L])

Which of the following is the most appropriate next step in this patient's management?
   A. Initiate an SGLT-2 inhibitor
   B. Increase the levothyroxine dosage
   C. Reduce the interval between testosterone injections
   D. Reduce the octreotide LAR dosage
   E. Refer for sleep assessment

108 A 37-year-old man with a 15-year history of type 1 diabetes mellitus presents for follow-up. He has had suboptimal glycemic control, with hemoglobin A$_{1c}$ levels ranging from 7.5% to 9.0% (58-75 mmol/mol). However, over the past year, his hemoglobin A$_{1c}$ levels have ranged from 6.5% to 6.7% (48-50 mmol/mol) despite persistent elevation in blood glucose values. Review of his blood glucose log reveals mean plasma glucose levels around 250 mg/dL (13.9 mmol/L).

His medical history also includes hypothyroidism, celiac disease, and dermatitis herpetiformis. He has been adherent to a gluten-free diet, and follow-up tissue transglutaminase antibody levels have normalized. Current medications are insulin aspart (via a pump), lisinopril, atorvastatin, aspirin, and dapsone for dermatitis herpetiformis.

On physical examination, he is afebrile, blood pressure is 139/66 mm Hg, and pulse rate is 84 beats/min. His height is 70 in (177.8 cm), and weight is 188 lb (85.5 kg) (BMI = 27 kg/m²). Oxygen saturation is 89%. The patient appears comfortable, but he is pale.

Laboratory test results (from his last visit):

Creatinine = 1.6 mg/dL (0.7-1.3 mg/dL) (SI: 159.1 µmol/L [61.9-114.9 µmol/L])

Estimated glomerular filtration rate = 92 mL/min per 1.73 m^2 (>60 mL/min per 1.73 m^2)

Metabolic panel, normal

Tissue transglutaminase antibodies, normal

TSH = 1.34 mIU/L (0.5-5.0 mIU/L)

Which of the following is the most likely cause of the discrepant (low) hemoglobin A$_{1c}$ level in this patient?

    A. Congenital hemoglobinopathy

    B. Renal insufficiency

    C. Celiac disease

    D. Medication-induced hemolysis

    E. Medication-induced nonenzymatic inhibition of glycation

109 A 52-year-old man with hypertension and a right thyroid nodule underwent total thyroidectomy 6 weeks ago after FNA biopsy revealed pathology suspicious for papillary thyroid cancer. He developed hoarseness several weeks ago. His pathology report documents a 3-cm medullary thyroid carcinoma confined to the right thyroid lobe with no capsular or vascular invasion. He experiences fatigue and shortness of breath due to the hoarseness. There is no family history of endocrinopathy, but his mother has a history of colon cancer. He has never smoked cigarettes. He had an unremarkable colonoscopy at age 50 years.

He currently takes lisinopril, 20 mg daily, and a daily multivitamin.

On physical examination, his blood pressure is 120/60 mm Hg and pulse rate is 50 beats/min. His height is 72 in (182.9 cm), and weight is 174 lb (79.1 kg) (BMI = 23.6 kg/m^2). He has a well-healed scar at the base of his neck with no palpable cervical lymphadenopathy. His lungs are clear to auscultation. There is no lower-extremity edema. The rest of the examination findings are normal.

Laboratory test results:

TSH = 135.0 mIU/L (0.5-5.0 mIU/L)

Free T$_4$ = 0.1 ng/dL (0.8-1.8 ng/dL) (SI: 1.3 pmol/L [10.30-23.17 pmol/L])

Carcinoembryonic antigen = 76 ng/mL (<2.5 ng/mL) (SI: 76 µg/L [<2.5 µg/L])

Calcitonin = <2 pg/mL (<16 pg/mL) (SI: <0.58 pmol/L [<4.67 pmol/L])

Calcium = 10.0 mg/dL (8.2-10.2 mg/dL) (SI: 2.5 mmol/L [2.1-2.6 mmol/L])

In addition to starting levothyroxine therapy, which of the following is the best next step in this patient's management?

    A. Radioactive thyroid scan

    B. Colonoscopy

    C. Neck ultrasonography

    D. PET-CT

    E. TSH measurement in 2 months

110 A 43-year-old man presents to his primary care physician with abdominal pain. Abdominal CT shows a 17 × 12 × 15-cm left adrenal mass. A radical adrenalectomy is performed, and pathologic examination reveals high-grade adrenocortical carcinoma (stage III). He is treated with local radiation and starts adjuvant mitotane therapy, 3 to 4 g daily. Surveillance imaging has not shown any evidence of recurrence. His mitotane levels have ranged from 18.0 to 31.6 µg/mL (recommended therapeutic range = 14-20 µg/mL). He is also treated with hydrocortisone for adrenal insufficiency and levothyroxine for hypothyroidism.

After 2 years of mitotane therapy, he has concerns of fatigue, low libido, and erectile dysfunction.

Laboratory test results:

Total testosterone = 185 ng/dL (300-900 ng/dL) (SI: 6.4 nmol/L [10.4-31.2 nmol/L])

LH = 24.3 mIU/mL (1.0-9.0 mIU/mL) (SI: 24.3 IU/L [1.0-9.0 IU/L])

Despite initiating testosterone enanthate and undergoing multiple dosage escalations over time, he continues to experience low libido. He is currently taking 200 mg of testosterone enanthate intramuscularly once weekly.

Laboratory test results:

Total testosterone (measured by liquid chromatography/tandem mass spectrometry) = 2430 ng/dL (300-900 ng/dL) (SI: 84.3 nmol/L [10.4-31.2 nmol/L])

Free testosterone (measured by equilibrium dialysis) = <0.04 ng/dL (9.0-30.0 ng/dL) (SI: 0.001 nmol/L [0.31-1.04 nmol/L])

Mitotane = 25.1 μg/mL (recommended therapeutic range 14-20 μg/mL)

Which of the following is the most likely explanation for the discrepancy between testosterone measurements?

A. Assay interference by circulating antibodies

B. Assay interference by mitotane metabolites

C. Mitotane-induced elevations in SHBG

D. Use of an aromatase inhibitor

E. Use of exogenous anabolic androgens

111 A 38-year-old woman is evaluated for hyperhidrosis by her primary care physician. She describes headaches, and a head CT is ordered, which shows a sellar lesion. Follow-up pituitary MRI documents a 1.4-cm pituitary adenoma with mass effect on the right cavernous sinus, but without chiasmatic compression (*see image*).

Review of systems is negative, other than headaches and excessive sweating. She has taken an oral contraceptive pill since age 20 years.

On physical examination, her blood pressure is 123/74 mm Hg, pulse rate is 65 beats/min, and temperature is 97.4°F (36.3°C). Her height is 68 in (172.7 cm), and weight is 139 lb (63.2 kg) (BMI = 21 kg/m²). She has no cushingoid features or coarse facial features. She has no expressible galactorrhea or breast masses. Her palms are sweaty.

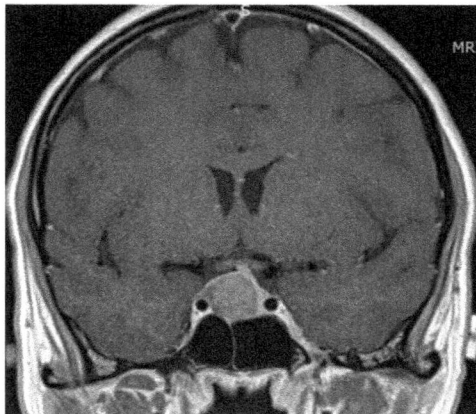

Laboratory test results (sample drawn at 7:30 AM):

Serum cortisol = 30.6 μg/dL (5-25 μg/dL) (SI: 844.2 nmol/L [137.9-689.7 nmol/L])

DHEA-S = 74 μg/dL (31-228 μg/dL) (SI: 2.0 μmol/L [0.84-6.78 μmol/L])

TSH = 2.8 mIU/L (0.5-5.0 mIU/L)

Free T$_4$ = 1.0 ng/dL (0.8-1.8 ng/dL) (SI: 12.9 pmol/L [10.30-23.17 pmol/L])

Prolactin = 47 ng/mL (4-30 ng/mL) (SI: 2.0 nmol/L [0.17-1.30 nmol/L])

IGF-1 = 261 ng/mL (106-277 ng/mL) (SI: 34.2 nmol/L [13.9-36.3 nmol/L])

Which of the following is the most appropriate next step in this patient's management?

A. Refer to neurosurgery

B. Perform a glucose-suppression test

C. Perform a 1-mg dexamethasone-suppression test

D. Measure prolactin after dilution

E. Measure chromogranin

112

A 28-year-old pregnant woman returns for continued management of diabetes mellitus. Type 1 diabetes was diagnosed at age 12 years. Insulin pump therapy and a continuous glucose sensor were initiated 2 years ago. Her hemoglobin A_{1c} level has ranged from 6.7% to 7.4% (50-57 mmol/mol) over the last 24 months. She has hypoglycemia unawareness, but the last time that she needed assistance to treat hypoglycemia was 2 years ago.

She is at 7 weeks' gestation with her second pregnancy and has nausea most days. She has had emesis twice in the last 2 weeks. She has lost 3 lb (1.4 kg) since becoming pregnant. She gained 24 lb (10.9 kg) during her last pregnancy 3 years ago and delivered a healthy baby girl at 38 weeks' gestation after induction. The baby had mild jaundice at birth but no other complications.

Ten days ago, she decreased several basal insulin rates to reduce hypoglycemia. Current basal insulin rates:

12 AM to 3 AM:	0.75 units per h
3 AM to 7 AM:	0.95 units per h
7 AM to 12 PM:	0.80 units per h
12 PM to 5:30 PM:	0.70 units per h
5:30 PM to 12 AM:	0.80 units per h

The insulin-to-carbohydrate ratio with insulin lispro is 1 unit per 12 g carbohydrate. She boluses insulin 10 to 15 minutes before she eats.

Laboratory test results:

Hemoglobin A_{1c} = 6.6% (4.0%-5.6%) (49 mmol/mol [20-38 mmol/mol])
Creatinine = 0.72 mg/dL (0.6-1.1 mg/dL) (SI: 63.6 μmol/L [53.0-97.2 μmol/L])
TSH = 1.21 mIU/L (0.5-5.0 mIU/L)
Albumin-to-creatinine ratio = 12.3 mg/g (<30 mg/g creat)

The 14-day continuous glucose sensor data are shown (*see image, black arrows indicate mealtimes*).

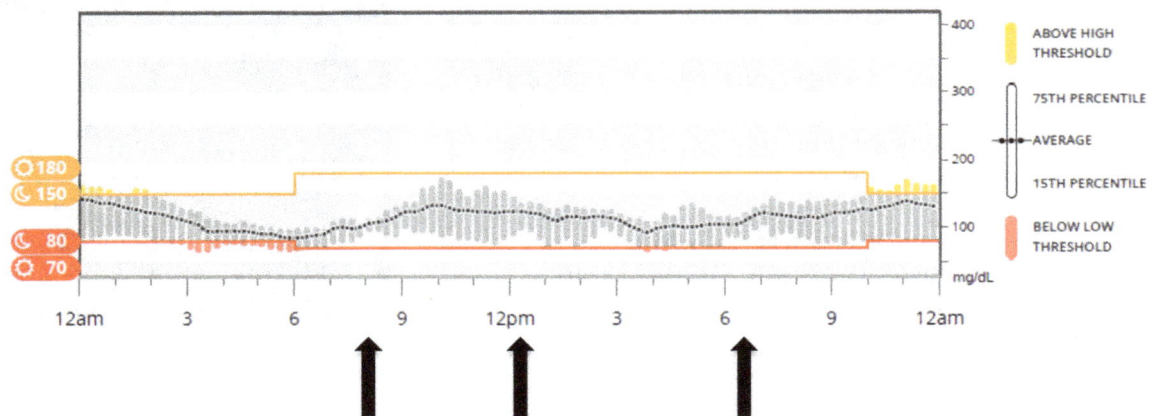

In addition to lowering the basal rate from 12 AM to 7 AM, which of the following is the best next step in managing diabetes in this pregnant patient?

    A. No additional changes needed
    B. Change the insulin-to-carbohydrate ratio to 1 to 10 at 8 AM
    C. Increase the basal rate from 5:30 PM to 12 AM, and change the insulin-to-carbohydrate ratio to 1 to 10 at 8 AM
    D. Increase the basal rate from 5:30 PM to 12 AM
    E. Decrease the basal rate from 12 PM to 5:30 PM

113 A 25-year-old woman is referred for evaluation of lower-extremity pain and abnormal x-rays. She reports bilateral lower leg pain that began approximately 10 years ago and has gradually progressed. She describes it as a chronic aching that is exacerbated by prolonged standing or walking. She has also developed intermittent aching of her upper arms and forearms, as well as severe fatigue that has worsened over the past few years. She had normal onset of menses at age 13 years and regular menstrual cycles. Her family members have commented that she seems to be experiencing hearing loss. She has no other medical problems and takes no medications. Family history is negative for musculoskeletal disorders except for osteoporosis in her mother (documented by bone density testing) without fragility fractures.

On physical examination, she is in mild distress due to self-reported bone pain. Her blood pressure is 100/65 mm Hg, and pulse rate is 92 beats/min. She has evidence of conductive hearing loss. There is no tibial tenderness to palpation. Findings on neurologic examination are normal except for a somewhat wide-based, nonantalgic gait. The rest of the examination findings are noncontributory.

Laboratory test results (serum):
  Calcium = 9.5 mg/dL (8.2-10.2 mg/dL) (SI: 2.4 mmol/L [2.1-2.6 mmol/L])
  Phosphate = 2.5 mg/dL (2.3-4.7 mg/dL) (SI: 0.8 mmol/L [0.7-1.5 mmol/L])
  Creatinine = 0.8 mg/dL (0.6-1.1 mg/dL) (SI: 70.7 µmol/L [53.0-97.2 µmol/L])
  Albumin = 4.0 g/dL (3.5-5.0 g/dL) (SI: 40 g/L [35-50 g/L])
  Intact PTH = 62 pg/mL (10-65 pg/mL) (SI: 62 ng/L [10-65 ng/L])
  25-Hydroxyvitamin D = 32 ng/mL (30-80 ng/mL [optimal]) (SI: 79.9 nmol/L [74.9-199.7 nmol/L])
  Alkaline phosphatase = 105 U/L (50-120 U/L) (SI: 1.75 µkat/L [0.84-2.00 µkat/L])

DXA documents the following values:
  Lumbar spine Z-score = +2.5
  Femoral neck Z-score = +4.2
  Total hip Z-score = +3.8

Radiographic images are shown (*see images*).

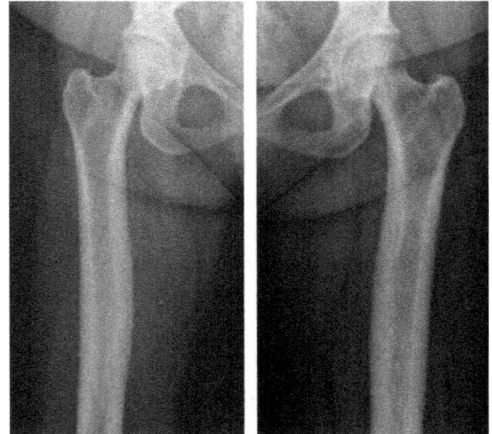

On the basis of the available clinical data, which of the following is this patient's most likely diagnosis?
  A. Hypophosphatasia
  B. Primary hyperparathyroidism
  C. Paget disease of bone
  D. X-linked hypophosphatemia
  E. Progressive diaphyseal dysplasia

114 A 65-year-old man seeks consultation regarding type 2 diabetes mellitus without known complications. Diabetes was diagnosed 12 years ago on routine blood testing with fasting glucose levels of 140 mg/dL (7.8 mmol/L). After engaging in lifestyle changes for 3 to 6 months, his glucose control remained above target (hemoglobin A_{1c} = 7.5% [58 mmol/mol]). Metformin was started with good results. Three years ago, glimepiride was added because his hemoglobin A_{1c} level was rising.

He feels well and has no specific concerns. He notes occasional dietary indiscretions. He exercises for 30 minutes 3 to 4 days per week. Recent ophthalmologic exam noted no evidence of retinopathy. Current medications include metformin, 1000 mg twice daily; glimepiride, 2 mg once daily; lisinopril, 20 mg once daily; and atorvastatin, 10 mg daily.

On physical examination, his blood pressure is 134/78 mm Hg and pulse rate is 82 beats/min. His height is 68 in (172.7 cm), and weight is 180 lb (81.8 kg) (BMI = 27.4 kg/m²). Notable features include the absence of acanthosis nigricans, good peripheral pulses, and mildly reduced vibratory sensation at the great toes.

Laboratory test results:

    Complete blood cell count, normal

    Basic metabolic panel, normal

    Hemoglobin A_{1c} = 6.9% (4.0%-5.6%) (52 mmol/mol [20-38 mmol/mol])

    Nonfasting lipid panel:

        Triglycerides = 175 mg/dL (<150 mg/dL [optimal]) (SI: 1.98 mmol/L [<1.70 mmol/L])

        Total cholesterol = 180 mg/dL (<200 mg/dL [optimal]) (SI: 4.66 mmol/L [<5.18 mmol/L])

        HDL cholesterol = 49 mg/dL (>60 mg/dL [optimal]) (SI: 1.27 mmol/L [>1.55 mmol/L])

        LDL cholesterol = 96 mg/dL (<100 mg/dL [optimal]) (SI: 2.49 mmol/L [<2.59 mmol/L])

In addition to a lab request for measurement of the urinary albumin-to-creatinine ratio, which of the following assessments should be done?

    A. Vitamin B_{12} measurement

    B. Fasting lipid panel

    C. Exercise stress test

    D. Serum 25-hydroxyvitamin D measurement

    E. Coronary artery calcium score

115

A 48-year-old woman is referred for a second opinion regarding possible Cushing syndrome. She was initially evaluated for weight gain of 10 lb (4.5 kg) over the past year. At that time, her morning cortisol concentration was 34 µg/dL (938.0 nmol/L) and urinary free cortisol excretion was 54 µg/24 h (149.0 nmol/d). The patient's primary care physician initially called you for advice, and you noted that the patient was on oral contraceptives and advised repeated testing after stopping them. The patient has now been referred to you for further evaluation.

For the past 6 months, she has had worsening hot flashes with increasing frequency and disrupted sleep at night. She has had only 2 menstrual periods in 6 months. She is experiencing "brain fog," and her work is significantly affected by this, as well as by the embarrassment of having hot flashes during presentations. She has no personal or family history of deep venous thrombosis or ovarian, endometrial, breast, or colon cancer. She has not been sexually active since her divorce 1 year ago.

On physical examination, her height is 60 in (152.4 cm) and weight is 175 lb (79.5 kg) (BMI = 34.2 kg/m^2). Her blood pressure is 134/95 mm Hg. She has no striae, facial plethora, or dorsocervical or supraclavicular fat pads. She has a hot flash during your visit with visible facial perspiration. The rest of her examination findings are normal.

Laboratory test results:

    TSH = 2.6 mIU/L (0.5-5.0 mIU/L)

    FSH = 43.5 mIU/mL (1.0-9.0 mIU/mL [luteal]) (SI: 43.5 IU/L [1.0-9.0 IU/L])

    ACTH = 25 pg/mL (10-60 pg/mL) (SI: 5.5 pmol/L [2.2-13.2 pmol/L])

    Cortisol (8 AM) = 12 µg/dL (5-25 µg/dL) (SI: 331.1 nmol/L [137.9-689.7 nmol/L])

    Urinary free cortisol = 32 µg/24 h (4-50 µg/24 h) (SI: 882.8 nmol/d [11-138 nmol/d])

Which of the following should be prescribed for this patient?

    A. Paroxetine

    B. Combined oral contraceptive pill

    C. Oral estradiol and micronized progesterone

    D. Venlafaxine

    E. Transdermal estradiol and micronized progesterone

116 A 21-year-old woman is referred for evaluation of an abnormal incidental finding on imaging. She sustained an injury to her right chest while playing rugby, and an x-ray showed an expansile appearance of multiple right-sided ribs (*see image, below left*). This was followed by a whole-body bone scan (*see image, below right*).

She reports being evaluated at age 4 years for vaginal bleeding and has had irregular menstrual cycles since age 14 years. She has several "birthmarks." She does not take any calcium or vitamin D supplements. She has no history of fractures or thyroid disease. She has no family history of bone disease.

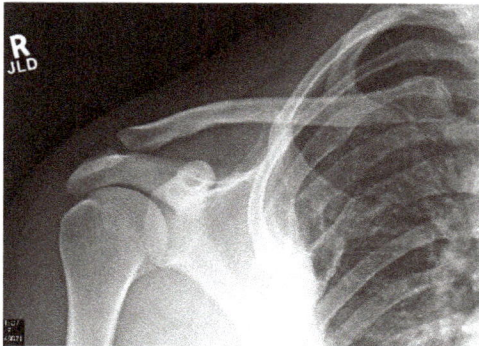

Plain x-ray of the right chest and shoulder (anteroposterior view).

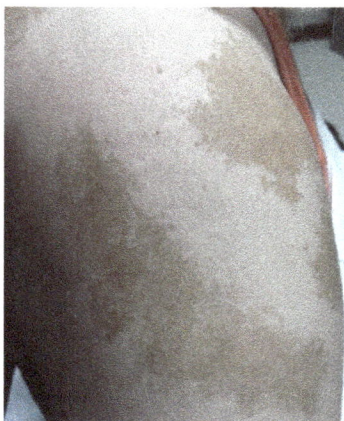

Photograph showing skin finding.

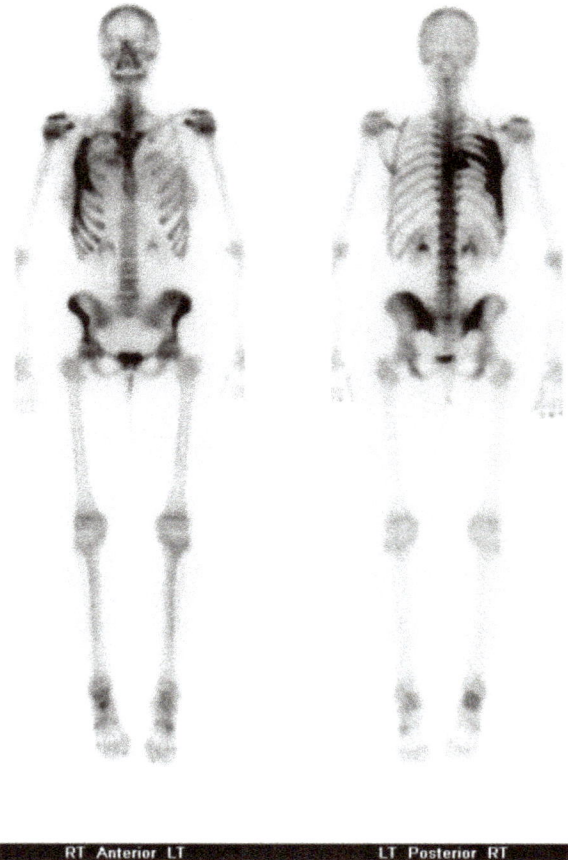

RT Anterior LT   LT Posterior RT

Bone scan.

On physical examination, there are no palpable bony abnormalities and she has no tenderness to palpation of her ribs. Her skin examination findings are shown (*see image, above*).

Laboratory test results:
  Serum 25-hydroxyvitamin D = 18 ng/mL (30-80 ng/mL [optimal]) (SI: 44.9 nmol/L [74.9-199.7 nmol/L])
  Complete blood cell count, normal
  Complete metabolic panel, normal
  TSH, normal

Which of the following is the most likely diagnosis?
  A. Multiple endocrine neoplasia type 1
  B. Carney complex
  C. Neurofibromatosis type 1
  D. Von Hippel-Lindau disease
  E. McCune-Albright syndrome

117 A 66-year-old man who was previously in good health was diagnosed with prostate cancer 6 months ago. He has been treated with the immune checkpoint inhibitor PD-L1 atezolizumab (anti-PD-L1 monoclonal antibody), and 3 days ago he completed cycle 4. On the morning of that office visit, he had blood drawn for a complete metabolic panel, and the results were normal except for a fasting blood glucose value of 195 mg/dL (10.8 mmol/L) with a hemoglobin A_{1c} level of 5.8% (40 mmol/mol). He has no history of hyperglycemia. He is currently not taking glucocorticoids. He reports no fevers, chills, or other symptoms that would suggest infection.

On physical examination, he is afebrile, blood pressure is 122/72 mm Hg, pulse rate is 98 beats/min, and respiratory rate is 18 breaths/min. His height is 72 in (183 cm), and weight is 160.5 lb (73 kg) (BMI = 22 kg/m²). He is alert and does not appear to be in distress. There are no signs of oral infection. On lung auscultation, he has good air movement. His heart rhythm is normal. His abdomen is soft and nontender to palpation. His skin shows no signs of breakdown.

Which of the following is the best next step in this patient's management?
    A. Recommend lifestyle changes
    B. Start metformin
    C. Start glimepiride
    D. Start a GLP-1 receptor agonist
    E. Start insulin

118 A 54-year-old man seeks a second opinion regarding testosterone treatment. He presented to his primary care physician 12 months ago with low libido and fatigue. At that time, his serum total testosterone concentration was 260 ng/dL (300-900 ng/dL) (SI: 9.0 nmol/L [10.4-31.2 nmol/L]). He was prescribed standard-dosage topical testosterone gel. At a follow-up appointment with his primary care physician 3 months later, he reported improved energy and libido. His serum testosterone concentration on treatment was approximately 550 ng/dL (19.1 nmol/L). At subsequent review 9 months after initiating testosterone gel, he reported that fatigue had returned and libido had declined, similar to how he felt before testosterone treatment. His serum testosterone concentration at that time was 530 ng/dL (18.4 nmol/L).

At today's appointment, he describes fatigue, low libido, and low mood. His serum testosterone concentration (sample drawn several days ago) is 520 ng/dL (18.0 nmol/L). Apart from testosterone gel, he takes no regular medications and has no notable medical history.

On physical examination, his height is 69 in (175.3 cm) and weight is 185 lb (84.1 kg) (BMI = 27 kg/m²). He has normal body hair and normal muscle bulk. There is mild gynecomastia that is tender to palpation. Testes are 20 mL bilaterally.

Results of routine blood tests, including complete blood cell count, metabolic panel, and renal and liver function, are unremarkable.

Which of the following is the best next step in this patient's management?
    A. Increase the testosterone gel dosage by 50%
    B. Change to intramuscular testosterone
    C. Add an aromatase inhibitor
    D. Add a selective estrogen receptor modulator
    E. Stop testosterone therapy

119 A 68-year-old woman with hypertension is noted to have hypokalemia. She currently takes diltiazem, 120 mg daily, and lisinopril, 40 mg daily, and her home systolic blood pressure ranges between 140 and 160 mm Hg. On routine blood testing, her serum potassium concentration was noted to be low at 3.3 mEq/L (3.3 mmol/L). Records indicate that she has had intermittent hypokalemia, with values as low as 3.1 mEq/L (3.1 mmol/L), for the last 2 years. She has never been treated with a diuretic and does not use laxatives. She does drink tea that contains some unknown amount of glycyrrhizic acid (also referred to as licorice) 4 to 5 times per week.

Abdominal CT from 2 months ago shows a normal right adrenal gland. The left adrenal gland has a 3.8-cm mass that is described as having a lobulated contour and heterogeneous lipid-poor content. The unenhanced attenuation of the left adrenal mass is 24 Hounsfield units, and the absolute washout of intravenous contrast after a 15-minute delay is 44%.

Laboratory test results:
  Serum potassium = 3.2 mEq/L (3.5-5.0 mEq/L) (SI: 3.2 mmol/L [3.5-5.0 mmol/L])
  Plasma aldosterone = 23 ng/dL (4-21 ng/dL) (SI: 638.0 pmol/L [111.0-582.5 pmol/L])
  Plasma renin activity = <0.6 ng/mL per h (normal depends on posture and diet)
  Morning cortisol after overnight 1-mg dexamethasone = 1.3 µg/dL (<1.8 µg/dL) (SI: 35.9 nmol/L [<49.7 nmol/L]
  DHEA-S = 45 µg/dL (15-157 µg/dL) (SI: 1.22 µmol/L [0.12-1.54 µmol/L])
  Plasma normetanephrine = 146.5 pg/mL (<165 pg/mL) (SI: 0.80 nmol/L [<0.90 nmol/L])
  Plasma metanephrine = 61.1 pg/mL (<99 pg/mL) (SI: 0.31 nmol/L [<0.50 nmol/L])

An incidentally discovered adrenal mass and primary aldosteronism are diagnosed. Spironolactone and supplemental potassium are initiated. When considering options such as medical or surgical therapy, she is open to either and is interested in pursuing whichever option you recommend to prolong a good quality of life.

Which of the following is the best recommendation now?
A. Perform left adrenalectomy without adrenal venous sampling
B. Continue spironolactone and perform adrenal venous sampling
C. Continue spironolactone and avoid teas containing glycyrrhizic acid
D. Stop spironolactone for 4 weeks and avoid teas containing glycyrrhizic acid
E. Stop spironolactone for 4 weeks and then proceed to adrenal venous sampling

120 A 35-year-old woman with obstructive sleep apnea and depression who underwent Roux-en-Y gastric bypass 3 months ago presents for follow-up. Her initial appointment was 9 months ago. At that time, her weight was 252 lb (114.5 kg) and BMI was 42 kg/m². Bariatric surgery was recommended, which she underwent. She did not have any immediate postsurgical complications. She is pleased with her weight loss of 35 lb (15.9 kg). Since surgery, she has had recurrent episodes of emesis that are partially resolved by antiemetics. Recently, she has noticed numbness in her feet and legs, which is leading to some balance problems and generalized fatigue.

On physical examination, her blood pressure is 100/70 mm Hg and pulse rate is 84 beats/min. Her height is 65 in (165 cm), and weight is 217 lb (98.6 kg) (BMI = 36 kg/m²). She has dry mucous membranes and dry skin. Her lungs are clear to auscultation bilaterally, and heart sounds are regular. She is oriented to person, place, and time. She does not have nystagmus or asterixis. She has normal strength in all extremities and no peripheral edema.

A deficiency of which of the following micronutrients is the most likely cause of this patient's symptoms?
A. Thiamine
B. Iron
C. Folic acid
D. Cobalamin
E. Copper

ENDOCRINE SELF-ASSESSMENT PROGRAM 2021

Part II

1 **ANSWER: C) Adrenocortical carcinoma**

Although this patient had a history of polycystic ovary syndrome and diabetes, she presents with rapidly worsening hyperandrogenism, hypertension, and glycemic control despite adherence to her insulin regimen. The pace of progression of these abnormalities should raise concern for Cushing syndrome. She has all the classic hallmarks of Cushing syndrome, and the severity of her myopathy is indicative of the severity and/or duration of the hypercortisolism.

When Cushing syndrome is ACTH-dependent (such as in the case of an ACTH-secreting pituitary adenoma or ectopic ACTH syndrome due to a neuroendocrine tumor [Answer D]), there may be hypercortisolism and hyperandrogenism because ACTH stimulates the secretion of cortisol and androgens from the adrenal glands. Although this patient has clear hypercortisolism, as evidenced by a markedly elevated cortisol level after dexamethasone and in the 24-hour urine collection, the circulating ACTH level is suppressed. Thus, this is a case of ACTH-independent Cushing syndrome. Although the use of exogenous glucocorticoids (Answer A) could cause Cushing syndrome and suppression of ACTH, adrenal androgens in the setting of suppressed ACTH would also be expected to be low, not high.

Benign causes of ACTH-independent Cushing syndrome include a cortisol-secreting adrenal adenoma (Answer B), primary pigmented nodular adrenocortical disease (Answer E) (often associated with Carney complex), and bilateral macronodular adrenal hyperplasia. When ACTH is suppressed in these benign neoplastic conditions, adrenal androgens are usually low. The severity of this patient's hyperandrogenism is marked, including diffuse hirsutism, 3-fold elevations in total testosterone, and 6-fold elevations in DHEA-S, despite the suppression of ACTH. Collectively, the rapid pace of the disease, its severity, and concomitant hypercortisolism and hyperandrogenism are most concerning for an adrenocortical carcinoma (Answer C). By the time of diagnosis, most patients with adrenocortical carcinoma have invasive or metastatic disease, and at least half of these patients present with some degree of Cushing syndrome or hyperandrogenism.

This patient was found to have a 10-cm right adrenocortical carcinoma with multiple hepatic and pulmonary metastases.

Educational Objective
Guide the investigation to diagnose Cushing syndrome and recognize features of adrenocortical carcinoma.

Reference(s)
Fassnacht M, Dekkers OM, Else T, et al. European Society of Endocrinology clinical practice guidelines on the management of adrenocortical carcinoma in adults, in collaboration with the European Network for the Study of Adrenal Tumors. *Eur J Endocrinol.* 2018;179(4):G1-G46. PMID: 30299884

2 **ANSWER: E) Teriparatide**

This postmenopausal woman has untreated worsening osteoporosis in the setting of osteonecrosis of the jaw (ONJ) after 1 year of alendronate therapy. As with any other patient with osteoporosis, she should be counseled on adequate calcium and vitamin D supplementation and fall prevention. She should also receive pharmacologic therapy for osteoporosis, with the most appropriate drug chosen given her ONJ.

ONJ is defined as exposed necrotic bone in the maxillofacial region, not healing after 8 weeks in patients with no history of craniofacial radiation. It appears as areas of exposed yellow or white hard bone with smooth or ragged borders. Risk factors for developing ONJ include dosage and duration of exposure to bisphosphonate therapy, intravenous administration of bisphosphonate therapy, glucocorticoids, cancer and anticancer therapy, cigarette smoking, poorly fitting dentures, and preexisting dental disease. ONJ can occur spontaneously but is generally associated with invasive dental procedures such as tooth extractions or dental implants. It has been estimated that the risk of ONJ is approximately 1 in 10,000 to 1 in 100,000 patient-years in patients taking oral bisphosphonates for osteoporosis, but it appears to be much more common in patients with cancer receiving bisphosphonates at much higher dosages than those used to treat osteoporosis. Given the active ONJ in this patient, it would be best to avoid initiating an intravenous bisphosphonate such as zoledronic acid (Answer B).

Denosumab (Answer C) is a fully human monoclonal antibody to the receptor activator of nuclear factor kappaB ligand (RANKL). By blocking the binding of RANKL to RANK, it reduces osteoclast formation, function, and survival, which results in decreased bone resorption and increased bone density. Romosozumab (Answer D) is a monoclonal antibody to sclerostin, an endogenous inhibitor of bone formation. Romosozumab was approved by the US FDA for the treatment of postmenopausal osteoporosis in 2019. ONJ has been reported with the use of both denosumab and romosozumab, which would eliminate these 2 options as the most appropriate drug for this patient.

Teriparatide (PTH 1-34) (Answer E), an osteoanabolic agent used in the treatment of osteoporosis, would be the most appropriate drug to treat her severe osteoporosis, especially given her active ONJ. Teriparatide may also promote ONJ healing (off-label use), but limited data support its efficacy in this regard. It is administered as a daily subcutaneous injection. Teriparatide has a black box warning for osteosarcoma and its use is limited to 2 years in a lifetime, although postmarketing surveillance has documented only 3 reported cases of osteosarcoma in more than 1 million patients worldwide treated with teriparatide, which does not exceed epidemiologic expectations. Contraindications to its use include history of skeletal irradiation, Paget disease of bone, or unexplained elevation in alkaline phosphatase. After discontinuation of teriparatide, there is a decrease in bone mineral density over the subsequent 12 months if an antiresorptive medication is not prescribed; however, fracture risk reduction appears to be maintained for at least 18 months.

Raloxifene (Answer A) is a selective estrogen receptor modulator approved for the treatment of postmenopausal osteoporosis; however, it is considered a second-line agent because it only decreases the risk of vertebral fractures and has no effect on hip or other nonvertebral fracture risk. This option would not be the best choice in this patient who is at high risk of future fracture, especially given her very low T-scores at the hips. There has been no link between ONJ and raloxifene, so this may be reserved as an alternative for women who cannot or choose not to take teriparatide. This may be also considered as an option after completing the 2-year course of teriparatide therapy. Similar to estrogen, safety concerns with raloxifene include an increased risk of venous thromboembolism and fatal stroke.

Educational Objective
Recommend the most appropriate osteoporosis therapy in a patient with declining bone mineral density and osteonecrosis of the jaw.

Reference(s)
Adler RA, El-Hajj Fuleihan G, Bauer DC, et al. Managing osteoporosis in patients on long-term bisphosphonate treatment: report of a task force of the American Society for Bone and Mineral Research. *J Bone Miner Res.* 2016;31(1):16-35. PMID: 26350171

Khan AA, Morrison A, Hanley DA, et al; International Task Force on Osteonecrosis of the Jaw. Diagnosis and management of osteonecrosis of the jaw: a systematic review and international consensus. *J Bone Miner Res.* 2015;30(1):3-23. PMID: 25414052

Cipriani C, Irani D, Bilezikian JP. Safety of osteoanabolic therapy: a decade of experience. *J Bone Miner Res.* 2012;27(12):2419-2428. PMID: 23165426

3 **ANSWER: C) Perform abdominal CT**

This elderly woman has rising hemoglobin A_{1c} levels, apparently in the absence of any changes in diet or health concerns. Although her dietary intake is not optimal, she has not made recent changes. The hemoglobin A_{1c} value appears to be accurate since the plasma glucose level is also elevated. Therefore, measuring serum fructosamine (Answer B) is not necessary. Although dietary counseling (Answer A) to help her make better food choices is a good idea, and the addition of glimepiride (Answer D) might lower her blood glucose, the unexpected rise in hemoglobin A_{1c} with no identifiable cause should prompt evaluation for a secondary etiology.

The patient's symptoms are nonspecific. She did not realize that she had lost weight; on review of her medical record, she had lost 20 lb (9.1 kg) in 3 years. She is unlikely to have a somatostatinoma, as these tumors are extremely rare (annual incidence of 1 in 40 million). They typically occur in the fourth to sixth decade of life with a mean age at diagnosis of 51 to 53 years. Measuring somatostatin (Answer E) is not the best next step. Adenocarcinoma of the pancreas, however, occurs in older patients, often in the seventh and eighth decades of life. Presentation can include weight loss, abdominal pain, jaundice, and hyperglycemia (diabetes can be the presenting feature). This patient had an abdominal CT (Answer C), which revealed a 3.6-cm lesion in the body of the pancreas.

Pancreatic cancer is associated with a number of risk factors, including race/ethnicity, family history, and diabetes. A meta-analysis demonstrated that patients with type 2 diabetes have an odds ratio of 1.82 for developing pancreatic cancer. There has been some concern that incretin therapy (GLP-1 receptor agonists and DDP-4 inhibitors) may be associated with pancreatic cancer, but this has been controversial with some studies suggesting increased risk, some no increased risk, and still others suggesting some protection against pancreatic cancer. More prospective studies are needed to determine the role of incretin therapy in the risk of pancreatic cancer. Additional risk factors include obesity, cigarette smoking, and high alcohol consumption (>30 g daily). Counseling patients about modifiable factors should be undertaken in an effort to reduce the risk of adenocarcinoma of the pancreas.

Educational Objective
Assess the underlying cause of uncontrolled hemoglobin A_{1c} in a patient with type 2 diabetes mellitus who had previously good glycemic control.

Reference(s)
McGuigan A, Kelly P, Turkington RC, Jones C, Coleman HG, McCain RS. Pancreatic cancer: a review of clinical, diagnosis, epidemiology, treatment and outcomes. *World J Gastroenterol.* 2018;24(3):4846-4861. PMID: 30487695

Huxley R, Ansary-Moghaddam A, Berrington de Gonzalez A, Barzi F, Woodward M. Type-II diabetes and pancreatic cancer: a meta-analysis of 36 studies. *Br J Cancer.* 2005;92(11):2076-2083. PMID: 15886696

4 ANSWER: D) Coronary artery calcium scoring

This patient is seeking advice on cardiovascular risk management in the setting of underlying genetic risk and the inability to take standard cholesterol-lowering therapy.

Apolipoprotein B (Answer A) is the protein signature carried on the surface of all atherogenic lipoproteins such as VLDL remnants, intermediate-density lipoprotein, and LDL. There is 1 apolipoprotein B molecule per lipoprotein particle. Therefore, the apolipoprotein B level reflects the total number of atherogenic particles. Most circulating apolipoprotein B is associated with LDL particles, and levels correlate strongly with LDL-cholesterol and non–HDL-cholesterol concentrations. Apolipoprotein B is an excellent predictor of cardiovascular events. However, measurement of apolipoprotein B in addition to traditional risk factors does not significantly alter treatment decisions according to data from several large studies. Therefore, apolipoprotein B measurement would not add helpful information in this case.

Apolipoprotein A-1 (Answer B) is the apoprotein carried on HDL particles. Most particles have 1 to 4 molecules of apolipoprotein A-1 per HDL particle. The apolipoprotein A-1 level is suggestive of the total number of HDL particles in the circulation. Epidemiologic studies have shown a consistent inverse association between HDL-cholesterol concentration and coronary artery disease. Recent evidence suggests that while HDL cholesterol is a helpful biomarker, functional testing, such as the cholesterol efflux capacity of HDL, may be more discriminating of cardiovascular risk. Apolipoprotein A-1 levels do not reflect HDL function and there is no evidence that apolipoprotein A-1 is a predictor of cardiovascular disease. Therefore, its measurement is not recommended.

Carotid intima media thickness (Answer C) is an ultrasonography evaluation of the common carotid artery to measure subclinical atherosclerotic burden. It measures the distance between the vessel lumen and the media-adventitia of the artery wall using B-mode vascular ultrasonography. Before symptomatic vascular disease develops in the coronary or carotid arteries, the arterial wall develops atherosclerosis. The intima-medial layer thickens and plaque forms before there is significant stenosis (subclinical atherosclerosis). Carotid ultrasonography can detect these alterations and is safe, noninvasive, widely available, and relatively inexpensive. Prospective epidemiologic studies have shown that carotid intima media thickness is a predictor of future cardiovascular events, independent of traditional risk factors. Limitations include reproducibility, the need for highly trained sonographers, and the lack of clinical evidence that carotid intima media thickness measurements translate into improved cardiovascular outcomes. Routine measurement of carotid intima media thickness is not advocated in any guidelines and is not recommended.

Coronary artery calcium (CAC) scoring (Answer D) is another measure of subclinical atherosclerosis determined by performing a noncontrast, limited chest CT obtained during a 3- to 5-second breath hold. It measures calcium in the epicardial coronary system. Radiation exposure is comparable to that of a mammogram. By comparing a patient's CAC score with that of others of the same age, sex, and ethnicity (through the use of large databases of asymptomatic patients), a calcium percentile is generated. Higher than the 75th percentile is considered high risk irrespective of the score, and this indicates premature or accelerated atherosclerosis. CAC is a marker of vascular calcification and is a good tool in decision making when the choice to initiate treatment remains uncertain for the provider or the patient. CAC scores increase with age and are higher in men. CAC improves risk prediction across the spectrum of age and risk factors. Coronary mortality risk is low among individuals with CAC scores of 0, even when multiple risk factors are present. Several retrospective and prospective studies and meta-analyses have shown that asymptomatic individuals with a CAC score of 0 are very unlikely to have clinically important coronary heart disease events despite the presence of clinical risk factors. Conversely, CAC scores higher than 100 or higher than the 75th percentile are associated with a high risk (>2% annual risk) of a coronary heart disease event and provide a rationale for aggressive LDL-cholesterol–lowering therapy. In this patient, determining the

CAC score can help with risk stratification and the decision of whether further or more aggressive lipid-lowering therapy should be pursued. CAC calcium measurement can be used as a decision aid in select adults to facilitate the clinician–patient risk discussion.

Stress echocardiography (Answer E) is a validated option for evaluating patients with symptoms of coronary artery disease. It evaluates myocardial function using exercise or pharmacologic agents such as dobutamine to induce myocardial stress. The patient in this vignette reported no symptoms, and stress testing in asymptomatic individuals, especially women, cannot be recommended because false-positive test results can occur.

Educational Objective
Guide the cardiovascular risk assessment in a patient with statin intolerance and genetic risk.

Reference(s)

Greenland P, Blaha MJ, Budoff MJ, Erbel R, Watson KE. Coronary calcium score and cardiovascular risk. *J Am Coll Cardiol*. 2018;72(4):434-447. PMID: 30025580

Stone NJ, Grundy SM. The 2018 AHA/ACC/mult-society cholesterol guidelines: looking at past, present and future. *Prog Cardiovasc Dis*. 2019;62(5):375-383. PMID: 31733217

Arnett DK, Blumenthal RS, Albert MA, et al. 2019 ACC/AHA guideline on primary prevention of cardiovascular disease: a report of the American College of Cardiology/American Heart Association Task Force on Clinical Practice Guidelines. *Circulation*. 2019;140(11):e596-e646. PMID: 30879355

5 ANSWER: D) Add a GLP-1 receptor agonist

This patient has class 3 obesity and suboptimally controlled type 2 diabetes. He is currently receiving a high dosage of daily insulin therapy and reports nonadherence to dietary recommendations. To date, the titration of this patient's insulin therapy to a total daily dose of greater than 500 units has not achieved his hemoglobin A_{1c} goal. For these reasons, adding an additional agent that may augment his current insulin regimen, and potentially assist with weight loss, would be a good option to consider. Regardless of the pharmacologic therapy that is chosen, a continued emphasis on dietary intake and nutrition should simultaneously occur.

Data in the literature describe the synergistic and complementary action of insulin therapy and GLP-1 receptor agonist therapy. There are data regarding the combination of insulin therapy and the most commonly used GLP-1 receptor agonists (exenatide, exenatide LAR, dulaglutide, and semaglutide). However, in patients receiving high-dosage insulin therapy, particularly U500, the data regarding liraglutide are perhaps the most well-documented. Data in the literature support the effectiveness of GLP-1 receptor agonist therapy (Answer D) in patients receiving large insulin doses, including U500. In a group of 15 patients with type 2 diabetes and high insulin requirements (mean daily insulin U500 insulin dose = 192 ± 77 units; initial mean weight = 300.9 ± 55.7 lb [136.5 ± 25.3 kg]; mean baseline hemoglobin A_{1c} = 8.48% [69 mmol/mol]), 12 weeks of liraglutide therapy resulted in a 1.4% reduction in hemoglobin A_{1c} (P = .0001) and an average decrease in body weight of 11.2 lb (5.1 kg) (P = .0001). The total daily insulin dose was reduced by 28% (P = .0001), and no severe episodes of hypoglycemia occurred. Similarly, in a prospective randomized trial, 37 patients with type 2 diabetes requiring more than 100 units of insulin daily administered either by continuous subcutaneous insulin infusion or multiple daily injections, with or without metformin, were randomly assigned to receive either liraglutide plus insulin (LIRA group) or intensive insulin only (control group). At 6 months, participants in the LIRA group experienced significant reductions in hemoglobin A_{1c}, weight, insulin dose, and glycemic variability as assessed by continuous glucose monitoring compared with the control group. Continuous glucose monitoring showed that the LIRA group experienced a significant 42% decrease in time spent in hyperglycemia (blood glucose >180 mg/dL [>10.0 mmol/L]), from 38% of the time at baseline to 22% of the time at 6 months (P < .0001). Participants in the control group did not experience any change in the amount of time spent in hyperglycemia. Both treatment groups had a significant reduction in hemoglobin A_{1c} from baseline after 6 months of treatment; however, the LIRA group experienced a greater hemoglobin A_{1c} reduction of 0.65%, from a mean baseline value of 7.80% (62 mmol/mol) (P < .0001), compared with the control group, which had a hemoglobin A_{1c} reduction of 0.39%, from a mean baseline value of 7.79% (62 mmol/mol) (P < .0001). The LIRA group experienced significant weight loss of 11.6 lb (5.27 kg) at 6 months (P < .0001), whereas the control group experienced a nonsignificant weight gain of 0.8 lb (0.37 kg) (P = .595). The total daily insulin dose in the LIRA group decreased significantly by 34%, from a mean baseline daily dosage of 200 units to a daily dosage of 132 units at 6 months (P < .0001). By contrast, the control group experienced an insignificant increase in total daily insulin dose of 4%, from a baseline of 171 units to 178 units at 6 months (P = .453).

In this patient with established cardiovascular disease, GLP-1 receptor agonist therapy may also help to reduce his cardiovascular risk.

As this patient's estimated glomerular filtration rate is less than 30 mL/min per 1.73 m^2, both metformin (Answer E) and SGLT-2 inhibitor therapy (Answer A) would be contraindicated; otherwise, these would have been options to consider. Use of pioglitazone (Answer C), particularly in patients receiving higher insulin doses, increases the risk of fluid retention and potentially congestive heart failure. Given this patient's insulin requirements, pioglitazone would not be the best option. Lastly, while further increases in the U500 insulin dosage (Answer B) might improve glycemic control, this would come at the expense of weight gain and increased risk of hypoglycemia. Moreover, dosage titrations over the past few years have been unsuccessful for this patient. Although a referral for metabolic surgery was not provided as a potential answer in this vignette, given his weight, suboptimally controlled type 2 diabetes, and insulin requirements, bariatric surgery may also be an intervention to consider.

Lastly, there is limited experience with GLP-1 receptor agonists in patients with mild, moderate, and severe renal impairment, including end-stage renal disease. Therefore, liraglutide (and other GLP-1 receptor agonists) should be used with caution in this patient population. No dosage adjustments are recommended for patients with renal impairment who are taking GLP-1 receptor agonists. The only exception is that exenatide (both short- and long-acting versions) should not be used in patients with severe renal impairment (creatinine clearance <30 mL/min).

Educational Objective
Determine when it is appropriate to add a GLP-1 receptor agonist to the regimen of a patient with suboptimally controlled type 2 diabetes who takes U500 insulin.

Reference(s)
Lane W, Weinrib S, Rappaport J. The effect of liraglutide added to U-500 insulin in patients with type 2 diabetes and high insulin requirements. *Diabetes Technol Ther.* 2011;13(5):592-595. PMID: 21406014

Lane W, Weinrib S, Rappaport J, Hale C. The effect of addition of liraglutide to high-dose intensive insulin therapy: a randomized prospective trial. *Diabetes Obes Metab.* 2014;16(9):827-832. PMID: 24589127

Meade LT, Mannka ML. The effect of glucagon-like peptide-1 receptor agonists and sodium-glucose cotransporter-2 inhibitors in patients prescribed regular U-500 insulin. *Ann Pharmacother.* 2019;53(11):111-1116. PMID: 31215219

Nesto RW, Bell D, Bonow RO, et al. Thiazolidinedione use, fluid retention, and congestive heart failure: a consensus statement from the American Heart Association and American Diabetes Association. *Diabetes Care.* 2004;27(1):256-263. PMID: 14693998

Pantalone KM, Faiman C. Liraglutide effective in the severely insulin-resistant patient with type 2 diabetes requiring U-500 insulin: a case report. *Diabetes Technol Ther.* 2013;15(4):342-343. PMID: 23379638

Brietzke SA. Oral antihyperglycemic treatment options for type 2 diabetes mellitus. *Med Clin North Am.* 2015;99(1):87-106. PMID: 25456645

6   ANSWER: D) Iron studies

This patient has clinical and biochemical evidence of acquired hypogonadotropic hypogonadism. Total testosterone concentrations are unequivocally and repeatedly low, and gonadotropin concentrations are inappropriately low-normal.

Several clues in this vignette point to a likely diagnosis of hemochromatosis. Despite his hypogonadism, the hemoglobin value is high-normal. Due to the erythropoietic actions of testosterone, hypogonadism due to other etiologies is typically associated with mild anemia. Moreover, while central adiposity and prediabetes are typically associated with a lowered SHBG level, his SHBG concentration is unexpectedly high-normal. This is a clue suggesting underlying liver disease/cirrhosis, which is also consistent with his hepatomegaly and abnormal liver function test results. With respect to extragonadal manifestations of hemochromatosis, he has evidence of "bronze diabetes" and possible joint involvement. Hemochromatosis-associated cardiomyopathy might have contributed to the premature death of his father. Therefore, ordering iron studies (Answer D), including transferrin saturation, is the most important initial investigation.

Hemochromatosis is often associated with hypogonadotropic hypogonadism (ie, inappropriately normal LH), because iron accumulates in the pituitary rather than in the testes. Within the pituitary, iron accumulation appears to be restricted to gonadotropic cells, explaining the selective involvement of the gonadal axis.

While obesity can cause functional hypogonadotropic hypogonadism, which is reversible with weight loss, this patient's BMI is not in the obese range. In general, modest obesity primarily leads to a decrease in total testosterone due to the obesity-associated decrease in SHBG, while the free testosterone level remains normal. More substantial obesity is associated with hypothalamic suppression, leading additionally to a decrease in free testosterone, while the LH level is inappropriately low to low-normal. Alcohol abuse can cause hypogonadism and cirrhosis, but this tends to be associated with primary hypogonadism. Moreover, alcohol abuse is typically associated with gynecomastia, whereas gynecomastia, interestingly, is typically absent in men with hemochromatosis-associated hypogonadism. This has been attributed to even higher SHBG concentrations (leading to an increased free estradiol-to-testosterone ratio) in alcoholic hypogonadism compared with hemochromatosis-associated hypogonadism, and to lower conversion of androgens to estrogens in the latter. Weight loss and alcohol abstinence (Answer A) are an important part of holistic clinical care, and these measures may decelerate the progression of hemochromatosis-associated liver disease. However, they are unlikely to reverse his hypogonadism. In a relatively young man with clear-cut hypogonadism, an underlying cause must be sought.

A pituitary-directed MRI (Answer B) can demonstrate evidence compatible with iron deposition such as decreased signal intensity of the pituitary gland on T2-weighted MRI. Pituitary imaging is part of the workup of secondary hypogonadism, especially if the total testosterone concentration is less than 150 ng/dL (<5.2 nmol/L). However, especially in the absence of a clinical mass effect, raised prolactin, or other pituitary function abnormalities, iron studies should be performed first because of the clinical suspicion for hemochromatosis.

There are no features of cortisol deficiency in this case, and the patient's tanned appearance is due to iron deposition in the skin. Of note, while glucocorticoid excess can cause secondary hypogonadism, there is no clinical evidence of Cushing syndrome. Therefore, evaluation of the pituitary-adrenal axis (Answer C) is not indicated.

While sarcoidosis can be associated with pituitary dysfunction and inflammatory arthropathy, the absence of other typical features makes this diagnosis less likely. Thus, serum ACE measurement (Answer E) is incorrect.

Educational Objective
Consider iron overload due to hemochromatosis as a cause of hypogonadotropic hypogonadism in middle-aged men.

Reference(s)
Kley HK, Niederau C, Stremmel W, et al; Conversion of androgens to estrogens in idiopathic hemochromatosis: comparison with alcoholic liver cirrhosis. *J Clin Endocrinol Metab*. 1985;61(1):1-6. PMID: 3998072

Cundy T, Bomford A, Butler J, et al; Hypogonadism and sexual dysfunction in hemochromatosis: the effects of cirrhosis and diabetes. *J Clin Endocrinol Metab*. 1989;69(1):110-6. PMID: 2732293

7 **ANSWER: B) Supplemental calcium and vitamin D and an oral bisphosphonate**
Although osteoporotic fractures are not often considered as significant a health issue in men as they are in women, approximately one-fifth of osteoporotic fractures and one-quarter of hip fractures occur in men. Vertebral fractures are actually more prevalent in younger men, although this is thought to be due, in part, to higher rates of spinal trauma. Nonetheless, vertebral fractures are common in older men but are frequently not recognized. In addition, when present clinically and/or radiographically, prevalent vertebral fractures predict a high risk of subsequent low-trauma fractures.

This patient presents with an acute vertebral fracture that occurred with low trauma (ie, ground level fall) and has DXA evidence of osteopenia, thereby confirming a clinical diagnosis of osteoporosis. Of note, even though L2 is excluded because of the presence of a compression fracture, his lumbar spine T-score most likely overestimates his true bone mineral density based on the known greater effect of artifactual degenerative changes in older men compared with women. Although his secondary biochemical workup is negative, his mother's history of vertebral fractures probably predisposes him to osteoporotic fractures as well. On the basis of his history, he most likely does not have a single gene pathogenic variant (eg, *WNT1*, *PLS3*, *CYP19A1*) and could be characterized instead as having aging-related osteoporosis. He does have evidence for hypercalciuria (urine calcium >4 mg/kg per day or urine calcium >250 mg/g of creatinine), which is a risk factor for osteoporosis in men and women, although the mechanisms underlying the association are poorly understood.

On the basis of his presentation and increased risk for additional fragility fractures, therapy should be considered, and recommending no treatment (Answer E) is inappropriate. Calcium and vitamin D (1000 IU daily)

(Answer A) are recommended for male osteoporosis, although when given alone they have limited benefit in fracture prevention based on an established meta-analysis that is heavily weighted by postmenopausal women. In this patient and others with evidence of hypercalciuria with or without concomitant nephrolithiasis, optimization of dietary calcium intake with an additional calcium supplement if required is appropriate, with a goal daily intake of 1200 mg of elemental calcium.

Although the listed FDA-approved antifracture therapies are approved for men as well as women and they most likely have comparable efficacy on vertebral fracture risk reduction, based on available evidence and lack of head-to-head studies, oral bisphosphonates (Answer B) would be the best choice for this patient. Intravenous zoledronic acid (Answer C) has been shown in 1 of 2 randomized controlled trials to reduce the risk of vertebral fractures, although it is associated with a higher risk of a more severe and prolonged acute-phase reaction (fever, myalgias) given that he is bisphosphonate naïve. More importantly, this patient has stage 4 chronic kidney disease, which is a contraindication to the use of zoledronic acid based on concerns over precipitation of worsening renal function. Indeed, his elevated intact PTH level is likely related to his degree of renal dysfunction. Teriparatide (Answer D) is also approved to increase bone mineral density in men with either idiopathic or hypogonadal osteoporosis, but it has not been demonstrated to reduce fracture risk in men. In addition, teriparatide increases urinary calcium excretion by approximately 40 mg daily, which is a concern in this patient with preexisting hypercalciuria.

Educational Objective
Recommend appropriate treatment in a man with a recent osteoporotic vertebral fracture.

Reference(s)
Adler RA. Update on osteoporosis in men. *Best Pract Res Clin Endocrinol Metab.* 2018;32(5):759-772. PMID: 30449553

Nayak S, Greenspan SL. Osteoporosis treatment efficacy for men: a systematic review and meta-analysis. *J Am Geriatr Soc.* 2017;65(3):490-495. PMID: 28304090

8 ANSWER: D) Order a celiac enteropathy panel

Celiac disease is a disorder of the small bowel characterized by inflammation of the gut mucosa, villous atrophy, and hyperplasia of the villous crypts. This occurs with chronic exposure to dietary gluten and improves or resolves by following a gluten-free diet. The diagnosis of celiac disease is made based on positive serology and is confirmed with duodenal biopsy, which demonstrates increased intraepithelial lymphocytes and crypt hyperplasia with or without villous atrophy.

Celiac disease is associated with type 1 diabetes and autoimmune polyglandular syndrome type 3. Patients with type 1 diabetes and celiac disease share the same genetic susceptibility subtypes, including HLA-DR3, HLA-DQ2, and other variants. Between 2.6% and 7.8% of adults with type 1 diabetes have IgA autoantibodies to endomysium or tissue transglutaminase, and most of these patients are confirmed to have celiac disease following small-bowel biopsy. Similarly, 2% to 5% of patients with autoimmune thyroid disease have celiac disease. The prevalence of hypothyroidism in patients with celiac disease is as high as 30%.

Clues to underlying celiac disease in asymptomatic patients include iron deficiency anemia, low vitamin D stores, menorrhagia, metabolic bone disease, and increased levothyroxine requirement in patients with hypothyroidism. One study demonstrated that patients who had hypothyroidism and asymptomatic celiac disease who were not adherent to a gluten-free diet required a nearly 50% higher dosage of levothyroxine than predicted based on weight.

The patient in this vignette has primary hypothyroidism and well-controlled type 1 diabetes. She does not have typical symptoms of celiac enteropathy, but she has developed iron-deficiency anemia. She is currently being treated with levothyroxine, 175 mcg daily, yet has an elevated TSH level. The levothyroxine dosage is higher than predicted based on her weight (2.3 mcg/kg daily) and is a clue that she may have underlying celiac disease.

Therefore, the best next step in her management is to screen for celiac disease (Answer D). If the serology is positive, the diagnosis can be confirmed by a small-bowel biopsy. Treatment with iron (Answer A) may be required, but it is not the best first step. If the diagnosis of celiac enteropathy is confirmed and the patient starts a gluten-free diet, iron absorption from the small bowel should improve and the anemia may correct on its own. Ordering a hemoglobin electrophoresis panel (Answer C) may be needed to assess for thalassemia, but this can be delayed for now.

If the patient is confirmed to have celiac disease and starts a gluten-free diet, increasing the levothyroxine dosage to 200 mcg daily (Answer B) may lead to overtreatment and iatrogenic thyrotoxicosis. The strategy of changing the administration of levothyroxine to bedtime (Answer E) may lead to a lower TSH level, but it would most likely not normalize TSH and is not the best answer.

Educational Objective
Evaluate for celiac disease in a patient with type 1 diabetes mellitus and hypothyroidism if levothyroxine dosage requirements increase.

Reference(s)

Kordonouri O, Dieterich W, Schuppan D, et al. Autoantibodies to tissue transglutaminase are sensitive serological parameters for detecting silent coeliac disease in patients with type 1 diabetes mellitus. *Diabet Med.* 2000;17(6):441-444. PMID: 10975212

Cerutti F, Bruno G, Chiarelli F, et al; Diabetes Study Group of the Italian Society of Pediatric Endocrinology and Diabetology. Younger age of onset and sex predict celiac disease in children and adolescents with type 1 diabetes: an Italian multicenter study. *Diabetes Care.* 2004;27(6):1294-1298. PMID: 15161778

Virili C, Bassotti G, Santaguida MG, et al. Atypical celiac disease as cause of increased need for thyroxine: a systematic study. *J Clin Endocrinol Metab.* 2012;97(3) E419-E422. PMID: 22238404

9 ANSWER: B) Measure prolactin after dilution

This patient has a very large sellar mass with chiasmatic compression. Therefore, she requires urgent measures to decompress the chiasm. The next step depends on the type of sellar mass she has. If she has a prolactinoma, then dopaminergic therapy could be started and surgery could possibly be avoided. However, if the tumor is not a prolactinoma, then surgical decompression is needed. In a prolactinoma of this size, the prolactin concentration would most likely be greater than 1000 ng/mL (>43.5 nmol/L). A mild increase such the one recorded here is probably caused by pituitary stalk compression (the stalk effect). If this value is confirmed, she would need surgical decompression. However, in some cases when prolactin is extremely elevated, the assay can be fooled and read low levels. This is known as the *hook effect*. This can occur in "sandwich" assays, which rely on the binding of 1 antibody (capturing) to 1 epitope of the analyte and a second antibody (capturing) to a different epitope. If there is vast antigen excess, the capturing and detecting antibodies may become saturated by the high analyte concentration. When this happens, no sandwich can be formed by the capturing antibody, the antigen, and the detection antibody. This yields a result that is lower than the real value. Thus, in this vignette, the prolactin should be re-measured after dilution (Answer B) to rule out macroprolactinoma. In this case, prolactin after dilution was unchanged, thus ruling out the hook effect, and the patient underwent surgical adenoma resection. Some laboratories routinely run dilution when a prolactin value is abnormal.

Pituitary glycoproteins (TSH, FSH, and LH) are composed of identical α-subunits and specific β-subunits that confer biologic specificity. Some pituitary adenomas produce the α-subunit, which may serve as a tumor marker and may differentiate TSH-secreting pituitary adenomas (in which the ratio of α- to intact TSH serum concentrations is >1) from thyroid hormone resistance syndromes. Gonadotropin-secreting pituitary adenomas can also produce excessive α-subunit, but its measurement (Answer A) would not change the therapeutic approach in this case. Macroprolactinemia (Answer C) is a condition in which prolactin binds to immunoglobulins, thereby generating a large molecular mass of prolactin (macroprolactin) as the main molecular form in sera, which causes elevated serum prolactin. The overall prevalence of macroprolactinemia in patients with hyperprolactinemia is 10% to 30%. In this case, however, even if the patient had macroprolactinemia, the surgical indication would not change. Referring to radiation oncology (Answer D) or neurosurgery (Answer E) would be premature before establishing whether this is a prolactin-secreting adenoma.

Educational Objective
Explain the concept of the "hook effect" and the need to measure prolactin after dilution in the setting of a giant pituitary adenoma.

Reference(s)

Delgrange E, Raverot G, Bex M, et al. Giant prolactinomas in women. *Eur J Endocrinol.* 2013;170(1):31-38. PMID: 24088550

Fleseriu M, Lee M, Pineyro MM, et al. Giant invasive pituitary prolactinoma with falsely low serum prolactin: the significance of 'hook effect'. *J Neurooncol.* 2006;79(1):41-43. PMID: 16598425

10

ANSWER: B) Ehlers-Danlos syndrome

The patient in this vignette presents with abnormally low bone mineral density for his age, sex, and race. In such a scenario, secondary contributors to low bone mineral density should be considered. There are numerous causes of secondary osteoporosis, including endocrine disorders, nutritional deficiencies, medications, genetic disorders (particularly of collagen metabolism), and other miscellaneous conditions (such as immobilization and HIV). His age, history of multiple joint dislocations as a child and adolescent, and physical exam findings of velvety skin and scoliosis are most consistent with classic Ehlers-Danlos syndrome (Answer B). Ehlers-Danlos syndrome refers to a group of rare genetic disorders of connective tissue characterized by joint hypermobility (the hallmark of most types of Ehlers-Danlos syndrome), skin hyperextensibility, and tissue fragility. Skeletal abnormalities, including thoracolumbar scoliosis, may be seen in some patients, and valvular heart disease is uncommon. In addition, there is evidence of reduced bone mass, reduced bone quality, and higher prevalence of vertebral and nonvertebral fragility fractures in patients with Ehlers-Danlos syndrome. Although there are very limited data to guide treatment for low bone mineral density in young adults with Ehlers Danlos syndrome, discussion of off-label osteoporosis therapy should be initiated in this case since this patient has already sustained a right hip fragility fracture. Classic Ehlers-Danlos syndrome is inherited in an autosomal dominant manner, with pathogenic variants found in the type V collagen genes *COL5A1* and *COL5A2* in about 90% of patients who are diagnosed clinically. The characteristic skin findings in classic Ehlers-Danlos syndrome include velvety or "doughy," hyperextensible, fragile skin, with increased bruising and delayed healing.

Osteogenesis imperfecta (Answer A) is a group of disorders characterized by fragile bones with recurrent fractures, which this patient does not have. There are many different subtypes of osteogenesis imperfecta based on genetic and clinical characteristics, and the mildest form (type I) is typically caused by pathogenic variants in genes encoding the α1 and α2 chains of type I collagen. Clinical manifestations of osteogenesis imperfecta may include blue-gray discoloration of the sclerae, short stature, scoliosis, bone deformities, hearing loss, and easy bruising.

Marfan syndrome (Answer C), one of the most common inherited disorders of connective tissue, is typically characterized by disproportionate tall stature and an increased arm span to height ratio, which this patient does not have. It is inherited in an autosomal dominant pattern due to pathogenic variants in the fibrillin 1 gene (*FBN1*). As in Ehlers-Danlos syndrome, joint hypermobility and scoliosis can be seen in patients with Marfan syndrome, but dislocation of the lens, pectus excavatum and/or carinatum, and aortic dilatation with a propensity for aortic rupture distinguish Marfan syndrome from Ehlers-Danlos syndrome. In addition, the skin findings seen in the classic form of Ehlers-Danlos syndrome are not typical for Marfan syndrome.

Hereditary hypophosphatemic rickets (Answer D) is characterized by hypophosphatemia, teeth defects, and rickets or osteomalacia. Pathogenic variants in the *PHEX* gene (phosphate-regulating endopeptidase on the X chromosome) lead to an increase in circulating FGF-23 and are responsible for the development of X-linked hypophosphatemia. Pathogenic variants in the *DMP1* gene (dentin matrix acidic phosphoprotein 1) lead to autosomal recessive hypophosphatemic rickets. This patient had an unremarkable complete metabolic panel, which is not consistent with such a diagnosis.

Finally, hypophosphatasia (Answer E) is a rare, autosomal disorder caused by a deficiency of tissue nonspecific alkaline phosphatase and characterized by abnormal mineralization of bone and dental tissues. Patients with hypophosphatasia have decreased serum concentrations of alkaline phosphatase, which this patient does not have.

Educational Objective

Diagnose classic Ehlers-Danlos syndrome as a cause of secondary osteoporosis in an adult presenting with low bone density.

Reference(s)

Formenti AM, Doga M, Frara S, et al. Skeletal fragility: an emerging complication of Ehlers-Danlos syndrome. *Endocrine.* 2019;63(2):225-230. PMID: 30554346

Camacho PM, Petak SM, Binkley N, et al. American Association of Clinical Endocrinologists and American College of Endocrinology clinical practice guidelines for the diagnosis and treatment of postmenopausal osteoporosis – 2016. *Endocr Pract.* 2016;22(Suppl 4):1-42. PMID: 27662240

Eller-Vainicher C, Bassotti A, Imeraj A, et al. Bone involvement in adult patients affected with Ehlers-Danlos syndrome. *Osteoporos Int.* 2016;27(8):2525-2531. PMID: 27084695

11 ANSWER: E) Branchial cleft cyst

The differential diagnosis of a neck mass is broad and can be categorized by the location of the mass in the neck. A lateral neck mass could be cervical lymphadenopathy, branchial cleft cyst, hemangioma, carotid body tumor, cystic hygroma, ectopic thyroid gland, or vascular neoplasm/malformation. A mid-neck mass could be a thyroid nodule/cyst or thyroglossal duct cyst. In this vignette, the patient has a mass on the left side of her neck at level II.

This patient's neck CT demonstrates a well-circumscribed, homogenously hypoattenuated mass surrounded by a thin wall. The location of the mass and its appearance on neck CT are most consistent with a left branchial cleft cyst (Answer E). Branchial cleft cysts are congenital anomalies arising from incomplete involution of branchial cleft structures. They are usually diagnosed in childhood but may not be evident for years. Branchial cleft cyst abnormalities account for approximately 20% of congenital head and neck abnormalities, and second branchial anomalies are the most common and account for approximately 95% of cases. Branchial cleft cysts are divided into 4 categories: first branchial cleft cyst, second branchial cleft cyst, third branchial cleft cyst, and fourth branchial cleft cyst (extremely rare). First branchial cleft cysts are located on the face near the auricle. Second branchial cysts are the most common type of branchial cleft anomaly. They are typically located just inferior to the angle of the mandible and anterior to the sternocleidomastoid muscle in the corresponding level II lymph node region. Third branchial cleft cysts are also located anterior to the sternocleidomastoid muscle, but they are typically lower in the neck than second branchial cleft cysts.

Imaging can be helpful in the diagnosis of these structures. Ultrasonography can be performed to determine the cystic characteristics of the lesion. In this setting, contrast-enhanced CT depicts a cystic, enhanced mass in the neck. FNA biopsy can be considered, as it is helpful in distinguishing a branchial cleft cyst from a malignant neoplasm. Recurrent infections of branchial cysts can occur, and a fistula tract to the skin may develop. Acute severe infections of third or fourth branchial cleft cysts can cause pharyngeal edema and airway and swallowing difficulties. Management of branchial cleft cysts begins with controlling infection, if present. Once the infection has resolved, the mass is usually excised. The surgical intervention has a risk of injury to important structures close by. After branchial cleft cysts are excised, recurrence is relatively uncommon. This patient should be referred to an otolaryngologist to perform surgery.

Cervical lymphadenopathy (Answer A) and paraganglioma (Answer C) have a different appearance on neck CT. Cervical lymph nodes appear as a soft-tissue density, and paragangliomas are well-circumscribed, heterogeneous, highly vascular tumors with avid contrast enhancement as shown (*see images*).

This patient does not have fever and the skin over the lump does not look inflamed. Therefore, neck abscess (Answer B) is less likely. In contrast to this patient's mass, thyroglossal duct cysts (Answer D) are located in the midline neck.

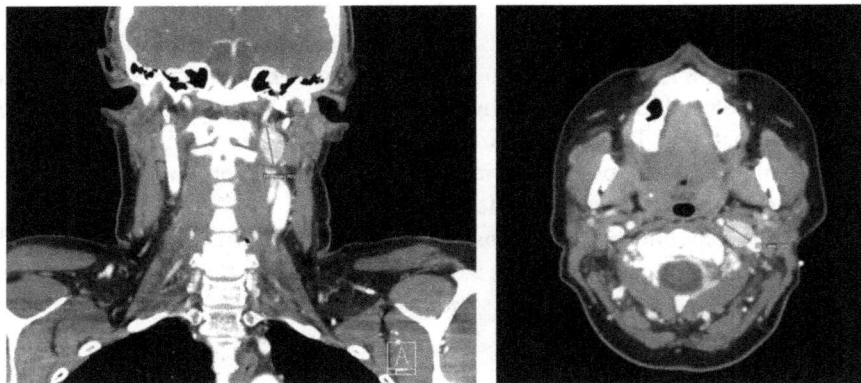

Educational Objective
Identify a branchial cleft cyst in a patient with a lateral neck mass.

Reference(s)

Prosser JD, Myer CM 3rd. Branchial cleft anomalies and thymic cysts. *Otolaryngol Clin North Am.* 2015;48(1):1-14. PMID: 25442127

Koeller KK, Alamo L, Adair CF, Smirniotopoulos JG. Congenital cystic masses of the neck: radiologic-pathologic correlation. *Radiographics.* 1999;19(1):121-146. PMID: 9925396

12 ANSWER: C) Refer for ovarian/adrenal venous sampling

This woman presented with a rapid pace of severe hair loss that warrants evaluation with measurements of testosterone and DHEA-S to determine whether further evaluation for a tumor is indicated. General guidelines for total testosterone concentrations suggest a threshold of 150 to 200 ng/dL (5.2-6.9 nmol/L), although more recent data suggest that a lower threshold of 147 ng/dL (5.1 nmol/L) is appropriate with more universal use of liquid chromatography–tandem mass spectrometry. These same data also suggest an even lower threshold of 63.5 ng/dL (2.2 nmol/L) for postmenopausal women. This patient, who would be evaluated with the postmenopausal range, has a total testosterone concentration above 60 ng/dL (>2.1 nmol/L) even while on oral contraceptives.

With the rising testosterone level on oral contraceptives and asymmetric ovaries on ultrasonography without a visible tumor, this patient was referred for ovarian/adrenal venous sampling (Answer C) and the results are shown in the table.

Measurements	Right ovarian vein	Left ovarian vein	Right adrenal	Left adrenal	Inferior vena cava
Total testosterone	271 ng/dL (SI: 9.4 nmol/L)	443 ng/dL (SI:15.4 nmol/L)	82 ng/dL (SI: 2.8 nmol/L)	76 ng/dL (SI: 2.6 nmol/L)	84 ng/dL (SI: 2.9 nmol/L)
DHEA-S	54 µg/dL (SI: 1.46 µmol/L)	51 µg/dL (SI: 1.38 µmol/L)	150 µg/dL (SI: 4.07 µmol/L)	124 µg/dL (SI: 3.36 µmol/L)	55 µg/dL (SI: 1.49 µmol/L)

Combined ovarian and adrenal venous sampling (selective venous sampling) is performed to help make treatment decisions in the evaluation of women with hyperandrogenism when clinical suspicion for an androgen-producing tumor is high, pelvic ultrasonography is normal, and adrenal imaging is either normal or identifies a nodule or mass with benign features. The procedure includes selective catheterization of the ovarian and adrenal veins to demonstrate a gradient in androgen concentrations and localize the source. This procedure is technically difficult and should only be performed by a highly experienced interventional radiologist. Unstimulated testosterone concentrations with a ratio greater than 3 from the ovarian or adrenal vein to the peripheral (inferior vena cava) measurement and a ratio greater than 1.4 from 1 side indicated unilateral source.

Although the right ovarian volume was greater than the left ovarian volume, this patient has greater secretion from the left ovary (1.6:1). The right ovary also has a gradient greater than 3 compared with the inferior vena cava, so it is also a significant source of androgen excess. Similar to the use of adrenal venous sampling for primary hyperaldosteronism, this case shows that the larger ovary might not be the source of greater androgen production, which is why referring for right oophorectomy (Answer D) is incorrect. Ovarian/adrenal venous sampling would be considered both to diagnose an ovarian source and determine whether the androgen production is bilateral, which would be more important in a premenopausal woman. However, in this case, the patient's gynecologist presented the options for unilateral left oophorectomy vs bilateral oophorectomy because she had premature ovarian insufficiency and there was evidence of excess androgen production from both ovaries. Because of the significant left-to-right gradient, left oophorectomy might be considered to significantly improve symptoms, although some androgen excess symptoms might persist. Additional data and considerations come from a study that showed increased morbidity from bilateral oophorectomy in premenopausal women. Although estrogen replacement lowered that risk, the gynecologist and patient both decided on a course of medical management intensification instead of unilateral oophorectomy and to pursue bilateral oophorectomy after age 50 years.

GnRH agonists such as leuprolide (Answer E) have been shown to significantly reduce androgens in women with hyperandrogenism and can decrease androgens and improve hirsutism scores as well as or better than oral contraceptives. However, since GnRH agonists can be expensive, require injections in a clinic setting, and result in estrogen deficiency often requiring estrogen add-back, they are recommended only for women with severe forms of hyperandrogenemia not controlled by oral contraceptives and/or antiandrogens.

Antiandrogen therapy such as spironolactone (Answer A) can be used as an alternative to treat hyperandrogenism when first-line oral contraceptives are contraindicated or not tolerated. Spironolactone can also be used as additive therapy to oral contraceptives if hirsutism has not improved after 6 months. Because of this patient's progressive symptoms and rise in total testosterone despite the addition of oral contraceptives, further diagnostic evaluation was indicated with ovarian/adrenal venous sampling before the addition of therapy.

In this case, the patient's FSH remained elevated despite being on oral contraceptives, which is different from what is observed in premenopausal women. Because of her premature ovarian insufficiency, her elevated FSH and LH resulted in increased androgen production, which worsened her hirsutism. To improve suppression of FSH and LH, her regimen was switched to a continuous oral contraceptive (Answer B), and in 3 months her symptoms improved and total testosterone concentrations decreased to 33 ng/dL (1.1 nmol/L).

Educational Objective
Diagnose and treat hirsutism in a woman with premature ovarian insufficiency.

Reference(s)
Martin KA, Anderson RR, Chang RJ, et al. Evaluation and treatment of hirsutism in premenopausal women: an Endocrine Society clinical practice guideline. *J Clin Endocrinol Metab.* 2018;103(4):1233-1257. PMID: 29522147

Rocca WA, Gazzuola-Rocca L, Smith CY, et al. Accelerated accumulation of multimorbidity after bilateral oophorectomy: a population-based cohort study. *Mayo Clin Proc.* 2016;91(11):1577-1589. PMID: 27693001

Levens ED, Whitcomb BW, Csokmay JM, Nieman LK. Selective venous sampling for androgen-producing ovarian pathology. *Clin Endocrinol (Oxf).* 2009;70(4):606-614. PMID: 18721192

Sharma A, Kapoor E, Singh RJ, Chang AY, Erickson D. Diagnostic thresholds for androgen-producing tumors or pathologic hyperandrogenism in women by using total testosterone concentrations measured by liquid-chromatography-tandem mass spectrometry. *Clin Chem.* 2018;64(11):1636-1645. PMID: 30068692

13 ANSWER: C) Start atorvastatin, 20 mg daily

Very little clinical trial evidence exists for guidance on primary cardiovascular prevention in patients with type 1 diabetes of any age. The patient in this vignette has no other additional cardiovascular risk factors besides type 1 diabetes. However, atherosclerotic cardiovascular disease is the leading cause of death in persons with type 1 diabetes, and this significantly increased risk is not completely accounted for by traditional cardiovascular risk factors.

The coronary artery calcium (CAC) score is determined by performing chest CT that visualizes the heart with multiple 3-mm slices obtained through the coronary arteries between heart beats during a held breath. Calcium in the coronary arteries is easily visualized and quantified with specific software. A total score is automatically calculated as the sum of scores for each of the 4 main coronary arteries, and the Agatston scoring system is most commonly used. The primary reason to obtain a CAC score is to help with the decision of whether to start statin therapy in an asymptomatic patient. The CAC score allows for an accurate prediction of future risk of atherosclerotic cardiovascular disease events. A positive score often motivates patients to initiate lipid-lowering therapy. In type 1 diabetes, there is now evidence that high CAC scores are associated with incident coronary artery disease. More recently, the American Heart Association and American Diabetes Association have suggested that recommendations for CAC screening in the general population should also apply to patients with type 1 diabetes. Such information can be useful for the clinician when considering whether to start or intensify preventive therapies such as statins, particularly in younger persons in whom assessment of other risk factors may not offer a definitive recommendation.

Until recently, cardiovascular risk management in younger adults with type 1 diabetes had not been addressed in any major guidelines due to paucity of data. The 2018 American Heart Association/American College of Cardiology multisociety cholesterol management guidelines recommend at least moderate-intensity statin therapy for all patients with diabetes 40 years and older and for those aged 20 to 39 years if risk enhancers are present (ie, diabetes of long duration [10 years for type 2 diabetes or 20 years for type 1 diabetes], microalbuminuria or macroalbuminuria, chronic kidney disease [estimated glomerular filtration rate <60 mL/min per 1.73 m²], retinopathy, neuropathy, or ankle brachial index <0.9). The American Diabetes Association has recently taken a similar approach, and the 2020 consensus guidelines state that even though the data are not definitive, statin treatment approaches for type 2 diabetes should be considered for patients with type 1 diabetes, especially in the presence of other cardiovascular risk factors. For patients who are younger than 40 years and/or have type 1 diabetes with other atherosclerotic cardiovascular disease risk factors, it is now recommended that the patient and health care provider discuss the relative benefits and risks and consider the use of moderate-intensity statin therapy.

The patient in this vignette has a long duration of diabetes and an elevated CAC score. Therefore, he should be started on at least moderate-intensity statin therapy such as atorvastatin, 20 mg daily (Answer C). Atorvastatin, 5 mg daily (Answer D) is low-intensity statin therapy and is not the best option for this individual. Recommending no therapy (Answer E) is incorrect.

There is no known direct relationship between total calcium intake, coronary artery calcium, and atherosclerotic cardiovascular disease. However, recent evidence from randomized controlled trials, including the Women's Health Initiative, has raised concern for an association between calcium supplement use and increased risk for cardiovascular disease events. Among calcium supplement users, a calcium intake greater than 1400 mg daily has been associated with higher death rates from all causes, including cardiovascular disease. Conversely, a recent analysis of a large, multiethnic study of men and women without history of clinical cardiovascular disease suggested a possible protective association for those with the highest daily dietary calcium intake (ie, those who achieved this without calcium supplements). Calcium supplement use and total calcium intake was in fact associated with an increased risk of incident CAC. Therefore, low dietary calcium (Answer A) cannot be recommended for cardiovascular risk reduction.

Empagliflozin (Answer B) is an SGLT-2 inhibitor that is approved for use in patients with type 2 diabetes. Drugs in this class lower plasma glucose via an insulin-independent mechanism by blocking SGLT-2 in the proximal convoluted tubule of the kidneys and preventing glucose reabsorption. SGLT-2 inhibitors have demonstrated distinct cardiovascular and renal benefits in patients with type 2 diabetes. However, these drugs are not currently approved for use in type 1 diabetes in the United States. Thus, empagliflozin is not the best option in this patient who has otherwise well-managed diabetes.

Educational Objective
Manage high coronary artery calcium in younger patients with type 1 diabetes mellitus.

Reference(s)

Burge MR, Eaton RP, Schade DS. The role of a coronary artery calcium scan in type 1 diabetes. *Diabetes Technol Ther*. 2016;18(9):594-603. PMID: 27585206

Guo J, Eroqou SA, Miller RG, Edmundowicz D, Orchard TJ, Costacou T. The role of coronary artery calcification testing in incident coronary artery disease risk prediction in type 1 diabetes. *Diabetologia*. 2019;62(2):259-268. PMID: 30426170

American Diabetes Association. 10. Cardiovascular disease and risk management: Standards of Medical Care in Diabetes. *Diabetes Care*. 2020;43(Suppl 1): S111-S134. PMID: 31862753

14 **ANSWER: C)** *KCNJ11*

The patient's personal and family histories are highly suggestive of neonatal diabetes, which is defined as onset of diabetes within 6 months of birth. It is frequently caused by a pathogenic variant in a single gene affecting pancreatic β-cell function. In about one-third of cases, the diabetes is permanent. In transient cases, many individuals often develop permanent diabetes mellitus later in life. Identifying these patients is important, as many can achieve glycemic control with sulfonylurea therapy, which can often negate the need for insulin or reduce insulin dependency. Accordingly, checking for pathogenic variants in the *KCNJ11* gene (Answer C), which encodes the Kir6.2 protein, would confirm the correct diagnosis. Kir6.2 is a major subunit of the ATP-sensitive potassium ion channel. Pathogenic variants result in reduced ATP sensitivity of the ATP-sensitive potassium channel. Increasing the current of the ATP-sensitive potassium channel inhibits β-cell electrical activity and insulin secretion. *KCNJ11* pathogenic variants are a common cause (53%) of permanent neonatal diabetes in individuals of European ancestry. Sulfonylurea therapy blocks the ATP-sensitive potassium channel, reducing the current and thereby overcoming the inhibition of insulin secretion. Accordingly, sulfonylureas are prescribed (generally at higher dosages than usually used in the management of type 2 diabetes). Transitioning a patient's regimen from insulin to a sulfonylurea should be done in a controlled setting (ie, by following a research protocol or during hospitalization) to avoid development of marked hyperglycemia.

Conducting a thorough family history and assessing for C-peptide, plasma glucose, and the autoimmune markers of diabetes should be completed before ordering genetic testing.

Pathogenic variants in the *HNF1A* (Answer D) or *HNF4A* gene (Answer B) result in maturity-onset diabetes of the young (MODY) type 3 and type 1, respectively. Pathogenic variants lead to abnormal or reduced insulin secretion. MODY is a disorder characterized by noninsulin-dependent diabetes diagnosed at a young age (<25 years) with autosomal dominant inheritance and lack of autoantibodies. There are numerous subtypes of MODY. MODY 3 usually presents after puberty. This form of diabetes is also more common among individuals of European ancestry. The clinical features of MODY type 1 are similar to those of MODY type 3, but macrosomia is very common and 20% have prolonged neonatal hypoglycemia. MODY type 1 is considerably less common than MODY type 3, and the age of diagnosis tends to be later. *HNF4A* pathogenic variants should be considered when *HNF1A* sequencing is negative but the clinical features are strongly suggestive of *HNF1A*-related MODY. In either case, patients are often sensitive to sulfonylurea therapy. The timing of diabetes onset in the patient and his siblings is consistent with neonatal diabetes. Thus, testing for *HNF1A* or *HNF4A* gene variants is not the best choice.

Congenital generalized lipodystrophy is an autosomal recessive disorder characterized by marked paucity of adipose tissue, extreme insulin resistance, hypertriglyceridemia, hepatic steatosis, and early onset of diabetes. Pathogenic variants in the *AGPAT2* gene (Answer E) or *BSCL2* gene (Answer A) account for most cases of congenital lipodystrophy. This patient does not have a history that is consistent with lipodystrophy, so it would not be appropriate to assess for a pathogenic variant in either of these genes.

Educational Objective
Suspect a diagnosis of neonatal diabetes in patients who have a personal history of insulin-dependent diabetes diagnosed shortly after birth and a strong family history of diabetes.

Reference(s)
Agarwal AK, Arioglu E, De Almeida S, et al. AGPAT2 is mutated in congenital generalized lipodystrophy linked to chromosome 9q34. *Nat Genet.* 2002;31(1):21-23. PMID: 11967537

Craveiro Sarmento AS, Ferreira LC, Lima JG, et al. The worldwide mutational landscape of Berardinelli-Seip congenital lipodystrophy. *Mutat Res.* 2019;781:30-52. PMID: 31416577

Fösel S. Transient and permanent neonatal diabetes. *Eur J Pediatr.* 1995;154(12):944-8. PMID: 8801100

Gloyn AL, Pearson ER, Antcliff JF, et al. Activating mutations in the gene encoding the ATP-sensitive potassium-channel subunit Kir6.2 and permanent neonatal diabetes [published correction appears in *N Engl J Med.* 2004;351(14):1470]. *N Engl J Med.* 2004;350(18):1838-1849. PMID: 15115830

Hattersley A, Bruining J, Shield J, Njolstad P, Donaghue KC. The diagnosis and management of monogenic diabetes in children and adolescents. *Pediatr Diabetes.* 2009;10(Suppl 12):33-42. PMID: 19754616

Pearson ER, Flechtner I, Njolstad PR, et al; Neonatal Diabetes International Collaborative Group. Switching from insulin to oral sulfonylureas in patients with diabetes due to Kir6.2 mutations. *N Engl J Med.* 2006;355(5):467-477. PMID: 16885550

Timsit J, Bellanné-Chantelot C, Dubois-Laforgue D, Velho G. Diagnosis and management of maturity-onset diabetes of the young. *Treat Endocrinol.* 2005;4(1):9-18. PMID: 15649097

Vaxillaire M, Populaire C, Busiah K, et al. Kir6.2 mutations are a common cause of permanent neonatal diabetes in a large cohort of French patients. *Diabetes.* 2004;53(10):2719-2722. PMID: 15448107

15   ANSWER: C) CT of the chest, mediastinum, and neck
This patient presents with excessive sweating, anxiety, and fatigue—symptoms that are not specific for, but may suggest, hyperadrenergic activity. Evaluation of plasma and urinary metanephrines shows dramatic elevations in the normetanephrine fraction along with elevations in urinary norepinephrine.

Pheochromocytomas are tumors arising from the adrenal medulla, which may secrete catecholamines that induce adrenergic symptoms and signs such as palpitations, anxiety, sweating, pallor, and elevated blood pressure and heart rate. Paragangliomas are tumors that arise from the ganglia of the autonomic nervous system and therefore can occur in any region from the base of the skull to the pelvic floor. Unlike pheochromocytomas, sympathetic paragangliomas can secrete norepinephrine and dopamine, but are unable to synthesize epinephrine.

Metanephrines are the stable and inactive metabolites of catecholamines that provide the highest sensitivity and specificity for diagnosing pheochromocytoma and paraganglioma. Metanephrine is the metabolite of epinephrine, and normetanephrine is the metabolite of norepinephrine. Thus, from a diagnostic perspective, functional pheochromocytomas may have elevated metanephrine and/or normetanephrine fractions, whereas functional paragangliomas usually only have an elevated normetanephrine fraction. Typically, pheochromocytomas and paragangliomas that induce clinical symptoms are associated with metanephrine and/or normetanephrine levels that are substantially higher than the upper limit of the reference range—usually 4 times or more (less commonly 2 or 3 times higher). Importantly, mild elevations above the upper limit of the metanephrines reference range (<2 times) are common and are usually attributed to enhanced sympathoadrenergic tone (eg, in a state of anxiety, stress, or illness) and/or the use of catecholamine reuptake inhibitors (eg, some antidepressant medications and cocaine or methamphetamines). These milder elevations are a frequent cause of false-positive values.

This patient's use of venlafaxine (a norepinephrine reuptake inhibitor) should be considered as a potential cause of a false-positive result. It is not uncommon for this medication, along with others in the same drug class, to cause 2-fold elevations in normetanephrine, and very rarely 3- to 4-fold elevations. This patient's greater than 6-fold elevation in plasma normetanephrine and greater than 20-fold elevation in urinary normetanephrines are extremely high and diagnostic for a norepinephrine-secreting tumor. Thus, pursuing no further testing (Answer E) is incorrect. Stopping the venlafaxine and repeating testing (Answer A) is not necessary, nor is additional testing for potential causes of metanephrine elevations (Answer D). Symptomatic and functional pheochromocytomas and paragangliomas are at least 1 to 2 cm in size and are easily seen on cross-sectional imaging. Therefore, imaging of the abdomen and pelvis (Answer B) in addition to what has already been done is not indicated.

The most likely location for the catecholamine-secreting tumor is the abdomen. However, the normal abdominal imaging suggests that there must be a norepinephrine-secreting paraganglioma in the chest, mediastinum, or neck (including the base of the skull) (Answer C). This patient was found to have a cardiac paraganglioma (6-cm mass in the atrioventricular groove of the heart) and a paravertebral paraganglioma near the sixth thoracic vertebra. These masses were successfully removed and confirmed to be paragangliomas. Genetic testing documented a pathogenic variant in the succinate dehydrogenase B gene (*SDHB*).

Educational Objective
Guide the diagnostic evaluation for pheochromocytoma and paraganglioma.

Reference(s)
Lenders LW, Duh QY, Eisenhofer G, et al; Endocrine Society. Pheochromocytoma and paraganglioma: an Endocrine Society clinical practice guideline. *J Clin Endocrinol Metab*. 2014;99(6):1915-1942. PMID: 24893135

16 ANSWER: A) β-hCG measurement
This patient presents with hyperthyroidism in the setting of a mediastinal mass. Lactate dehydrogenase is markedly elevated. Gonadotropins are fully suppressed, but testosterone is only modestly reduced. While central gonadal axis suppression could be due to acute illness, the serum testosterone should be lower in that setting. The low-normal serum testosterone suggests a gonadotropin-independent stimulus, or an exogenous source. Moreover, the prepubertal testicular size is not consistent with an acute illness effect, instead indicating organic hypogonadism. The diagnosis that best explains the clinical presentation is a β-hCG–producing mediastinal germ-cell tumor with β-hCG–induced thyrotoxicosis and undiagnosed Klinefelter syndrome as an underlying risk factor. Measuring β-hCG (Answer A) is the best next step in this patient's management. His initial β-hCG concentration was greater than 225,000 mIU/mL (>225,000 IU/L). Following tumor resection and postoperative chemotherapy, his β-hCG level decreased to 4 mIU/mL (4 IU/L) and hyperthyroidism resolved. Histologic examination demonstrated a nonseminomatous germ-cell tumor. The major tissue type was choriocarcinoma, which is commonly associated with β-hCG secretion.

Due to structural homology with TSH, β-hCG can, at high concentrations, stimulate the TSH receptor. This is exemplified by reduced TSH concentrations commonly seen in the first trimester of pregnancy, when β-hCG concentrations are at their peak. Tumor-produced β-hCG is structurally different from pregnancy-produced β-hCG, especially with respect to glycosylation patterns. These structural changes increase its affinity to the TSH receptor. In a case series of nonseminomatous germ-cell tumors, the prevalence of paraneoplastic hyperthyroidism was 3.5%, and hyperthyroidism occurred in 50% of patients with a β-hCG concentration greater than 50,000 mIU/mL (>50,000 IU/L).

Graves disease is a less likely diagnosis and would not explain the entire clinical presentation. Thus, TRAb assessment (Answer B) is not the best next step. A thyroid uptake scan (Answer C) would not distinguish β-hCG–induced hyperthyroidism from Graves disease, as thyroid uptake is diffusely increased in both conditions. Moreover, the patient had intravenous iodine contrast, which can suppress thyroid uptake.

Although karyotype analysis (Answer D) would confirm the underlying diagnosis of Klinefelter syndrome, it is not the most important test to order in the initial workup. The small testicular size makes Klinefelter syndrome very likely, and the diagnosis of primary hypogonadism is supported by the fact that despite the very high β-hCG concentrations (due to close structural homology with LH, β-hCG is an equipotent stimulator of the Leydig-cell

LH receptor), serum testosterone is clearly subnormal. Of note, Klinefelter syndrome, subsequently confirmed by karyotyping in this patient, is the only known risk factor for germ-cell tumors. The lifetime risk of mediastinal germ-cell tumors in men with Klinefelter syndrome is about 1%, which is much higher than the risk in the general male population.

While anabolic steroid abuse can present with gonadal suppression and gynecomastia and could be detected with a urinary androgen screen in some cases (Answer E), anabolic steroid use would not explain this patient's entire clinical picture.

Two interesting features in this case not yet addressed are the marked gynecomastia, evident on CT, and the marked suppression of gonadotropins despite the underlying primary hypogonadism due to Klinefelter syndrome. Both are explained by an increase in endogenous estradiol bioactivity. This is due to the combined effect of the hyperthyroidism and elevated β-hCG. Thyroid hormones increase circulating SHBG, leading to a higher free estradiol-to-testosterone ratio, especially in the context of an already low serum testosterone level. Thyroid hormones also stimulate the aromatase enzyme, leading to increased estradiol production. β-hCG promotes gynecomastia by stimulating ductal development via the LH receptor, which is known to be expressed in male breast tissue, and also stimulates estradiol production by the Leydig cells. Indeed, due to the combined effect of thyroid hormone and β-hCG action, this patient's serum estradiol was markedly elevated at presentation (423 pg/mL [10-40 pg/mL] [SI: 1553 pmol/L (36.7-146.8 pmol/L)]). The high estradiol explains not only the prominent gynecomastia, but also his suppressed gonadotropins via negative hypothalamic-pituitary feedback. Following treatment of the tumor, reduction of β-hCG, and consequent normalization of thyroid function, estradiol normalized. His LH concentration then increased to 28.6 mIU/mL (28.6 IU/L), while serum testosterone remained low at 280 ng/dL (9.7 nmol/L), unmasking primary hypogonadism due to Klinefelter syndrome.

Educational Objective
Diagnose hCG-induced hyperthyroidism in a man with an hCG-producing mediastinal germ-cell tumor and undiagnosed Klinefelter syndrome.

Reference(s)
Oosting SF, de Haas EC, Links TP, et al. Prevalence of paraneoplastic hyperthyroidism in patients with metastatic non-seminomatous germ-cell tumors. *Ann Oncol.* 2010;21(1):104-108. PMID: 19605510

Hasle H, Jacobsen BB, Asschenfeldt P, Andersen K. Mediastinal germ cell tumour associated with Klinefelter syndrome. A report of case and review of the literature. *Eur J Pediatr.* 1992;151(10):735-739. PMID: 1425792

17 ANSWER: A) Necrobiosis lipoidica diabeticorum

Dermatologic complications are estimated to occur in 30% to 90% of patients with diabetes over their lifetime. These complications can vary in intensity from cosmetic to severe and potentially life-threatening. Some dermatologic findings are specific to diabetes such as necrobiosis lipoidica diabeticorum (Answer A), generalized granuloma annulare (Answer C), diabetic bullae (Answer D), scleroderma diabeticorum (Answer B), acanthosis nigricans, eruptive xanthomatosis, acquired perforating dermatoses, and diabetic dermopathy (Answer E). A brief summary of each condition, including prevalence, histology, progression, and treatment, is provided (*see tables*).

Table 1. Diabetes-Related Dermatologic Complications: Prevalence, Location, Number, Initial Presentation, and Progression of Lesions

Characteristics	Necrobiosis lipoidica diabeticorum	Scleroderma diabeticorum	Granuloma annulare	Diabetic bullae	Diabetic dermopathy
Prevalence	• 0.3% to 1.6% of patients with type 2 diabetes; can be seen in patients with type 1 diabetes, although prevalence is less clear • 3rd to 4th decades of life in patients with type 2 diabetes • Might be associated with suboptimal glycemic control • Female predominance (75%-80% of cases)	• 2.5% to 14% of patients with type 2 diabetes • 10 times more prevalent in men than in women • Higher prevalence with suboptimal control	• Granuloma annulare has 5 variants; the generalized form is associated with diabetes • 0.3% to 4% of patients with diabetes • Average age of diagnosis is 50 years • Twice as common in women than in men	• 0.5% of patients with type 1 diabetes • Usually seen in patients with other diabetes-related complications such as neuropathy, nephrology, etc	• 40% to 50% of patients with type 2 diabetes • More common in men than in women • More common in patients with diabetes-related complications
Location	• Mostly lower extremities (pretibial), but can occur on the face, trunk, and arms	• Posterior neck, back, and shoulders	• Symmetric on extremities and sun-exposed portion of trunk	• Usually distal extremities	• Pretibial
Solitary/multiple	• Either solitary or multiple	• Diffuse	• Multiple	• Either solitary or multiple	• Small, multiple
Initial presentation	• Small, firm erythematous papule with gradual growth	• Skin hard, thick, and indurated	• Small, skin-colored or reddish papule	• Acute onset as painless bullous lesion	• Circular, red, scaly lesions
Progression	• Grows, well-demarcated, indurated, yellow-brown atrophic centers with ectatic vessels, reddish brown or violaceous granulomatous margins	• Same as initial but more profound	• Lesions gradually increase in size, have central involution, annular rings, and raised borders	• Progresses and rapidly becomes tense and blisters	• Well-circumscribed, brown macule • Atrophic • New lesions appear after old ones resolve

Table 2. Histopathology, Clinical Symptoms, and Treatment

Characteristics	Necrobiosis lipoidica diabeticorum	Scleroderma diabeticorum	Granuloma annulare	Diabetic bullae	Diabetic dermopathy
Histopathology	• Necrobiosis with palisading granulomas	• Thickened reticular dermis, thick collagen bundles with small amounts of mucin in dermis	• Lymphohistiocytic granulomatous changes; increased presence of mucin and lack of plasma cells help separate this entity from necrobiosis lipoidica diabeticorum	• Cleavage can be either intraepidermal or subepidermal with acantholysis; another form shows cleavage at dermoepidermal junction	• Usually does not need biopsy; findings can be nonspecific
Clinical presentation	• Varied (asymptomatic, painful, pruritic, decreased sensation over lesion)	• Often asymptomatic, can have some pain and decreased mobility when severe	• Asymptomatic or pruritic	• Can be uncomfortable when tense, usually heals in 2 to 6 weeks; can have secondary infection and ulceration	• Usually asymptomatic
Treatment	• Treatment can be challenging; topical and intralesional steroids, calcineurin inhibitors, compression therapy, psoralen, and ultraviolet A radiation are the most commonly tried therapies	• No clearly effective therapy; psoralen and ultraviolet A radiation with physical therapy may help with mobility; improved glycemic control is also advised	• Patients with diabetes often have relapsing courses; first-line therapies are ultraviolet A phototherapy, oral psoralen with ultraviolet A radiation, systemic retinoids, and dapsone	• Skin protection to avoid secondary infection	• Usually no specific therapy; avoid secondary infection; may be a marker for cardiovascular disease

In the case described, the lesion is not bullous, making the diagnosis of diabetic bullae (Answer D) incorrect. Because the lesion is distinct and present on the patient's extremity, scleroderma diabeticorum (Answer B) is an unlikely diagnosis, as this presents as skin thickening on the neck and back. Although diabetic dermopathy (Answer E) does present on the pretibial area, it often appears as multiple hyperpigmented "spots" in middle-aged men. More images can be reviewed in the listed reference (Murphy-Chutorian et al). Distinguishing between granuloma annulare (Answer C) and necrobiosis lipoidica (Answer A) can be difficult. Both have a similar prevalence rate, as well as a female predominance and lesions commonly located on the extremities. The presence of a solitary lesion with a yellow center, however, makes necrobiosis lipoidica more likely than granuloma annulare. A photograph of granuloma annulare is shown (*see image*). In patients with diabetes, the generalized variant of granuloma annulare is the most likely diagnosis, and multiple lesions would be expected. Although clinically necrobiosis lipoidica seems most likely, biopsy and histologic evaluation are required to determine diagnosis with certainty.

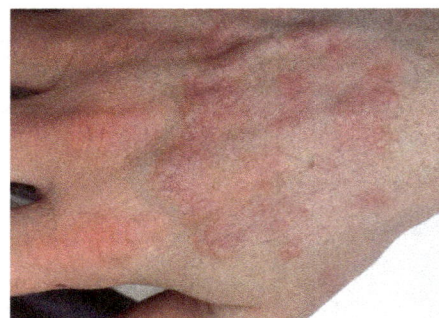

Educational Objective
Identify skin findings associated with type 2 diabetes mellitus.

Reference(s)

Murphy-Chutorian B, Han G, Cohen SR. Dermatologic manifestations of diabetes mellitus: a review. *Endocrinol Metab Clin North Am.* 2013;42(4):869-898. PMID: 24286954

Erfurt-Berge C, Seitz AT, Rehse C, Wollina U, Schwede K, Renner R. Update on clinical and laboratory features in necrobiosis lipoidica: a retrospective multicentre study of 52 patients. *Eur J Dermatol.* 2012;22(6):770-775. PMID: 23114030

18   ANSWER: D) Measure TSH and free T₄ again in 3 to 6 months

This patient has subclinical hyperthyroidism, which is defined as low or undetectable serum TSH with T_3 and free T_4 levels in the reference range. Subclinical hyperthyroidism affects nearly 2% of the US population and is most often caused by toxic multinodular goiter. Symptoms can be present, but they tend to be milder than those associated with overt hyperthyroidism.

Unless a patient is at high risk for complications related to subclinical hyperthyroidism, TSH and free T_4 should be measured again in 3 to 6 months (Answer D) to confirm that the biochemical abnormality is persistent before considering treatment. Approximately 0.5% to 7% progress to overt hyperthyroidism per year and 5% to 12% revert to normal thyroid function.

Subclinical hyperthyroidism is associated with an increased risk of atrial fibrillation and cardiovascular mortality, particularly in older patients with TSH concentrations below 0.1 mIU/L. Although younger patients with subclinical hyperthyroidism also appear to have an increased relative risk of adverse cardiovascular outcomes, the absolute risk is very low in this population and thus the benefits of treatment in younger patients are less clear. Subclinical hyperthyroidism is associated with reductions in bone mineral density in postmenopausal women, but this has not been established for other populations. A large meta-analysis by Blum and colleagues demonstrated higher rates of hip fracture with subclinical hyperthyroidism (7% in subclinical hyperthyroidism vs 4.5% in euthyroid patients), but it remains uncertain whether treatment reduces fracture risk.

Treatment of subclinical hyperthyroidism is indicated when serum TSH is persistently below 0.1 mIU/L in all patients 65 years and older; in younger patients with symptoms, known cardiac disease, or significant risk factors; in patients with osteoporosis; and in postmenopausal women who are not taking estrogen, bisphosphonates, or other antiresorptive agents. Treatment should be considered in all patients 65 years and older and in those with the described comorbidities and risk factors in the setting of persistent mild TSH suppression (0.1-0.4 mIU/L), as well as in younger asymptomatic patients if the serum TSH concentration is below 0.1 mIU/L. The underlying disorder should be determined to guide management.

This 40-year-old premenopausal woman without known cardiovascular disease or low bone density does not have specific signs or symptoms of hyperthyroidism. Persistent TSH suppression has also yet to be confirmed. Even if persistent subclinical hyperthyroidism is confirmed with laboratory testing in 3 to 6 months, treatment would not be recommended if the serum TSH concentration remains above 0.1 mIU/L. There is currently no indication to prescribe methimazole (Answer A) or recommend radioactive iodine therapy (Answer C).

Diagnostic testing, such as measuring TRAb (Answer B), to determine the etiology of subclinical hyperthyroidism would only be considered if treatment were planned.

Thyroid ultrasonography (Answer E) is not routinely recommended to evaluate patients with hyperthyroidism except in very specific clinical situations, such as amiodarone-induced thyrotoxicosis, or when it is needed to correlate with findings on nuclear imaging in the setting of thyroid nodular disease.

Educational Objective
List the indications for treatment of subclinical hyperthyroidism.

Reference(s)

Blum MR, Bauer DC, Collet TH, et al; Thyroid Studies Collaboration. Subclinical thyroid dysfunction and fracture risk: a meta-analysis. *JAMA.* 2015;313(20):2055-2065. PMID: 26010634

Ross DS, Burch HB, Cooper DS, et al. 2016 American Thyroid Association guidelines for diagnosis and management of hyperthyroidism and other causes of thyrotoxicosis. *Thyroid.* 2016;26(10):1343-1421. PMID: 27521067

Selmer C, Olesen JB, Hansen ML, et al. Subclinical and overt thyroid dysfunction and risk of all-cause mortality and cardiovascular events: a large population study. *J Clin Endocrinol Metab.* 2014;99(7):2372-2382. PMID: 24654753

19 **ANSWER: A) Order genetic testing for pathogenic variants in the *HNF1A* gene**

Only genetic testing for pathogenic variants in the *HNF1A* gene (Answer A) will confirm the correct diagnosis. Monogenic diabetes results from the inheritance of a pathogenic variant or variants in a single gene. It may be dominantly or recessively inherited or may be due to a de novo mutation and hence a spontaneous case. Almost all cases of monogenic diabetes result from pathogenic variants in genes that regulate β-cell function, although diabetes can rarely be caused by pathogenic variants resulting in very severe insulin resistance (lipodystrophy). The main forms of monogenic diabetes are classified into 2 groups: neonatal diabetes and familial diabetes (also called maturity-onset diabetes of the young [MODY]). Neonatal diabetes is usually diagnosed in the first 6 months of life, and familial diabetes is typically diagnosed in late childhood through early adulthood. Conducting a thorough family history and obtaining an assessment of C-peptide, plasma glucose, and the autoimmune markers of diabetes should preclude ordering of genetic testing. Monogenic diabetes should be considered if the features listed below are present in patients initially thought to have type 1 diabetes:

1. A diagnosis of diabetes before 6 months of age
2. Family history of diabetes with a parent affected
3. Evidence of endogenous insulin production outside the "honeymoon" phase (after 3 years of diabetes) with detectable C peptide (>0.6 ng/mL [>200 pmol/L]) when glucose >72 mg/dL (>4 mmol/L)
4. Absent pancreatic islet autoantibodies, especially if measured at diagnosis

This patient's family history is highly suggestive of MODY. MODY is a disorder characterized by noninsulin-dependent diabetes diagnosed at a young age (<25 years) with autosomal dominant inheritance and lack of autoantibodies. There are numerous subtypes of MODY. Pathogenic variants in the *HNF1A* gene (Answer A) and the *GCK* gene (Answer B) are most commonly identified, occurring in 52% to 65% and 15% to 32% of MODY cases, respectively. Cases of MODY type 3 (due to *HNF1A* pathogenic variants) usually present after puberty. This form of diabetes is also more common among patients of European ancestry. While *GCK* pathogenic variants also cause MODY (MODY type 2), affected patients rarely require treatment, usually have only mild fasting hyperglycemia, and do not commonly develop complications of diabetes. Thus, given the available information (presence of diabetes-related complications, current therapies, etc), *HNF1A* genetic testing is the best choice of the 2 answer options pertaining to MODY.

Pathogenic variants associated with monogenic diabetes result in abnormal or reduced insulin secretion; thus, C-peptide (Answer C) could be low or undetectable in both cases of monogenic diabetes or type 1 diabetes. It is important to remember that C-peptide should always be assessed with a corresponding glucose value, as the C-peptide level may be appropriately low in the setting of a low serum glucose. The C-peptide level (and corresponding glucose value) will provide an assessment of the patient's underlying insulin-producing capacity/reserve, which will be helpful when an attempt is being made to transition the patient to noninsulin therapies (ie, sulfonylurea therapy). Assessing for insulin-producing capacity before fully withdrawing insulin therapy is a must. It is important to note that low or undetectable C-peptide would not necessarily preclude a trial of sulfonylurea therapy; rather, this finding would require this trial to be completed in a more controlled manner/safe setting.

If autoimmune markers of diabetes were detected, that would be very consistent with a diagnosis of type 1 diabetes. However, the antibody markers that are often detected in patients with autoimmune forms of diabetes (type 1 diabetes) may not always be identified during laboratory evaluation. Glutamic acid decarboxylase (GAD) is an enzyme found in islet cells (among other tissues). Antibodies to GAD (Answer D) are found in approximately 70% of patients with type 1 diabetes at the time of diagnosis. ZnT8 is an islet β-cell secretory granule membrane protein. ZnT8 antibodies are found in up to 80% of patients with newly diagnosed type 1 diabetes. In addition, 26% of patients with antibody-negative type 1 diabetes (insulin, GAD, insulinoma-associated protein 2 [IA-2], and islet-cell [ICA] autoantibodies) have ZnT8 autoantibodies. Insulin autoantibodies (Answer E) are often the first to appear in children followed from birth through progression to diabetes and are highest in young children developing diabetes. It is important to recognize that once insulin is administered subcutaneously for a few weeks, nearly all individuals develop insulin antibodies. Accordingly, measurement of insulin autoantibodies after patients have initiated insulin injections is of little value and cannot be used as a marker of immune-mediated diabetes.

Educational Objective

Identify patients with maturity-onset of diabetes of the young on the basis of their personal and family history of diabetes and order the most appropriate diagnostic testing.

Reference(s)

Achenbach P, Koczwara K, Knopff A, Naserke H, Ziegler AG, Bonifacio E. Mature high-affinity immune responses to (pro)insulin anticipate the autoimmune cascade that leads to type 1 diabetes. *J Clin Invest.* 2004;114(4):589-597. PMID: 15314696

Awa WL, Thon A, Raile K, et al; DPV-Wiss Study Group. Genetic and clinical characteristics of patients with *HNF1A* gene variations from the German-Austrian DPV database. *Eur J Endocrinol.* 2011;164(4):513-520. PMID: 21224407

Baekkeskov S, Aanstoot HJ, Christgau S, et al. Identification of the 64K autoantigen in insulin-dependent diabetes as the GABA-synthesizing enzyme glutamic acid decarboxylase. *Nature.* 1990;347(6289):151-156. PMID: 1697648

Fajans SS, Bell GI. MODY: history, genetics, pathophysiology, and clinical decision making. *Diabetes Care.* 2011;34(8):1878-1884. PMID: 21788644

Hattersley A, Bruining J, Shield J, Njolstad P, Donaghue KC. The diagnosis and management of monogenic diabetes in children and adolescents. *Pediatr Diabetes.* 2009;10(Suppl 12):33-42. PMID: 19754616 [*Due to a typographical error, incorrect C-peptide units are used on page 34 of this article; the correct units are pmol/L.*]

Taplin CE, Barker JM. Autoantibodies in type 1 diabetes. *Autoimmunity.* 2008;41(1):11-18. PMID: 18176860

Wenzlau JM, Walter M, Gardner TJ, et al. Kinetics of the post-onset decline in zinc transporter 8 autoantibodies in type 1 diabetic human subjects. *J Clin Endocrinol Metab.* 2010;95(10):4712-4719. PMID: 20610599

Yamagata K, Oda N, Kaisaki PJ, et al. Mutations in the hepatocyte nuclear factor-1alpha gene in maturity-onset diabetes of the young (MODY3). *Nature.* 1996;384(6608):455-458. PMID: 8945470

Hope SV, Knight BA, Shields BM, et al. Random non-fasting C-peptide testing can identify patients with insulin-treated type 2 diabetes at high risk of hypoglycemia. *Diabetologia.* 2018;61(1):66-74. PMID: 28983693

Hope SV, Knight BA, Shields BM, et al. Random non-fasting C-peptide: bringing robust assessment of endogenous insulin secretion to the clinic. *Diabet Med.* 2016;33(11):1554-1558. PMID: 27100275

20   ANSWER: C) Measure sodium

This patient with a nonfunctioning macroadenoma was discharged after surgery on a replacement hydrocortisone dosage. He did well for the first few postoperative days; therefore, even if he has adrenal insufficiency, he should not be symptomatic on hydrocortisone replacement. One week after surgery is the typical timeframe when symptomatic and, almost invariably, transient syndrome of inappropriate antidiuretic hormone secretion (SIADH) occurs, even in the absence of immediate postoperative diabetes insipidus. Indeed, the typical triphasic pattern (transient diabetes insipidus-SIADH-permanent diabetes insipidus) is quite rare. No reliable predictors of SIADH after pituitary surgery have been identified, although SIADH has been reported to be more prevalent in patients with cardiac, renal, and/or thyroid disease and in female patients. SIADH causing hyponatremia is common after pituitary surgery (up to 18%), but it is often mild and manageable with observation or fluid restriction. Sometimes, however, it can be severe and appear quite abruptly. When severe, it can be life-threatening. For this reason, many centers thoroughly educate patients about the signs and symptoms of hyponatremia and routinely measure serum sodium 1 week after pituitary surgery. To reduce the risk of hyponatremia, some centers fluid restrict all patients during the first postoperative week. Therefore, in this patient, sodium should be measured urgently (Answer C), and if severe hyponatremia is confirmed, he should be treated with hypertonic fluid or with an aquaretic agent (vasopressin receptor antagonist).

If the sodium concentration is normal, MRI imaging (Answer A) could be performed to rule out postsurgical bleeding. Administering intravenous hydrocortisone (Answer B) would be appropriate for acute adrenal insufficiency, but this patient is already on replacement therapy and his vital signs are normal, which rules out an adrenal crisis. Measuring cortisol (Answer D) in a patient on hydrocortisone would generate a result that would be difficult to interpret. There is no indication for a lumbar puncture (Answer E) in the absence of symptoms of meningitis.

Educational Objective

Consider hyponatremia in the differential diagnosis of urgent complications of pituitary surgery.

Reference(s)

Krogh J, Kistorp CN, Jafar-Mohammadi B, Pal A, Cudlip S, Grossman A. Transsphenoidal surgery for pituitary tumours: frequency and predictors of delayed hyponatraemia and their relationship to early readmission. *Eur J Endocrinol*. 2018;178(3):247-253. PMID: 29263154

Barber SM, Liebelt BD, Baskin DS. Incidence, etiology and outcomes of hyponatremia after transsphenoidal surgery: experience with 344 consecutive patients at a single tertiary center. *J Clin Med*. 2014;3(4):1199-1219. PMID: 26237599

21 ANSWER: A) Continue alendronate

Bone mineral density assessment by DXA is the best test to diagnose osteoporosis. In addition, it is an effective means with which to predict an individual's risk of low-trauma fracture, particularly when combined with fracture risk prediction tools such as FRAX. DXA is also a robust tool to follow response to therapy longitudinally over time, although the ability to achieve this is predicated on establishment of the in vivo precision of the DXA machine. Completion of in vivo precision testing, which involves scanning either 30 patients twice or 15 patients 3 times, allows the clinician to determine with 95% confidence whether a truly significant change in bone density has occurred at the lumbar spine, total hip, or proximal one-third radius. While such an approach is recommended and is ideal in the care of patients with osteoporosis, real-world challenges often supervene to undermine this approach. Specifically, it may be necessary for patients to undergo follow-up DXA testing at a different facility because of insurance changes or a move to another city or state. As such, patients may have DXA testing on a completely different DXA platform (Hologic vs GE-Lunar vs Norland). This is problematic, given that the bone mineral density results are not comparable based on differences in DXA scanning technology among manufacturers (bone mineral density values are higher with GE-Lunar vs Hologic, and Norland values are between the other two).

Fortunately, determination of standardized bone mineral density can be used to provide some clinical guidance in patients who switch between DXA platforms (http://courses.washington.edu/bonephys/opBMDs.html). Even so, the use of standardized bone mineral density comparison does necessarily introduce additional error such that, in general, patients have to exceed at least an 8% to 10% change in standardized bone mineral density at the lumbar spine or total hip for a provider to be reasonably certain that a significant change has occurred.

In this vignette, although the actual bone mineral density value on the follow-up DXA is substantially lower, very little change in standardized bone mineral density has occurred (*see image*).

Given this result and based on evidence that vertebral fracture risk reduction is similar in a patient who either gains significant bone mineral density or remains stable on follow-up DXA testing, it would be reasonable to continue alendronate (Answer A). The absence of a true decline in bone mineral density argues against treatment failure in this patient and would therefore not warrant a change to a parenteral antiresorptive or anabolic agent (Answers B and C). While the presence of secondary disease processes may undermine the effectiveness of FDA-approved therapies for osteoporosis, this patient does not have clinical evidence for primary hyperparathyroidism based on a normal calcium value corrected for albumin:

LUMBAR SPINE	
First Measurement	Second Measurement
○ Hologic	● Hologic
● Lunar	○ Lunar
○ Norland	○ Norland
0.838 g / cm2	0.707 g / cm2
click to convert	
790 mg/cm2	764 mg/cm2
-3.3 % change	

$$(10.4 - ([\text{albumin}_{\text{patient}} - \text{albumin}_{\text{mid-normal}}] \times 0.8) = 10.4 - ([4.8\text{-}4.2] \times 0.8) = 9.9 \text{ mg/dL}$$

Therefore, neck ultrasonography (Answer D) to evaluate for possible parathyroid adenoma is not appropriate. Finally, although this patient's 25-hydroxyvitamin D level is borderline insufficient, the normal PTH level argues against clinically significant secondary hyperparathyroidism, which would potentially benefit from pharmacologic (ie, prescription strength) vitamin D_2 replacement (Answer E).

Educational Objective

Use standardized bone mineral density comparison to determine appropriate management for a woman with postmenopausal osteoporosis.

Reference(s)

Hui SL, Gao S, Zhou XH, et al. Universal standardization of bone density measurements: a method with optimal properties for calibration among several instruments. *J Bone Miner Res.* 1997;12(9):1463-1470. PMID: 9286763

Fan B, Lu Y, Genant H, Fuerst T, Shepherd J. Does standardized BMD still remove differences between Hologic and GE-Lunar state-of-the-art DXA systems? *Osteoporos Int.* 2010;21(7):1227-1236. PMID: 19859644

22 ANSWER: A) Refer to a dietitian to review her current meal plan

Roux-en-Y gastric bypass is a type of bariatric surgery indicated for individuals with a BMI of 40 kg/m^2 or higher or a BMI of 35 kg/m^2 or higher with a comorbidity. Late complications of this procedure include stomal stenosis, marginal ulcers, bowel obstruction, dumping syndrome, gallstones, hernias, malnutrition, and postbariatric hypoglycemia. The symptoms described by this patient are consistent with postbariatric hypoglycemia.

Postbariatric hypoglycemia is a rare complication that usually presents 1 year after surgery. A population-based study revealed the prevalence of postbariatric hypoglycemia to be 2% in patients who underwent Roux-en-Y gastric bypass. Episodes of hypoglycemia occur 1 to 3 hours after consumption of simple carbohydrates, and patients can present with autonomic symptoms (tremors, palpitations, hunger, or sweating) or neuroglycopenic symptoms (weakness, confusion, and altered level of consciousness).

The mechanism responsible for this condition is most likely multifactorial and includes increased levels of GLP-1 and gastric inhibitory peptide, increased sensitivity of β-cells to GLP-1, increased pancreatic islet-cell mass, increased insulin sensitivity after weight loss, inappropriate secretion of insulin, and an abnormal counterregulatory response to hypoglycemia.

It is important to distinguish postbariatric hypoglycemia from dumping syndrome. In the latter, symptoms start a few minutes up to 60 minutes after ingestion of a calorie-dense food. A detailed history, which includes symptoms during the episode, frequency of episodes, temporal relationship between the episode and the last meal, the presence or absence of nocturnal symptoms, and dietary history, is needed to make the diagnosis.

Fingerstick glucose measurements are not accurate for readings below 70 mg/dL (<3.9 mmol/L) and should not be used for diagnosis. Confirmation of the diagnosis is made by measuring plasma glucose that is drawn postprandially. A mixed-meal test is the preferred provocative test to diagnose postbariatric hypoglycemia. There is not a single standardized meal, as each institution uses their own version. In most practices, patients are asked to bring the food that triggers their symptoms, which is usually a food high in simple carbohydrates, and insulin and glucose levels are checked every 30 minutes. A positive result shows normal fasting glucose and hyperglycemia within the first 30 minutes of the test followed by hypoglycemia (plasma glucose <50 mg/dL [<2.8 mmol/L]).

The cornerstone for management of postprandial hypoglycemia is dietary modification. Patients should be referred to a registered dietitian (Answer A), so they can be counseled on following a low-simple carbohydrate, high-protein, high-fiber diet and eating multiple small meals. In most cases, dietary changes resolve hypoglycemia episodes. Medical management is usually second-line treatment, with acarbose (an a-glucosidase inhibitor) (Answer C) being the preferred initial agent. The starting dosage is 25 mg with each meal. Other medications that have been used include nifedipine, diazoxide, and octreotide (Answer B). If dietary changes do not decrease the frequency of hypoglycemia episodes, then pharmacotherapy should be considered. Surgical options such as gastrostomy tube placement, gastric outlet restriction, and Roux-en-Y gastric bypass reversal have been reported in case series when postbariatric hypoglycemia is not corrected with medical therapies.

A 72-hour fast is a supervised fast during which patients are monitored for the development of symptoms in the presence of hypoglycemia. Measurement of plasma glucose, insulin, C-peptide, proinsulin, and β-hydroxybutyrate is performed at regular intervals or when the patient has hypoglycemic symptoms. A 72-hour fast (Answer D) would be indicated if the patient presented with atypical symptoms; for example, if episodes only happened during the fasting state or more than 4 hours after a meal, or if her symptoms started less than 1 year after surgery.

During an oral glucose tolerance test (Answer E), glucose is measured at intervals after administration of 75 to 100 g of glucose. This test is not well tolerated by patients with a history of bariatric surgery, as the glucose load provokes dumping syndrome. It has been reported that up to 10% of healthy individuals have glucose levels less than 50 mg/dL (<2.8 mmol/L) during this test without associated symptoms. Therefore, oral glucose tolerance testing should not be used during the evaluation of postbariatric hypoglycemia.

Educational Objective

Identify and manage patients with hypoglycemia after gastric bypass surgery.

Reference(s)

Eisenberg D, Azagury DE, Ghiassi S, Grover BT, Kim JJ. ASMBS position statement on postprandial hyperinsulinemic hypoglycemia after bariatric surgery. *Surg Obes Relat Dis.* 2017;13(3):371-378. PMID: 28110984

Salehi M, Vella A, McLaughlin T, Patti ME. Hypoglycemia after gastric bypass surgery: current concepts and controversies. *J Clin Endocrinol Metab.* 2018;103(8):2815-2826. PMID: 30101281

Cryer PE, Axelrod L, Grossman AB, et al; Endocrine Society. Evaluation and management of adult hypoglycemic disorders: an Endocrine Society clinical practice guideline. *J Clin Endocrinol Metab.* 2009;94(3):709-728. PMID: 19088155

23 ANSWER: E) Secondary lymphoproliferative disease

Adrenal incidentalomas are common and are identified on 4% to 7% of abdominal CT or MRI scans in patients older than 40 years. While many of these are truly incidental and not associated with endocrine dysfunction, it is important to adopt a systematic approach to assessment. When faced with a patient with an adrenal incidentaloma, the clinician must answer 2 important questions: (1) what is the nature of the lesion and is there any possibility of a primary malignant tumor (eg, adrenocortical carcinoma) or secondary malignant tumor (eg, metastasis from bronchogenic carcinoma)? and (2) is the lesion functioning?

With modern imaging techniques (triple-phase CT, in-phase and out-of-phase MRI), most adrenal incidentalomas are readily classified as benign adrenal adenomas. However, in this case, there are several concerning features that suggest a more sinister cause: (1) it has been reported as a new 3-cm adrenal lesion and was presumably not evident on earlier surveillance imaging, which the patient would almost certainly have undergone within the last 12, and likely 6, months; (2) the lesion has relatively high density based on Hounsfield units at baseline and does not show washout following intravenous contrast; and (3) the patient has a history of malignancy and is on long-term immunomodulatory therapy.

Exclusion of a functioning adrenal lesion typically involves screening for adrenocortical and adrenomedullary causes. Measurement of plasma free metanephrines or 24-hour urinary fractionated metanephrines is the preferred investigation to detect an adrenal pheochromocytoma, although some clinicians reason that this is not required if the imaging assessment clearly demonstrates features of an adrenal adenoma. In this case, although the imaging characteristics could be compatible with a pheochromocytoma (Answer C), the plasma normetanephrine level is only mildly elevated (with normal plasma metanephrine) and is not in the range typically seen with pheochromocytoma. Indeed, the mild elevation in plasma normetanephrine in this case is explained by the concomitant use of amitriptyline. Moreover, it would be unusual for a pheochromocytoma to develop in such a short time interval.

The radiologic characteristics are not consistent with those of an adrenal adenoma (Answer A), which typically has a density less than 10 Hounsfield units on unenhanced imaging, and/or demonstrates significant contrast washout on triple-phase CT (absolute washout >60%, relative washout >40%). Here there is no washout even on delayed imaging. However, an adrenocortical carcinoma must be considered in this clinical context. Although the 24-hour urinary steroid profile and dexamethasone-suppressed cortisol are normal and there is no evidence of hypokalemia (unremarkable aldosterone-to-renin ratio, accepting the confounding effect of ramipril therapy), these findings do not completely exclude adrenocortical carcinoma, which would need to be carefully considered in the differential diagnosis. Similarly, the possibility of an adrenal metastasis (Answer D) from a previously undiagnosed independent primary tumor is a possibility. However, the absence of any other abnormality on PET-CT, in particular bronchogenic or renal carcinoma, makes this less likely.

The radiologic appearance is not typical of cytomegalovirus adrenalitis (Answer B), where bilateral adrenal involvement would be anticipated.

Importantly, this patient has a history of allogenic stem-cell transplant requiring immunosuppression, which was complicated by either newly acquired or reactivated Epstein-Barr infection. In this context, secondary lymphoproliferative disease (Answer E) is a well-recognized complication and may arise within the adrenal glands. In this patient, of the options offered, this is the most likely explanation for the development of a new adrenal mass with no clinical or biochemical features of adrenal dysfunction.

Educational Objective
Consider less common causes of adrenal incidentalomas.

Reference(s)
Fassnacht M, Arlt W, Bancos I, et al. Management of adrenal incidentalomas: European Society of Endocrinology clinical practice guideline in collaboration with the European Network for the Study of Adrenal Tumors. *Eur J Endocrinol*. 2016;175(2):G1-G34. PMID: 27390021

Shannon-Lowe C, Rickinson A, Bell AI. Epstein-Barr virus-associated lymphomas. *Philos Trans R Soc Lond B Biol Sci*. 2017;372(1732). PMID: 28893938

24 ANSWER: E) Refer for a Sistrunk procedure

Thyroglossal duct cysts are the most common cause of midline neck masses and are present in about 7% of the population worldwide. A thyroglossal duct cyst is formed due to failed closure of the thyroglossal duct extending from the foramen cecum in the tongue to the thyroid's location in the neck. They are typically located inferior to the hyoid bone, adjacent to the thyrohyoid membrane. They usually present as an asymptomatic neck mass but can also present with the infection of the cyst. Other causes of midline neck masses include lymphadenopathy, sebaceous cysts, epidermoid cysts, dermoid cysts, and ectopic thyroid gland.

On physical examination, thyroglossal duct cysts move upon swallowing or protrusion of the tongue. Affected patients can have other symptoms, including pain, sore throat, dysphagia, dysphonia, and the globus sensation. These cysts may cause airway obstruction in cases of rapid enlargement. The preferred imaging studies to diagnose thyroglossal duct cysts are neck ultrasonography and CT. Findings on CT include a well-circumscribed lesion with a thin rim enhancement. CT can provide information regarding the size, extent, and location of the cyst. Ultrasonography of a thyroglossal duct cyst reveals a well-defined, thin-walled, anechoic or hypoechoic mass with posterior acoustic enhancement in the midline anterior neck, but it does not provide information about the relationship to surrounding structures, including the hyoid bone.

FNA biopsy of the thyroglossal duct cyst is sometimes recommended to exclude other diagnoses, including malignancy when the cyst is not entirely cystic and contains a solid component. This patient's lesion seems to be a simple cyst with no worrisome features, so FNA biopsy (Answer C) is not necessary. Thyroid function tests should be performed in the workup of thyroglossal duct cysts, as hypothyroidism can be present in these patients. Patients with thyroglossal dust cysts often have ectopic thyroid and this must be determined before any surgery. In addition, an evaluation for normal thyroid tissue in the inferior neck should be completed by thyroid ultrasonography. The treatment for thyroglossal duct cysts is surgical removal. Simple excision (Answer D) of thyroglossal duct cysts is associated with recurrence. The Sistrunk procedure (Answer E) remains the standard of surgical management and has dramatically reduced recurrence rates. This procedure requires resection of the cyst and the midportion of the hyoid bone in continuity and resection of a tissue core from the hyoid upwards toward the foramen cecum. In the case of acute infection, surgery should be performed after the infection is treated with antibiotics.

The incidence of primary carcinoma of the thyroglossal duct is less than 1%, with most cases being papillary thyroid cancer. Several studies suggest that among patients with carcinoma in thyroglossal duct cysts, 11% to 33% have carcinoma within the thyroid gland. Thyroglossal duct cyst carcinoma is adequately treated by the Sistrunk procedure. However, thyroidectomy is performed if primary thyroid malignancy cannot be excluded or when secondary thyroid malignancy is detected.

In this patient, there are no clinical findings worrisome for infection, so initiating antibiotic treatment (Answer A) is incorrect. Starting levothyroxine (Answer B) would not affect the thyroglossal duct cyst.

Educational Objective
Manage a thyroglossal duct cyst.

Reference(s)
Thompson LD, Herrera HB, Lau SK. A clinicopathologic series of 685 thyroglossal duct remnant cysts. *Head Neck Pathol*. 2016;10(4):465-474. PMID: 27161104

Ross J, Manteghi A, Rethy K, Ding J, Chennupati SK. Thyroglossal duct cyst surgery: a ten-year single institution experience. Int J Pediatr. *Otorhinolaryngol*. 2017;101:132-136. PMID: 28964283

Patel S, Bhatt AA. Thyroglossal duct pathology and mimics. *Insights Imaging*. 2019;10(1):12. PMID: 30725193

25 ANSWER: A) Initiate cabergoline

In this case, hyperprolactinemia is associated with irregular menses and galactorrhea. The elevated prolactin is also associated with low estradiol levels due to suppression of FSH and LH, resulting in secondary hypogonadism. The ultrasonographic appearance is consistent with estrogen deficiency with an endometrial lining less than 4 mm. Therefore, although cyclic progesterone (Answer C) could be used to induce a period in cases of anovulatory oligomenorrhea, it is less likely to be effective with insufficient endogenous estradiol to promote the development of the endometrial lining. Cyclic progesterone would not restore estrogen status, and it would not treat the galactorrhea.

Since the cause of her secondary amenorrhea is secondary hypogonadism, metformin (Answer E) would not increase ovulatory frequency because she does not have polycystic ovary syndrome. Although pelvic ultrasonography did document an antral follicle count that could be consistent with polycystic ovarian morphology, this is not specific to the diagnosis of polycystic ovary syndrome, as healthy women with regular menses can also have this finding. In addition, more recent guidelines recommend a higher antral follicle count (≥20 with ultrasound transducer frequency now typically ≥8 mHz) to meet the criteria of polycystic ovarian morphology.

A persistent prolactin elevation of 50 ng/mL (2.2 nmol/L) with secondary hypogonadism is high enough to consider performing pituitary MRI (Answer D). However, given that her prolactin normalized just by switching to quetiapine, an anatomic lesion or adenoma is unlikely to have normalized. Therefore, the antipsychotic medication is the most likely cause because of the correlation of medication change with normalization of prolactin, as well as the recurrence of symptoms and the hyperprolactinemia when she restarted the medication.

Antipsychotic medications are a common cause of medication-induced hyperprolactinemia, especially dopamine receptor antagonists, which inhibit prolactin release by anterior pituitary lactotroph cells. The normalization of her prolactin after the change from risperidone to quetiapine is consistent with medication-induced hyperprolactinemia. However, this resulted in worsening of her psychiatric symptoms. The addition of aripiprazole was another reasonable treatment approach with the combined dopamine agonist/antagonist effect demonstrated to normalize prolactin when added to antipsychotic therapy. However, her symptoms did not resolve with a trial of this medication. Because she has already tried some alternatives in the management of her schizophrenia, referring back to psychiatry (Answer B) is less likely to be helpful at this stage. However, it will be important for her to continue attending regular follow-up psychiatry appointments.

Although it is generally not ideal to start an additional medication to treat the adverse effects of another, this patient has tried alternative medications, oral contraceptives, and switching to another antipsychotic agent (which worsened her schizophrenia). Studies have demonstrated the safety of cabergoline therapy (Answer A) in patients with psychotic disorders, although in limited sample sizes. After informed consent and discussion with her psychiatrist, this patient began a regimen of 0.25 mg twice weekly with subsequent normalization of prolactin, resolution of galactorrhea, and resumption of regular menses.

Educational Objective
Evaluate and treat a woman with hyperprolactinemia due to antipsychotic medication.

Reference(s)
Melmed S, Casanueva FF, Hoffman AR, et al; Endocrine Society. Diagnosis and treatment of hyperprolactinemia: an Endocrine Society clinical practice guideline. *J Clin Endocrinol Metab*. 2011;96(2):273-288. PMID: 21296991

Murphy MK, Hall JE, Adams JM, Lee H, Welt CK. Polycystic ovarian morphology in normal women does not predict the development of polycystic ovary syndrome. *J Clin Endocrinol Metab*. 2006;91(10):3878-3884. PMID: 16882750

Yunilaynen O, Starostina E, Dzeranova L, Baranov P, Dedov I. Efficacy and safety of long-term cabergoline treatment of antipsychotic-induced hyperprolactinemia (naturalistic study). *Eur Psychiatry*. 2016;33:S230.

26 ANSWER: B) Continue cabergoline at the current dosage

This patient has a macroprolactinoma as evidenced by markedly elevated serum prolactin at presentation and MRI findings of a macroadenoma with compression of the optic chiasm (more so on the right side than the left), thereby explaining the bitemporal hemianopia. His initial laboratory profile shows evidence of partial hypogonadotropic hypogonadism, but otherwise well-preserved anterior pituitary function.

Following treatment with cabergoline (titrated up to 750 mcg twice weekly), his serum prolactin has fully normalized, with correction of the associated hypogonadism without the need for exogenous testosterone replacement. His headaches and visual field defects have fully resolved. Repeated imaging reveals limited change in the overall appearance of the macroadenoma, which still fills the sella and extends superiorly into the suprasellar cistern.

This apparent disconnect between the clinical/laboratory and radiologic responses is not unusual in the early phase of dopamine agonist therapy. The decision regarding further escalation of treatment can be challenging and may be compounded by a patient's concern upon learning that the tumor has not changed significantly in appearance. Indeed, current Endocrine Society guidelines suggest further up-titration of medical therapy when both "response criteria" (correction of hyperprolactinemia and >50% tumor shrinkage) have not been met. In a study comparing conventional and more intensive cabergoline titration, an increase in dosage despite achieving normalization of serum prolactin was associated with an additional reduction in tumor volume by approximately one-third in just over 25% of patients.

Although some patients experience rapid tumor shrinkage following commencement of dopamine agonist therapy, tumor shrinkage in other patients can lag behind the improvement/normalization in serum prolactin by several weeks or even months. Therefore, when all other markers of disease activity have shown a clear improvement in a short timeframe, as in this vignette, it is reasonable to pause further dosage titration and arrange for imaging in 3 to 6 months to confirm the anticipated tumor shrinkage. Thus, no change in the patient's regimen is recommended now (Answer B). The patient's clinical symptoms have fully resolved (headache and visual disturbance); the serum prolactin is now in the lower half of the reference range; and the previously documented partial hypogonadism has fully resolved. Importantly, there were no other pituitary deficits on the baseline endocrine profile, although GH status was not assessed dynamically. Furthermore, on closer inspection of the images, there is evidence of a small reduction in the suprasellar component on the posttreatment scan (note the concave as opposed to convex upper margin on the right), which most likely explains the visual field improvement.

Although further up-titration of cabergoline (Answer C) could be considered, this is not necessary now and, importantly, it would put the patient at increased risk of developing unwanted adverse effects, including impulse control disorder.

As bromocriptine (Answer A) is less effective than cabergoline and is associated with greater adverse effects (eg, nausea, hypotension), it would not be appropriate to change dopamine agonist therapy in this context.

Transsphenoidal surgery (Answer E) may be indicated in the management of macroprolactinomas (eg, when there is visual compromise that does not respond rapidly to medical therapy or in a patient with dopamine agonist intolerance), but it may result in hypopituitarism and is not always curative.

Radiotherapy is generally reserved for aggressive or recurrent tumors. Stereotactic radiosurgery (Answer D) would not be appropriate in this case given the overall size of the tumor and its close proximity to the optic chiasm.

Educational Objective
Describe how the radiologic response to dopamine agonist therapy in macroprolactinomas may lag behind clinical and laboratory responses.

Reference(s)

Melmed S, Casanueva F, Hoffman AR, et al; Endocrine Society. Diagnosis and treatment of hyperprolactinemia: an Endocrine Society Clinical Practice Guideline. *J Clin Endocrinol Metab*. 2011;96(2):273-288. PMID: 21296991

Rastogi A, Bhansali A, Dutta P, et al. A comparison between intensive and conventional cabergoline treatment of newly diagnosed patients with macroprolactinoma. *Clin Endocrinol (Oxf)*. 2013;79(3):409-415. PMID: 23347435

Barake M, Klibanski A, Tritos NA. Impulse control disorder in patients with hyperprolactinemia treated with dopamine agonists: how much should we worry? *Eur J Endocrinol*. 2018;179(6):R287-R296. PMID: 30324793

Chanson P, Maiter D. The epidemiology, diagnosis and treatment of prolactinomas: the old and the new. *Best Pract Res Clin Endocrinol Metab*. 2019;33(2):101290. PMID: 31326373

27

ANSWER: E) Stop glyburide, start NPH insulin at bedtime and insulin lispro before dinner

Diagnosis and appropriate treatment of gestational diabetes mellitus lowers the risk of preeclampsia, macrosomia, and shoulder dystocia. Women with gestational diabetes should receive nutritional counseling as soon as possible following diagnosis. The goal of nutrition therapy is to improve glycemic control, limit weight gain in the mother and fetus, improve fetal well-being, and prevent ketosis. Glucose monitoring allows women to monitor the effects of diet on glycemic control and prompts the appropriate initiation of pharmacologic treatment to control hyperglycemia in the subset of women for whom diet therapy is unsuccessful.

The goals put forth by the American Diabetes Association and American College of Obstetricians and Gynecologists for glucose control in gestational diabetes are as follows:

Fasting glucose values <95 mg/dL (<5.3 mmol/L)
1-Hour postmeal glucose values <140 mg/dL (<7.8 mmol/L)
2-Hour postmeal glucose values <120 mg/dL (<6.7 mmol/L)

A key randomized controlled trial in women with gestational diabetes has shown that control of postprandial glucose compared with fasting glucose leads to better glycemic control overall, a lower incidence of large-for-gestational-age infants, and a lower rate of cesarean delivery.

The patient in this vignette follows a diabetes diet plan and started glyburide treatment and yet has suboptimal glycemic control. Contributing factors to the hyperglycemia in this case include her age, obesity, and history of having a large-for-gestational-age infant despite treatment with glyburide in her first pregnancy.

The American Diabetes Association and American College of Obstetricians and Gynecologists list insulin as the preferred treatment of choice for women with gestational diabetes for whom nutrition therapy fails. The Society for Maternal-Fetal Medicine has concluded that metformin is a safe first-line alternative to insulin. However, the Society for Maternal-Fetal Medicine guidelines state that insulin is presumed to be the most effective means to control hyperglycemia in gestational diabetes due to the ability to titrate doses to control glucose levels. Use of glyburide has not resulted in better pregnancy outcomes compared with insulin and some outcomes may be worse. In a review and meta-analysis comparing glyburide with insulin in women with gestational diabetes (published in 2015), women treated with glyburide had a higher rate of macrosomia (relative risk, 2.62; 95% CI, 1.35-5.08), higher mean birth weight (mean difference, +109 g; 95% CI, 36-182 g), and a higher rate of neonatal hypoglycemia (relative risk, 2.04; 95% CI, 1.30-3.20).

The greatest glucose-lowering effects of glyburide occur with the initial dosage of 5 to 10 mg daily. Doubling this patient's glyburide dosage (Answer D) or starting metformin (Answer A) would be unlikely to improve fasting glucose below 90 or 95 mg/dL (<5.0 or 5.3 mmol/L) or to control postprandial hyperglycemia.

Fast-acting insulin analogues such as insulin lispro or insulin aspart have been demonstrated to improve glycemic control in women with gestational diabetes and to limit the risk of hypoglycemia compared with treatment with human recombinant regular insulin. Starting insulin lispro before dinner (Answer B) should improve postmeal hyperglycemia but would not improve fasting hyperglycemia. Starting NPH insulin at bedtime (Answer C) should lead to control of fasting hyperglycemia but would not improve the postprandial hyperglycemia after dinner.

Therefore, the best next step is to start insulin lispro before dinner and NPH insulin at bedtime (Answer E). This should lead to rapid control of hyperglycemia and may lower the risk of maternal and neonatal morbidity. Glyburide should be stopped.

Educational Objective
Recommend glycemic goals for women with gestational diabetes mellitus and determine the optimal time to start insulin to prevent neonatal and maternal complications.

Reference(s)

American Diabetes Association. 14. Management of diabetes in pregnancy: standards of medical care in diabetes-2019. *American Diabetes Association. Diabetes Care.* 2019;42(Suppl 1):S165-S172. PMID: 30559240

Committee on Practice Bulletins—Obstetrics. ACOG practice bulletin No. 190: gestational diabetes mellitus. *Obstet Gynecol.* 2018;131(2):e49-e64. PMID: 29370047

Society of Maternal-Fetal Medicine (SMFM) Publications Committee. SMFM statement: pharmacological treatment of gestational diabetes. *Am J Obstet Gynecol.* 2018;218(5):B2-B4. PMID: 29409848

de Veciana M, Major CA, Morgan MA, et al. Postprandial versus preprandial blood glucose monitoring in women with gestational diabetes requiring insulin therapy. *N Engl J Med*. 1995;333(19):1237-1241. PMID: 7565999

Balsells M, Garcia-Patterson A, Solal Roque M, Gich I, Corcoy R. Glibenclamide, metformin, and insulin for treatment of gestational diabetes: a systematic review and meta-analysis. *BMJ*. 2015;350:h102. PMID: 25609400

28 ANSWER: E) Start empiric glucocorticoid therapy

Successful removal of an ACTH-secreting pituitary adenoma is invariably followed by adrenal insufficiency. The current practice in many centers is to withhold glucocorticoid therapy during and immediately after adenomectomy until there is clinical or biochemical evidence of ACTH deficiency. Serum cortisol and ACTH concentrations have been reported to predict cure after surgery for Cushing disease. In general, a serum cortisol level less than 3.0 µg/dL (<82.8 nmol/L) during the first 48 hours after pituitary adenoma resection is a reliable biochemical marker of ACTH deficiency and is associated with clinical remission of Cushing disease. A plasma ACTH concentration greater than 20 pg/mL (>4.4 pmol/L) has been associated with higher recurrence in 1 article, but it is not routinely measured. Some centers prefer to treat every patient with glucocorticoid therapy for presumptive adrenal insufficiency, deferring to a later time the assessment of whether the patient is in remission.

Serum cortisol usually reaches its nadir 24 to 36 hours after completion of curative surgery for Cushing disease, but some patients experience "late cure." Therefore, one should be very cautious in sending patients home on no glucocorticoid therapy even when cure seems unlikely (particularly if serum cortisol is not frankly low but is trending downward). If this is done, patients should be educated about the signs and symptoms of adrenal insufficiency. In this vignette, adrenal insufficiency should be suspected and glucocorticoids should be administered immediately (Answer E), while waiting for the serum cortisol measurement to return. This patient had severe postoperative adrenal insufficiency. Another possible explanation for her symptoms could be hyponatremia, and sodium should also be measured in the emergency department.

Measuring free T$_4$ (Answer A) would not be necessary in this case, as it would take weeks for postsurgical central hypothyroidism to be reflected by a low free T$_4$ value. Additionally, hypothyroidism would not explain her symptoms. Pituitary-directed MRI (Answer B) would not help, although it could be a consideration if adrenal insufficiency (and hyponatremia) are excluded to rule out rare postoperative bleeding. Plasma ACTH measurement (Answer C) could confirm the diagnosis of secondary adrenal insufficiency, but the result would probably not be available until several days later. Administering hypertonic fluid (Answer D) would be appropriate therapy for acute hyponatremia, but it should not be considered in the absence of a documented low sodium value.

Educational Objective

Consider the possibility of late cure after transsphenoidal surgery for Cushing disease.

Reference(s)

Simmons NE, Alden TD, Thorner MO, Laws ER Jr. Serum cortisol response to transsphenoidal surgery for Cushing disease. *J Neurosurg*. 2001;95(1):1-8. PMID: 11453376

El Asmar N, Rajpal A, Selman WR, Arafah BM. The value of perioperative levels of ACTH, DHEA, and DHEA-S and tumor size in predicting recurrence of Cushing disease. *J Clin Endocrinol Metab*. 2018;103(2):477-485. PMID: 29244084

Prete A, Corsello SM, Salvatori R. Current best practice in the management of patients after pituitary surgery. *Ther Adv Endocrinol Metab*. 2017;8(3):33-48. PMID: 28377801

29 ANSWER: E) Autoantibody status

Type 1 diabetes is an autoimmune disease, and genetic, autoimmune, and environmental factors all contribute to its development. However, the presence of β-cell autoimmunity (glutamic acid decarboxylase 65 antibodies, insulin autoantibodies, insulinoma antigen 2 antibodies, zinc transporter 8 antibodies, islet-cell antibodies) is highly predictive of the risk of type 1 diabetes. In addition to the presence of antibodies, the timing of their appearance has a strong role in predicting risk. β-Cell antibodies rarely appear before 6 months of age. Insulin autoantibodies appear early and might disappear. The rest of the β-cell antibodies tend to appear later and be more persistent. The presence of more than 1 antibody increases the risk of type 1 diabetes to greater than 70% (thus, Answer E is correct).

Table. Progression Rates to Type 1 Diabetes (In Children) Based on Number of Autoantibodies Present

Number of autoantibodies present	20-year risk
1 autoantibody	20%
2 autoantibodies	70%
3 autoantibodies	>80%

Data derived from Ziegler AG, Rewers M, Simell O, et al. Seroconversion to multiple islet autoantibodies and risk of progression to diabetes in children. JAMA. 2013;309(23):2473-2479.

There is no clear pattern of genetic inheritance for type 1 diabetes; however, variance in the HLA region of chromosome 6 is an important factor. Alterations in this region appear to contribute about 50% of the familial genetic risk in type 1 diabetes. Approximately 13% of patients with type 1 diabetes have a first-degree relative with a history of the condition. Having a parent with type 1 diabetes confers a risk of 3% to 5%, while having an affected sibling (as in this case) confers a risk of 8% to 12%. Having an affected monozygotic twin confers a risk of 30% to 50%. The greater the similarity of the high-risk HLA haplotype between the proband and the family member, the higher the risk of developing type 1 diabetes. Thus, the family history of type 1 diabetes in his fraternal twin (Answer A) does indicate higher risk than if he had no pertinent family history, but it is not the greatest risk indicator. The genetic risk is equal between sexes, and male sex (Answer C) is not associated with increased risk of progression to type 1 diabetes.

There has long been an interest in the role of environmental factors such as viruses (enterovirus, rubella, etc) and the relationship with β-cell autoimmunity, but causality has been hard to prove. His recent infection with mononucleosis (Answer D) is not a risk factor for progression to type 1 diabetes.

Although patients with 1 autoimmune disease are at higher risk for other autoimmune diseases, the relative impact of this risk is low. Patients with type 1 diabetes have 5% rates of concomitant autoimmune thyroid dysfunction. Thus, Hashimoto thyroiditis (Answer B) is not the greatest risk factor.

The development of type 1 diabetes is thought to occur in stages:

Stage 1: Asymptomatic β-cell autoimmunity
Stage 2: β-Cell autoimmunity with dysglycemia
Stage 3: Symptomatic type 1 diabetes

When the first appearance of β-cell antibodies is early, the progression through these stages is rapid. When the appearance is later in childhood or in adulthood, the progression through these stages can take decades. Other factors that affect seroconversion are genetic markers, sex (earlier in females), and type of antibody (eg, earlier with insulinoma antigen A2 than with glutamic acid decarboxylase 65 antibodies).

A recent study of the anti-CD3 antibody teplizumab has shown promising results in slowing the progression to type 1 diabetes in patients at high risk. Patients with at least 1 family member with type 1 diabetes and 2 β-cell autoantibodies and abnormal results on oral glucose tolerance testing were given a single course (14 days) of teplizumab. The hazard ratio for the diagnosis of type 1 diabetes (teplizumab vs placebo) was 0.41 (95% CI, 0.22-0.78; P = .006). If approved for use in high-risk individuals, anti-CD3 therapy might offer a mechanism to delay the onset of type 1 diabetes.

Educational Objective
Counsel patients regarding risk prediction for development of type 1 diabetes mellitus.

Reference(s)

Ziegler AG, Rewers M, Simell O, et al. Seroconversion to multiple islet autoantibodies and risk of progression to diabetes in children. *JAMA*. 2013;309(23):2473-2479. PMID: 23780460

Regnell SE, Lernmark A. Early prediction of autoimmune (type 1) diabetes. *Diabetologia*. 2017;60(8):1370-1381. PMID: 28550517

Herold KC, Bundy BN, Long SA, et al; Type 1 Diabetes TrialNet Study Group. An anti-CD3 antibody teplizumab in relatives at risk for type 1 diabetes. *N Engl J Med*. 2019;381(7):603-613. PMID: 31180194

30

ANSWER: D) Add purified icosapent ethyl

This patient presents for secondary prevention of atherosclerotic cardiovascular disease and persistent dyslipidemia characterized by moderate elevations of triglycerides and non-HDL cholesterol. He has intolerance to high-intensity statin therapy and has tried multiple statin dosages with resultant adverse effects. Statin-associated adverse effects commonly present as muscle symptoms. Switching to rosuvastatin, 20 mg daily (Answer A), a high-intensity statin dosage, in this patient who has documented evidence of intolerance to higher dosages could potentially result in discontinuation of statin therapy and elevations in LDL cholesterol, further increasing his cardiovascular risk. Thus, this approach is not recommended at this time.

Niacin (Answer B), or nicotinic acid, is a water-soluble B vitamin that at pharmacologic dosages can decrease triglycerides and LDL cholesterol and increase HDL cholesterol. Early trials in the prestatin era used immediate-release niacin monotherapy in men with previous myocardial infarction and showed reduced cardiovascular morbidity and mortality. Two large cardiovascular disease outcome trials (AIM-HIGH [Atherothrombosis Intervention in Metabolic Syndrome with Low HDL/High Triglycerides: Impact on Global Health Outcomes] and HPS2-THRIVE [Heart Protection Study 2-Treatment of HDL to Reduce the Incidence of Vascular Events]), studied the use of extended-release niacin formulations added to statins, and both failed to show clinical atherosclerotic cardiovascular disease benefit. These studies were conducted in individuals with known atherosclerotic cardiovascular disease who were on statin therapy with the goal of raising HDL cholesterol, and they highlighted several safety effects of niacin. Worsening insulin resistance can develop with high niacin dosages. Consequently, the US FDA withdrew the indication for use of extended-release niacin in combination with statins in 2016. Therefore, addition of extended-release niacin cannot be recommended for this patient who has impaired fasting glucose.

Bile-acid sequestrants such as colesevelam (Answer C) bind to bile salts within the intestinal lumen, preventing their enterohepatic reuptake. These agents up-regulate hepatic LDL receptors and result in increased clearance of circulating LDL cholesterol, thereby decreasing levels by 15% to 20%. An important adverse effect of bile acid resins is hypertriglyceridemia. In this individual with moderate hypertriglyceridemia, these agents are relatively contraindicated, as they can result in marked triglyceride elevations and risk of pancreatitis.

Until recently, marine fish oil supplementation trials did not demonstrate benefit from the standpoint of cardiovascular outcomes. The recently published Reduction of Cardiovascular Events with Icosapent Ethyl–Intervention Trial (REDUCE-IT) evaluated the benefit of using purified icosapent ethyl (Answer D) in individuals with known coronary artery disease or with diabetes and multiple risk factors for atherosclerotic cardiovascular disease. Icosapent ethyl is a highly purified and stable eicosapentaenoic acid ethyl ester. Compared with placebo, the addition of purified icosapent ethyl, 2 g twice daily, reduced cardiovascular events by 25% and cardiovascular mortality by 20% among patients who were already on statin therapy and had well-controlled LDL cholesterol (median LDL cholesterol, 86 mg/dL [2.23 mmol/L]). Also observed were statistically significant reductions in a variety of prespecified endpoints, such as a 31% reduction in myocardial infarction, 28% reduction in stroke, 32% reduction in hospitalization for unstable angina, and 35% reduction in urgent or emergent coronary revascularization. The magnitude of relative risk reduction was consistent across the range of triglyceride levels. The mechanisms underlying this cardiovascular benefit are not yet clear, since triglyceride lowering was only approximately 22% from baseline in these individuals. Beneficial effects on endothelial function, cell-membrane stability, and anti-inflammatory effects are potential mechanisms. Icosapent ethyl increased the risk of serious bleeding, atrial fibrillation, and peripheral edema. In this patient who is on maximum tolerated cholesterol-lowering therapy, addition of icosapent ethyl is the best option. Reasonable alternatives include further targeting the LDL-cholesterol pathway using a PCSK9 inhibitor, but this was not offered as an answer choice.

Dulaglutide (Answer E) is a GLP-1 receptor agonist that is approved for once-weekly treatment of type 2 diabetes. GLP-1 receptor agonists enable glucose lowering and weight loss by decreasing energy intake and inducing appetite suppression. Dulaglutide has significant hemoglobin A_{1c}–reducing and weight-loss effects. Dulaglutide can decrease triglycerides and LDL cholesterol and has demonstrated cardiovascular benefit in individuals with type 2 diabetes and known atherosclerotic cardiovascular disease or those with risk factors. However, data in individuals without diabetes or with prediabetes are lacking. Hence dulaglutide is not the best choice.

Educational Objective
Manage moderate hypertriglyceridemia using purified icosapent ethyl.

Reference(s)

Bhatt DL, Miller M, Brinton EA, et al; REDUCE-IT Investigators. REDUCE-IT USA: results from the 3146 patients randomized in the United States. *Circulation.* 2020;141(5):367-375. PMID: 31707829

Bhatt DL, Steg PG, Miller M, REDUCE-IT Investigators. Cardiovascular risk reduction with icosapent ethyl for hypertriglyceridemia. *N Engl J Med.* 2019;380(1):11-22. PMID: 30415628

31 ANSWER: C) Cholecalciferol

Patients with end-stage renal disease (ESRD) may have a number of bone and mineral disturbances. Notably, these patients usually have some degree of hyperparathyroidism based on the presence of hypocalcemia, hyperphosphatemia, and reduced endogenous production of calcitriol. In addition, patients with ESRD often develop renal bone disease or osteodystrophy, which may present as 1 or even a combination of specific skeletal disturbances (osteitis fibrosa cystica, osteomalacia, adynamic bone disease, or osteoporosis). Although a tetracycline-labeled iliac crest bone biopsy is required for definitive diagnosis of the underlying skeletal disease in these patients, clinical clues to the bone and mineral disorder can be obtained through noninvasive biochemical assessment.

This patient presents with low 25-hydroxyvitamin D, elevated PTH, and low bone density, which could be consistent with both osteitis fibrosa cystica and osteomalacia. Indeed, the pattern of bone mineral density deficit is consistent with both entities, with preferential loss of cortical-rich bone mineral density in the proximal one-third radius. The distinguishing feature in this patient, however, is the degree of 25-hydroxyvitamin D deficiency (11 ng/mL [27.5 nmol/L]). As such, one would expect a reasonable response to vitamin D replacement (Answer C), which is generally given as 50,000 IU once or twice per month.

Although calcitriol (Answer D) would also reduce PTH levels, there is no evidence that it would adequately treat underlying osteomalacia if present. Additionally, this patient has a borderline serum calcium level when corrected for albumin, as well as borderline hyperphosphatemia. Treatment with calcitriol would enhance both intestinal calcium and phosphorus absorption, thereby further increasing this patient's calcium × phosphorus product (currently 57) and possible risk of cardiovascular calcification based on available, albeit limited, evidence.

Alendronate (Answer A) is an effective treatment that reduces fracture risk in postmenopausal women, but it is contraindicated in the setting of advanced renal dysfunction, including ESRD, because of lack of clearance and concerns over increased risk of adverse events such as hypocalcemia and osteonecrosis of the jaw.

Teriparatide (Answer B) is approved for the treatment of osteoporosis in postmenopausal women, hypogonadal men, and both women and men with glucocorticoid-induced osteoporosis. It is unclear, however, what the true nature of this patient's bone disorder is based on available clinical data. In addition, she has evidence of secondary hyperparathyroidism, which may be evolving towards autonomous disease (primary or tertiary hyperparathyroidism) based on a borderline-high serum calcium level adjusted for albumin (10.3 mg/dL [2.6 mmol/L]). Treatment with teriparatide could potentially precipitate frank hypercalcemia in this patient.

Finally, while sevelamer hydrochloride (Answer E) is proven to reduce the serum phosphate level and calcium × phosphorus product in patients with ESRD, it would not address secondary hyperparathyroidism due to vitamin D deficiency in this patient and has not been shown to reduce the risk for skeletal events, including fractures.

Educational Objective

Recommend appropriate treatment in a patient with low bone density, end-stage renal disease, and vitamin D deficiency.

Reference(s)

Kandula P, Dobre M, Schold JD, Schreiber MJ Jr, Mehrotra R, Navaneethan SD. Vitamin D supplementation in chronic kidney disease: a systematic review and meta-analysis of observational studies and randomized controlled trials. *Clin J Am Soc Nephrol.* 2011;6(1):50-62. PMID: 20876671

Coen G, Mantella D, Manni M, et al. 25-hydroxyvitamin D levels and bone histomorphometry in hemodialysis renal osteodystrophy. *Kidney Int.* 2005;68(4):1840-1848. PMID: 16164662

32

ANSWER: E) Venlafaxine

Vasomotor symptoms such as hot flashes are a very common adverse effect of androgen-deprivation therapy (ADT) due to the severe reduction in sex steroids to castrate levels. Such vasomotor symptoms are associated with reduced quality of life in survivors of prostate cancer. Vasomotor instability is primarily due to estradiol (rather than testosterone) deficiency. Obese men are more susceptible. They have higher circulating estradiol because aromatase is expressed in adipose tissue, and consequently they have a more marked decrement with ADT. Hot flashes can interrupt sleep, leading to fatigue and low energy. Low energy associated with sex steroid deprivation is, however, multifactorial, and anemia (lack of erythropoietic cations of testosterone), changes in body composition (sarcopenic obesity), and effects on mood may contribute. In this patient, the anemia is relatively mild, and he screens negative for evidence of clinical depression. He most likely has sarcopenic obesity, and encouraging regular exercise is an important part of holistic clinical care.

There are 2 main reasons not to recommend testosterone therapy (Answers B and D) for this patient now. First, reactivation of the endogenous gonadal axis after a course of ADT takes time. ADT was only stopped 6 months before presentation and starting testosterone therapy now could suppress endogenous gonadal axis recovery. Indeed, his serum testosterone is above the castrate range and LH is detectable, suggesting incipient gonadal axis recovery. In one study of 88 older men with localized prostate cancer prospectively followed after completing a short course (6 months) of adjuvant ADT, actuarial rates of serum testosterone normalization at 3, 6, 12, and 24 months were 10%, 26%, 38%, and 59%, respectively. In a more recent prospectively maintained database study following 300 older men after cessation of longer-term ADT (median duration 17 months), serum testosterone levels increased slowly to 216 ng/dL (7.5 nmol/L) 6 to 12 months after ADT cessation and to 312 ng/dL (10.8 nmol/L) 24 months after ADT cessation. Twenty-four months after ADT cessation, 76% had a serum testosterone concentration greater than 300 ng/dL (>10.4 nmol/L), and 51% had returned to their baseline testosterone. However, in 8%, serum testosterone remained in the castrate range (<50 ng/dL [<1.7 nmol/L]). In general, older age, longer duration of ADT and a larger comorbid burden (including obesity) are predictors of slower testosterone recovery. Before starting ADT, patients should be counseled that posttreatment recovery of the gonadal axis can be delayed, or that rarely recovery may never occur.

The second reason for not commencing testosterone treatment is the uncertainty regarding its safety in survivors of prostate cancer. Endocrine Society guidelines recommend against testosterone therapy in men with a history of prostate cancer (grade 2 [ie, low-quality evidence recommendation]). The European Association of Urology suggests that symptomatic men with a history of low- to intermediate-risk prostate cancer who have no evidence of active prostate cancer 12 months after definitive treatment may be cautiously considered for testosterone treatment. However, evidence for safety is still limited and largely restricted to observational studies reporting outcomes in small, carefully selected, convenience samples. A recent review summarized 11 observational studies (mostly uncontrolled) comprising 700 survivors of prostate cancer receiving testosterone therapy after radical prostatectomy or radiation treatment or during active surveillance. Testosterone-treated men were followed up to 5 years. Overall, the review concluded that there was no evidence suggesting an increased recurrence risk. However, true risks are unknown, given methodologic shortcomings of these studies.

A trial of testosterone therapy may be considered in carefully selected symptomatic patients with persistently low testosterone and poor quality of life (but no evidence of active prostate cancer) after discussing the lack of safety data, obtaining informed consent, and consulting with the treating urologist/radiation oncologist. Patients should be monitored carefully, and testosterone should be stopped if there is no clinical benefit. While there are no data, initiation of short-acting topical testosterone therapy rather than long-acting intramuscular testosterone appears prudent.

In this patient, testosterone is not currently appropriate for the reasons discussed. Instead, a trial of low-dosage venlafaxine (Answer E), or alternatively a selective serotonin reuptake inhibitor, is the most appropriate initial therapy given that hot flashes are the predominant symptom. Such agents are generally well tolerated and are modestly effective (reducing hot flash frequency by 30% to 50%) and may improve sleep, energy, and quality of life. Of note, prescribing venlafaxine or a selective serotonin reuptake inhibitor is off-label use, as these drugs are not FDA approved for the treatment of hot flashes in men.

Estradiol (Answer A) is more effective against hot flashes than first-line agents, but it is generally reserved as a second-line treatment. Often, worsening of gynecomastia (already present) can be a limiting adverse effect. The history of venous thromboembolism is a contraindication to estradiol.

Selective estrogen receptor modulators such as tamoxifen (Answer C) do not improve hot flashes. There is no evidence that they hasten gonadal axis recovery. Also, this patient's history of venous thromboembolism is a contraindication.

Educational Objective
Counsel patients that recovery from androgen-deprivation therapy can be prolonged and describe the limited evidence regarding risks and benefits of testosterone treatment in this scenario.

Reference(s)

Grossmann M, Zajac JD. Management of side effects of androgen deprivation therapy. *Endocrinol Metab Clin North Am.* 2011;40(3):655-671. PMID: 21889727

Padula GD, Zelefsky MJ, Venkatraman ES, et al. Normalization of serum testosterone levels in patients treated with neoadjuvant hormonal therapy and three-dimensional conformal radiotherapy for prostate cancer. *Int J Radiat Oncol Biol Phys.* 2002;52(2):439-443. PMID: 11872290

Nascimento B, Miranda EP, Jenkins LC, Benfante N, Schofield EA, Mulhall JP. Testosterone recovery profiles after cessation of androgen deprivation therapy for prostate cancer. *J Sex Med.* 2019;16(6):872-879. PMID: 31080102

Bell MA, Campbell JD, Joice G, Sopko NA, Burnett AL. Shifting the paradigm of testosterone replacement therapy in prostate cancer. *World J Mens Health.* 2018;36(2):103-109. PMID: 29623698

33 ANSWER: B) Measure fructosamine

This patient has end-stage renal disease and anemia for which she is receiving iron supplements and epoetin alfa therapy. Anemia and a high reticulocyte count can result in falsely low hemoglobin A_{1c} values. This patient reports limited point-of-care blood glucose values (some of which were noted to be in the range of 200 mg/dL [11.1 mmol/L]) and blurred vision over the past few weeks. Her glycemic control is most likely worse than is suggested by her hemoglobin A_{1c} level. In this setting, checking another marker of glycemic control, such as glycated serum protein (fructosamine [Answer B]) can help to identify inadequate glycemic control and the need for therapeutic adjustment. Fructosamine reflects the level of glycated serum proteins (mostly albumin). It has a shorter half-life of about 2 to 3 weeks compared with the half-life of hemoglobin A_{1c}, which is dependent on the lifecycle of a mature red blood cell in the circulation (100 to 120 days in a healthy individual). Thus, fructosamine measurement represents a shorter period of preceding blood glucose levels, and it is also quicker to respond to treatment (changes in blood glucose control) compared with hemoglobin A_{1c}. In the opposite situation, where serum protein levels are markedly decreased, such as in nephrotic syndrome, using fructosamine as a marker of glycemic control would not be appropriate.

Sickle-cell trait, or the hemoglobin S variant (Answer A), occurs when an individual is heterozygous for a pathogenic variant in the β-globin gene (*HBB*). As many as 100 million individuals have sickle-cell trait worldwide. The hemoglobin S variant is associated with a higher hemoglobin A_{1c} level, and this elevation is not an artifact. While hemoglobin S disease (homozygous genotype) can make hemoglobin A_{1c} unreliable (falsely low), the patient in this vignette is of European ancestry and has no history to suggest sickle-cell disease. Sickle-cell trait and sickle-cell disease are far more common in individuals of African American ancestry. The hemoglobin A_{1c} test is not used in patients with diabetes who have sickle-cell disease because of the shortened lifespan of red blood cells in this condition, which yields inaccurately lower hemoglobin A_{1c} values. Assessing for the presence of the hemoglobin S variant may have been an appropriate test to obtain in a black patient (particularly if there were a known family history of sickle-cell trait or disease), in the setting of elevated hemoglobin A_{1c}, or after identifying a discordance between an elevated hemoglobin A_{1c} value and fructosamine concentration, thereby confirming the unreliability of the hemoglobin A_{1c} measurement.

Measuring C-peptide (Answer E) would not help to determine the need to intensify therapy or ascertain her current level of glycemic control.

Changing her therapy (Answers C or D) would only be appropriate after the current degree of glycemic control is reliably determined and/or if hypoglycemia were reported or suspected.

Referral of this patient for professional continuous glucose monitoring is another option to consider. However, the accuracy of continuous glucose sensors in persons with diabetes undergoing hemodialysis remains uncertain. There are ongoing clinical trials that are attempting to assess the accuracy of continuous glucose monitoring in such patients.

Educational Objective
Identify situations in which hemoglobin A_{1c} may not accurately reflect a patient's glycemic control.

Reference(s)

Goldsmith JC, Bonham VL, Joiner CH, Kato GJ, Noonan AS, Steinberg MH. Framing the research agenda for sickle cell trait: building on the current understanding of clinical events and their potential implications. *Am J Hematol*. 2012;87(3):340-346. PMID: 22307997

Johnson RN, Metcalf PA, Baker JR. Fructosamine: a new approach to the estimation of serum glycosylprotein. An index of diabetic control. *Clin Chim Acta*. 1983;127(1):87-95. PMID: 6825313

Klonoff DC. Hemoglobinopathies and hemoglobin A1c in diabetes mellitus. *J Diabetes Sci Technol*. 2020;14(1):3-7. PMID: 30897962

Lacy ME, Wellenius GA, Sumner AE, et al. Association of sickle cell trait with hemoglobin A1c in African Americans. *JAMA*. 2017;317(5):507-515. PMID: 28170479

Radin MS. Pitfalls in hemoglobin A1c measurement: when results may be misleading. *J Gen Intern Med*. 2014;29(2):388-394. PMID: 24002631

Ziemer DC, Kolm P, Weintraub WS, et al. Glucose-independent, black-white differences in hemoglobin A1c levels: a cross-sectional analysis of 2 studies. *Ann Intern Med*. 2010;152(12):770-777. PMID: 20547905

34 ANSWER: A) CT chest imaging in 6 months

This patient has a homogeneous-appearing anterior mediastinal mass without evidence of calcifications or invasion. These findings are consistent with thymic hyperplasia, which can sometimes be seen in association with Graves hyperthyroidism. There are 2 subtypes of thymic hyperplasia: true hyperplasia, in which the normal architecture is preserved but the thymus is grossly enlarged, and lymphoid hyperplasia, which is defined by the presence of an increased number of lymphoid follicles and germinal centers. The latter is most often seen in association with autoimmune disorders, including myasthenia gravis, rheumatoid arthritis, and systemic lupus erythematosus. However, both types of thymic hyperplasia have been reported in patients with Graves disease. Although the exact mechanism for thymic hyperplasia in Graves disease is unknown, animal studies suggest that true hyperplasia is secondary to T_3 excess, while lymphoid hyperplasia is thought to be related to autoimmunity.

The most appropriate initial management of the patient's anterior mediastinal mass would be to repeat CT chest imaging in 6 months (Answer A). Treatment with either antithyroidal drugs or radioactive iodine has been associated with thymic involution in patients with thymic hyperplasia related to Graves hyperthyroidism.

In contrast to what has been observed with myasthenia gravis, thymectomy does not ameliorate hyperthyroidism in Graves disease. Performing surgical resection via median sternotomy (Answer E) would not be recommended at this time due to risk of perioperative complications and lack of benefit.

Mediastinoscopy with biopsy (Answer B) to evaluate the cause of the patient's mediastinal mass is not needed now given the radiographic appearance characteristic of thymic hyperplasia and association with Graves hyperthyroidism. If the mediastinal mass has not decreased in size by more than 50% on the 6-month follow-up imaging after treatment of hyperthyroidism, then additional diagnostic testing, such as biopsy or surgery, would be considered. Further diagnostic testing would also have been indicated if the initial CT had demonstrated calcifications, evidence of invasion, or other suspicious findings.

In the absence of suspicious radiographic findings and signs and symptoms suggestive of a germ-cell tumor, measurement of serum β-hCG, α-fetoprotein, and lactate dehydrogenase (Answer C) would not be the most appropriate next step in this patient's management. The elevated thyroid-stimulating immunoglobin activity, a finding that is diagnostic of Graves disease, also makes hCG-mediated hyperthyroidism unlikely. PET-CT scan (Answer D) would also not be indicated unless malignancy is suspected.

Note: Image is reprinted from Kirkeby KM, Pont A. Image in endocrinology: thymic hyperplasia in a patient with Graves' disease. *J Clin Endocrinol Metab*. 2006;91(1):1.

Educational Objective

Identify the association between Graves hyperthyroidism and thymic hyperplasia.

Reference(s)

Kirkeby KM, Pont A. Image in endocrinology: thymic hyperplasia in a patient with Graves' disease. *J Clin Endocrinol Metab*. 2006;91(1):1. PMID: 16401829

Haider U, Richards P, Gianoukakis AG. Thymic hyperplasia associated with Graves' disease: pathophysiology and proposed management algorithm. *Thyroid*. 2017;27(8):994-1000. PMID: 28578595

Jinguji M, Nakajo M, Nakajo M, Koriyama C, Yoshiura T. Thymic involution after radioiodine therapy for Graves disease: relationships with serum thyroid hormones and TRAb. *J Endocr Soc*. 2017;1(7):852-860. PMID: 29264536

35 ANSWER: D) Initiation of intramuscular testosterone

Because of the significant dysphoria associated with menses, the best next step is to initiate intramuscular testosterone injections (Answer D), which would be more likely to induce amenorrhea in the shortest amount of time and will likely be the lowest cost to the patient. In one comparative study of different testosterone treatment routes in transgender men, testosterone enanthate injections were associated with a shorter time to amenorrhea vs gel or testosterone undecanoate, although the difference was not statistically significant (29.8 ± 18.4, 40.4 ± 10.6, and 41.0 ± 10.4 weeks). All participants became amenorrheic by week 54. In another study of testosterone enanthate injections, a dose-dependent difference was observed in the percentage of transgender men who achieved amenorrhea after 1 month (62.1% at the higher dose of 250 mg every 2 weeks, 50% with 250 mg every 3 weeks, and 47.3% with 125 mg every 2 weeks). By 6 months, 96.6%, 92.7%, and 92.7% of the highest to lowest dosage groups had achieved amenorrhea.

Transdermal testosterone (Answer C) would be considered if the patient had a fear of needles or self-injection or developed polycythemia. Although future fertility might decrease after testosterone therapy, the patient can be counseled that there are reports of successful pregnancies in transgender men, with return of menses within 6 months off testosterone and successful oocyte collection and in vitro maturation after gender-affirming surgery (even after at least 1 year of testosterone therapy).

Before initiation of gender-affirming hormone therapy, it is important to review fertility preservation options, as such therapy that can decrease future fertility. Surveys demonstrate that most patients think that fertility preservation should be offered to them, but only a minority consider options before gender-affirming hormone or surgical therapy. For transgender men, fertility preservation options include oocyte cryopreservation, embryo cryopreservation, or ovarian tissue cryopreservation. In the future, the oocytes or embryos can either be transferred to the patient's uterus or that of a female partner or gestational carrier. Controlled ovarian stimulation is required for both oocyte and embryo cryopreservation with transvaginal ultrasonography monitoring, which can trigger dysphoria in many patients. This patient has demonstrated suicidality provoked by menses, so he is less likely to tolerate ovarian stimulation. Therefore, embryo cryopreservation (Answer A) would not be recommended for this patient even though it is the best method to ensure future fertility. The stimulation, retrieval, and cryopreservation expenses would also be associated with significant cost to the patient.

Ovarian tissue cryopreservation (Answer B) is still experimental in United States and is associated with high cost, so it is not the best next step given this patient's financial concerns. Live births have been reported in cisgender women after ovarian tissue autotransplant. While ovarian tissue autotransplant might not be desirable for this patient due to the need to stop testosterone treatment for optimal in vivo follicular development, in vitro maturation of immature oocytes from the cryopreserved ovarian tissue might be possible. At this time, the patient can be counseled that in the future, at the time of gender-affirming hysterectomy, ovarian tissue cryopreservation could be performed with less cost. The cryopreserved ovarian tissue could possibly be used for in vitro maturation of oocytes in conjunction with in vitro fertilization with his fiancé's sperm and a gestational carrier.

Given the significant dysphoria this patient is experiencing, gender-affirming hormone therapy should not be delayed for the possibility of ovarian tissue cryopreservation. While GnRH agonist therapy (Answer E) is used in transgender and gender-diverse adolescents to delay pubertal secondary sex characteristics until age 16 years when gender-affirming hormone therapy would be considered, it is not standard of care in adults unless there is difficulty suppressing testosterone in transgender women or there are contraindications to testosterone therapy.

Educational Objective
Counsel a transgender man on fertility preservation options.

Reference(s)

Ainsworth AJ, Allyse M, Khan Z. Fertility preservation for transgender inidividuals: a review. *Mayo Clin Proc.* 2020;95(4):784-792. PMID: 32115195

Center of Excellence for Transgender Health, Department of Family and Community Medicine, University of California San Francisco. Guidelines for the Primary and Gender-Affirming Care of Transgender and Gender Nonbinary People. 2nd edition. Deutsch MB, ed. June 2016. www.transhealth.ucsf.edu/guidelines. Accessed for verification January 2020.

Hembree WC, Cohen-Kettenis PT, et al. Endocrine treatment of gender-dysphoric/gender-incongruent persons: an Endocrine Society clinical practice guideline. *J Clin Endocrinol Metab.* 2017;102(11):3869-3903. PMID: 28945902

Nakamura A, Watanabe M, Sugimoto M, et al. Dose-response analysis of testosterone replacement therapy in patients with female to male gender identity disorder. *Endocr J.* 2013;60(3):275-281. PMID: 23117148

Pelusi C, Constantino A, Martelli V, et al. Effects of three testosterone formulations in female-to-male transsexual persons. *J Sex Med.* 2014;11(12):3002-3011. PMID: 25250780

36

ANSWER: C) Repeat laboratory tests and neck imaging in 1 year

Primary hyperparathyroidism affects 0.1% to 0.3% of the population and is due to a benign parathyroid adenoma in 80% to 85% of cases. Parathyroid carcinoma and atypical parathyroid adenomas (APAs) are exceptionally rare causes of primary hyperparathyroidism (<1%). These typically present with marked hypercalcemia, very high PTH levels, and a neck mass. APAs represent a group of parathyroid neoplasms of uncertain malignant potential that show some atypical histologic features such as fibrous bands and cellular atypia but lack evidence of local invasion and/or distant metastasis seen in parathyroid carcinoma. There are no specific genetic tests or immunostains that can distinguish the two. Most cases of parathyroid carcinoma are due to pathogenic variants in the *CDC73* gene, but APAs can also be associated with the same pathogenic variants. Both APAs and parathyroid carcinoma can express immunohistochemical markers such as p27, bcl2, Ki-67, and parafibromin.

This patient was diagnosed with APA given there was no invasion of adjacent tissue, vasculature, lymphatics, or nerves on pathology, which is the only criterion that can definitively indicate parathyroid carcinoma over APA. Hence, referral for radiotherapy (Answer D) or chemotherapy (Answer E) is not indicated. Nonsurgical therapies have had disappointing results, even for patients with parathyroid carcinoma, and surgery is the mainstay of therapy for both the initial treatment and for the treatment of locally recurrent or metastatic disease in cases of parathyroid malignancy.

Further imaging with sestamibi scintigraphy (Answer A) or whole-body PET-CT (Answer B) is also not indicated at this time given that this patient's hypercalcemia has resolved and there is no evidence of residual disease on subsequent neck CT, consistent with a cure of his primary hyperparathyroidism.

There are no clear guidelines for long-term APA surveillance or management. APAs usually have a benign course and low recurrence risk. However, there is loss of similar gene loci in APAs and parathyroid carcinoma, which suggests that the molecular pathogenesis may be similar. Since definitive differentiation between APA and parathyroid carcinoma can only be based on findings of local invasion or distant metastasis, long-term surveillance of patients with APA is prudent. Therefore, repeating laboratory tests and neck imaging in 1 year (Answer C) is the best next step in this patient's management.

Educational Objective

Identify the clinical features of an atypical parathyroid adenoma in a patient with primary hyperparathyroidism and recommend the most appropriate intervention.

Reference(s)

Silva-Figueroa AM, Bassett R Jr, Christakis I, et al. Using a novel diagnostic nomogram to differentiate malignant from benign parathyroid neoplasms. *Endocr Pathol.* 2019;30(4):285-296. PMID: 31734935

Cetani F, Marcocci C, Torregrossa L, Pardi E. Atypical parathyroid adenomas: challenging lesions in the differential diagnosis of endocrine tumors. *Endocr Relat Cancer.* 2019;26(7):R441-R464. PMID: 31085770

Christakis I, Bussaidy N, Clarke C, et al. Differentiating atypical parathyroid neoplasm from parathyroid cancer. *Ann Surg Oncol.* 2016;23(9):2889-2897. PMID: 27160525

McCoy K, Seethala RR, Armstrong MJ, et al. The clinical importance of parathyroid atypia: is long-term surveillance necessary? Surgery. 2015;158(4):929-936. PMID: 26210223

Kim SS, Jeon YK, Lee SH, et al. Distant subcutaneous recurrence of a parathyroid carcinoma: abnormal uptakes in the (99m)Tc-sestamibi scan and (18)F-FDG PET/CT imaging. *Korean J Intern Med.* 2014;29(3):383-387. PMID: 24851075

37

ANSWER: E) Stop current regimen and start premixed insulin (NPH/regular) twice daily

Glucocorticoid-induced hyperglycemia is a common problem, and in patients with diabetes, glycemic control can be particularly difficult. The pathophysiology of glucocorticoid-induced hyperglycemia is complex, but it is generally accepted to be characterized by increased hepatic glucose production, reduced glucose uptake by muscle and adipose tissue, and compromised pancreatic β-cell insulin production and secretion.

Typically, after a dose of prednisone or prednisolone, the hyperglycemic effect onsets in 4 hours, with a peak effect at about 8 hours and total duration of 12 to 16 hours. In patients without preexisting diabetes, fasting plasma glucose is often normal. However, patients with preexisting diabetes often develop fasting hyperglycemia.

The pharmacology of NPH insulin, with peak effect in 6 to 8 hours, seems to match the peak hyperglycemic effect of prednisone very well. Patients can be managed with once-daily or twice-daily NPH insulin, depending on whether fasting hyperglycemia is present. Another option is to use a basal-bolus regimen (eg, insulins glargine and aspart). Studies do not confirm whether one regimen is better than the other, except for one prospective trial of hospitalized patients, which found that adding NPH insulin to a basal-bolus regimen achieved better glycemic control at hospital day 3 than did a basal-bolus regimen alone. However, the insulin dose was 16% higher in the NPH + usual regimen group. Another retrospective study suggested that NPH-based regimens were associated with similar glycemic control to that of a basal-bolus regimen with a 20% lower total insulin dosage.

GLP-1 receptor agonists (Answer C) augment glucose-stimulated insulin release and therefore may be an attractive option for patients with postprandial hyperglycemia. One study showed intravenous exenatide was effective in controlling glucocorticoid-induced hyperglycemia. However, beyond case reports, substantial data suggesting that GLP-1 receptor agonists are superior to insulin-based regimens are lacking.

In a basal-bolus regimen, administering a rapid-acting insulin analogue every 4 hours and not missing any doses of bolus insulin is critical because of the relatively short duration of action of rapid-acting analogues. In this patient, who admits to difficulty taking multiple daily injections, basal-bolus regimens (Answers A, B, and D) are not likely to be successful. A twice-daily NPH/regular insulin-based regimen (Answer E) would better match his lifestyle without sacrificing glycemic control because of NPH's favorable pharmacologic profile. Institutions may have different protocols for managing steroid-induced hyperglycemia. Examples include regular insulin with meals only (for prandial hyperglycemia) + NPH at bedtime (for fasting hyperglycemia), NPH once or twice daily, or NPH/regular (70/30) once or twice daily. Factors such as patient convenience help to guide the choice.

Indeed, this patient initiated a regimen of NPH/regular insulin twice daily and experienced markedly improved glycemic control with the added advantage that insulin titration was straightforward, as his prednisone dosage was reduced. An important clinical point is that the evening dose of NPH/regular in such a scenario is often less than the morning dose if prednisone is dosed once daily in the mornings, as the hyperglycemic effect of steroids has worn off by the evening.

Finally, another consideration is that NPH and regular insulin are far less expensive than analogue insulins and can deliver comparable glycemic control at a fraction of the cost. In research studies, the main downside of NPH-based regimens as compared with analogue basal insulins is a modestly increased risk of nocturnal hypoglycemia with NPH. Recent real-world data suggest that rates of hypoglycemia-related emergency department visits or hospital admissions and glycemic control are not significantly different when comparing basal insulin analogues and NPH in a clinical practice setting. Appropriate choice of patients and provider education may help mitigate any risks associated with NPH.

Educational Objective
Recommend use of NPH/regular insulin in patients with glucocorticoid-induced diabetes and review data supporting its use.

Reference(s)
Radhakutty A, Burt M. Management of endocrine disease: critical review of the evidence underlying management of glucocorticoid-induced hyperglycaemia. *Eur J Endocrinol*. 2018;179(4):R207-R218. PMID: 30299889

Crowley MJ, Maciejewski ML. Revisiting NPH insulin for type 2 diabetes: is a step back the path forward? *JAMA*. 2018;320(1):38-39. PMID: 29936528

38   ANSWER: B) Genetic testing for a *PTEN* germline pathogenic variant

Cowden syndrome (also known as Cowden disease) is part of a spectrum of clinical disorders that have been associated with germline pathogenic variants in the *PTEN* gene. The *PTEN* gene is a negative regulator of the phosphoinositide 3-kinase (PI3K)-AKT and the mechanistic target of rapamycin (mTOR) signaling pathways—critical for cell proliferation, cell-cycle progression, and apoptosis. Loss of function of this gene contributes to oncogenesis, and somatic variants are frequently identified in various malignancies. Germline pathogenic variants in the *PTEN* gene have been described in a variety of rare syndromes with different clinical presentations that are collectively known as *PTEN* hamartoma tumor syndromes. *PTEN* hamartoma tumor syndromes are inherited in an autosomal dominant fashion, and affected individuals have an increased risk of both benign and malignant tumors. The main clinical phenotypes are Cowden syndrome and Bannayan-Riley-Ruvalcaba syndrome.

Patients with Cowden syndrome have typical clinical findings such as macrocephaly; trichilemmomas (typically in the nasolabial folds as in this patient); acrokeratosis (small plaquelike hyperkeratotic areas on hands and feet);

oral mucosal cobble-stoning; penile pigmentation (macular speckling); lipomas and vascular anomalies; fibromas; esophageal acanthosis glycans; intestinal hamartomatous polyposis (eg, ganglioneuromas); goiter or multinodular goiter; cerebellar gangliocytomas (Lhermitte-Duclos syndrome) and vascular malformations; benign breast disease (including fibrocystic breast disease, intraductal papillomas, and fibroadenomas); and uterine leiomyoma (fibroids). They also have an increased cancer risk, mainly for breast, uterine, and thyroid (follicular thyroid cancer more so than papillary thyroid cancer), and to a lesser degree kidney cancer, melanoma, and colon cancer. Bannayan-Riley-Ruvalcaba syndrome is a more severe childhood-onset phenotype that includes autism spectrum disorder and delayed neuropsychomotor development.

There are at least 2 proposed diagnostic or operational criteria: the International Cowden Consortium diagnostic criteria from 1996 (updated in 2000) and the diagnostic criteria published by Pilarski et al in 2013. The latter contains major criteria and minor criteria (*see Box*).

Major criteria	Minor criteria
• Breast cancer	• Autism spectrum disorder
• Endometrial cancer	• Colon cancer
• Follicular thyroid cancer	• Esophageal glycogenic acanthosis
• Gastrointestinal hamartomas	• Lipomas (≥3)
• Lhermitte-Duclos disease (adult)	• Mental delay
• Macrocephaly (≥97th percentile: ≥22.8 in [≥58 cm] for women and ≥23.5 in [≥60 cm] for men)	• Renal cell carcinoma
• Macular pigmentation of the glans penis	• Testicular lipomatosis
• Multiple mucocutaneous lesions (≥3): trichilemmomas, acral keratoses, mucocutaneous neuromas, and oral papillomas	• Papillary thyroid cancer or follicular variant of papillary thyroid cancer
	• Benign thyroid disease
	• Vascular anomalies (intracranial venous anomalies)

Per Pilarski et al, 3 or more major criteria (1 must be macrocephaly, Lhermitte-Duclos disease, or gastrointestinal hamartomas) or 2 major criteria and 3 minor criteria are needed for clinical diagnosis of Cowden syndrome in an individual. However, despite the efforts to formulate a clinical diagnosis definition, criteria are sensitive, but not specific, and genetic testing is needed to confirm the diagnosis.

The National Comprehensive Cancer Network (NCCN) provides updated guidelines related to cancer surveillance programs for both men and women with Cowden syndrome. In addition to genetic counseling and education regarding this syndrome, recommendations related to cancer screening have been established. Due to the increased cancer risk, women with *PTEN* hamartoma tumor syndromes should have screening for breast cancer and endometrial cancer. For both men and women, screening for thyroid cancer, colon cancer, melanoma, and kidney cancer is recommended. Annual thyroid ultrasonography should be started at the time that a *PTEN* pathogenic variant is identified.

The patient in this vignette has a history of hamartomatous polyposis, lipomas, follicular thyroid cancer, and skin-colored papules with slightly rough surfaces in the nasolabial folds. These findings are consistent with Cowden syndrome, and genetic testing for a *PTEN* germline pathogenic variant (Answer B) should be recommended. He also has macrocephaly, but this finding was not provided in the vignette's stem. This condition is not associated with the *BRAF* V600 variant (Answer A). The *BRAF* V600E variant accounts for 60% of pathogenic variants in papillary thyroid cancer. He has a history of follicular thyroid cancer, and his thyroglobulin antibodies have significantly decreased compared with their level before radioiodine treatment. Therefore, neck CT (Answer D) is not the best option at this time. Once the diagnosis of Cowden syndrome is confirmed, he should have kidney ultrasonography (Answer C), but not yet. Thyroid ultrasonography for the patient's son (Answer E) is premature. If the patient has a *PTEN* pathogenic variant and additional testing confirms that his son has inherited the variant, thyroid ultrasonography in his son should be performed at the time of diagnosis and thereafter depending on initial findings.

Educational Objective

Diagnose Cowden syndrome.

Reference(s)

Pilarski R. Cowden syndrome: a critical review of the clinical literature. *J Genet Counsel.* 2009;18:13-27. PMID: 18972196

Pilarski R, Burt R, Kohlman E, Pho L, Shannon KM, Swisher E. Cowden syndrome and the PTEN hamartoma tumor syndrome: systematic review and revised diagnostic criteria. *J Natl Cancer Inst.* 2013;105(21):1607-1616. PMID: 24136893

39   ANSWER: B) Start lisinopril

Maturity-onset diabetes of the young (MODY) is the most common form of monogenic diabetes and may account for 2% to 5% of all diabetes cases. MODY is a heterogeneous disorder, and pathogenic variants in at least 13 different genes have been characterized. The phenotype is typified by diagnosis of diabetes at an early age (usually <25 years), intact C-peptide levels, and a lack of autoimmune diabetes antibodies. MODY has an autosomal dominant inheritance pattern. Patients with MODY are usually normal weight or overweight and are often misdiagnosed as having either type 1 or type 2 diabetes.

Pathogenic variants in the *HNF1A* gene and the *GCK* gene account for the most common subtypes of MODY and represent up to 65% of cases depending on the country and the patient's ethnicity.

Pathogenic variants in the *HNF1A* gene, associated with MODY type 3, lead to impaired insulin secretion and a low renal threshold for glucose. Patients with *HNF1A*-related diabetes have enhanced insulin sensitivity and often respond well to sulfonylurea treatment initially. However, there is progression of the secretory defect in many patients, and treatment with insulin is often required. Patients with an *HNF1A* pathogenic variant are at risk for developing microvascular and macrovascular complications, similar to patients with type 1 or type 2 diabetes.

The patient in this vignette has MODY type 3 and has had reasonable glycemic control on basal-bolus insulin analogue treatment. She has developed microalbuminuria. If left untreated, this could progress to overt diabetic nephropathy. Standard treatment of microalbuminuria in patients with diabetes consists of maintaining good glycemic and blood pressure control and use of ACE inhibitors or angiotensin-receptor blockers. The best treatment option for this patient is to start lisinopril (Answer B). As she has normal blood pressure, a low starting dosage of 2.5 or 5 mg daily would be warranted.

This patient has had good glucose control in general, and intensifying insulin therapy (Answer D) would be unlikely to lower her albumin excretion. Monitoring only (Answer A) is incorrect as most patients with MODY, other than those with *GCK* pathogenic variants, can develop microvascular complications and should be treated accordingly. Patients with *GCK* pathogenic variants (MODY 2) have an elevated set point for insulin secretion by the β cell. These patients have lifelong, mild hyperglycemia that is stable over time and does not require antihyperglycemic treatment except in unusual circumstances. These patients rarely if ever develop microvascular complications.

Canagliflozin (Answer C) was shown to significantly reduce the risk of a composite of development of end-stage renal disease (or sustained estimated glomerular filtration rate <15 mL/min per 1.73 m^2), doubling of creatinine, or death of renal or cardiovascular causes in the CREDENCE trial, a double-blind, randomized controlled trial of patients with type 2 diabetes and albuminuric renal disease (hazard ratio, 0.70; 95% CI, 0.59-0.82; $P = .00001$). However, use of canagliflozin and SGLT-2 inhibitors should be considered a second-line treatment option in patients with diabetes and albuminuria. There are no data on the treatment of albuminuria with SGLT-2 inhibitors in patients with MODY.

For patients with non–dialysis-dependent diabetic kidney disease, protein intake should be approximately 0.8 g/kg body weight per day. Further restriction of dietary protein intake (Answer E) has not been shown to alter the decline in renal function, improve glycemic control, or lower cardiovascular risk.

Educational Objective

Assess for microvascular complications in patients with monogenic diabetes and appropriately treat microalbuminuria.

Reference(s)

American Diabetes Association. 11. Microvascular complications and foot care: standards of medical care in diabetes-2019. *Diabetes Care.* 2019;42(Suppl 1):S124-S138. PMID: 30559237

Perkovic V, Jardine MJ, Neal B, et al. Canagliflozin and renal outcomes in type 2 diabetes mellitus and nephropathy. *N Engl J Med.* 2019;380(24):2295-2306. PMID: 30990260

Bellane-Chantelot C, Levy DJ, Carette C, et al; French Monogenic Diabetes Study Group. Clinical characteristics and diagnostic criteria of maturity-onset diabetes of the young (MODY) due to molecular anomalies of the HNF1A gene. *J Clin Endocrinol Metab.* 2011;96(8):E1346-E1351. PMID: 21677039

McDonald TJ, Colclough K, Brown R, et al. Islet autoantibodies can discriminate maturity-onset diabetes of the young (MODY) from type 1 diabetes. *Diabet Med.* 2011;28(9):1028-1033. PMID: 21395678

40 ANSWER: B) Naltrexone/bupropion

Pharmacotherapy for obesity should be considered for patients with a BMI of 27 kg/m² or greater who have comorbidities or for patients with a BMI greater than 30 kg/m² who, despite lifestyle modifications, continue to struggle to lose weight. One of the factors to consider when deciding which medication is best for a given patient is the patient's eating behavior.

Eating behavior in obese individuals is associated with overconsumption, and it is related to a reduced satiety response, higher reward with palatable foods, and disinhibited eating. Restricting calories in this setting increases the responsivity to food cues and cravings.

Naltrexone/bupropion extended-release (Answer B) is a combination pill with an opioid antagonist and a reuptake inhibitor of dopamine and norepinephrine. Bupropion stimulates proopiomelanocortin neurons that release α-melanocyte–stimulating hormone, which binds to melanocortin-4 receptors and induces satiety. Naltrexone blocks mu-opioid receptors, which blocks the binding of β-endorphins. β-Endorphins are responsible for providing inhibitory feedback and limiting the release of α-melanocyte–stimulating hormone. The Contrave Obesity Research trials I and II showed that the combination of naltrexone/bupropion increased patients' ability to resist and reduce food cravings. Given that this patient's main struggle is cravings, naltrexone/bupropion extended-release would be an ideal first choice.

Liraglutide (Answer A) is a long-acting GLP-1 receptor agonist approved for long-term weight loss. This medication decreases food intake by slowing gastric emptying and by activating hypothalamic and extrahypothalamic nuclei in the brain. Liraglutide has been shown to increase postmeal satiety and fullness ratings; however, it has no effect on control of cravings.

Metformin (Answer C) is first-line therapy for patients with type 2 diabetes. Metformin does not cause weight gain and could lead to modest weight loss (<5%); however, there are no published data describing its effects on cravings, which is this patient's main problem.

Phentermine/topiramate extended-release (Answer D) reduces appetite by increasing norepinephrine in the hypothalamus (phentermine) and through its action on GABA receptors (topiramate). There are no data on how this combination affects cravings.

Orlistat (Answer E) is an intestinal lipase inhibitor, and its use leads to fat malabsorption, which contributes to weight loss. Orlistat is not a centrally acting drug, and it has no known direct behavioral effects related to satiety or impulse control.

A figure describing the mechanism of action of weight-loss medications can be found in Apovian CM, Aronne LJ, Bessesen DH, et al; Endocrine Society. Pharmacological management of obesity: an Endocrine Society clinical practice guideline. *J Clin Endocrinol Metab.* 2015;100(2):342-362.

Educational Objective

Prescribe an appropriate weight-loss medication, bearing in mind the patient's eating behavior.

Reference(s)

Roberts CA, Christiansen P, Halford JCG. Tailoring pharmacotherapy to specific eating behaviours in obesity: can recommendations for personalised therapy be made from the current data? *Acta Diabetol.* 2017;54(8):715-725. PMID: 28421338

Apovian CM, Aronne LJ, Bessesen DH, et al; Endocrine Society. Pharmacological management of obesity: an Endocrine Society clinical practice guideline. *J Clin Endocrinol Metab.* 2015;100(2):342-362. PMID: 25590212

Apovian CM, Aronne L, Rubino D, et al; COR-II Study Group. A randomized, phase 3 trial of naltrexone SR/bupropion SR on weight and obesity-related risk factors (COR-II). *Obesity (Silver Spring).* 2013;21(5):935-943. PMID: 23408728

Greenway FL, Fujioka K, Plodkowski RA, et al; COR-I Study Group. Effect of naltrexone plus bupropion on weight loss in overweight and obese adults (COR-I): a multicentre, randomised, double-blind, placebo-controlled, phase 3 trial. *Lancet.* 2010;376(9741):595-605. PMID: 20673995

Martin CK, Redman LM, Zhang J, et al. Lorcaserin, a 5-HT(2C) receptor agonist, reduces body weight by decreasing energy intake without influencing energy expenditure. *J Clin Endocrinol Metab.* 2011;96(3):837-845. PMID: 21190985

41 ANSWER: A) Anticonvulsant drug therapy

This patient has a known diagnosis of primary hypothyroidism and is receiving long-term oral levothyroxine therapy. He was recently diagnosed with focal (partial) seizures and initiated treatment with carbamazepine. Anticonvulsant drug therapy (Answer A) with carbamazepine has been shown to increase the levothyroxine dosage requirement of patients with hypothyroidism. It is thus recommended that serum TSH be measured following initiation of this medication.

The metabolism of T_4 and T_3 is primarily through sequential deiodination; however, hepatic glucuronidation and sulfation pathways also contribute. Carbamazepine, phenytoin, and phenobarbital are all anticonvulsant drugs that have been shown to induce glucuronidation enzymes. Patients with hypothyroidism who were previously euthyroid on medical therapy may be unable to compensate for the increased metabolism of T_4 and T_3 that results from the initiation of anticonvulsant drugs, resulting in hypothyroidism. An increase in the levothyroxine dosage can restore a euthyroid state.

Carbamazepine use has also been associated with abnormal thyroid function in persons without hypothyroidism. When administrated to patients without thyroid disease, carbamazepine can be associated with low serum total T_4 and free T_4 concentrations, but TSH and (usually) T_3 levels remain normal. Low serum T_4 results from drug-induced displacement of thyroid hormone from its binding proteins, particularly thyroxine-binding globulin, transiently increasing free T_4 and suppressing TSH until a new steady-state is reached. Contrary to the drug-induced changes in physiology, measured levels of free T_4 may be artifactually reduced, mimicking central hypothyroidism. When evaluating for thyroid dysfunction in patients taking carbamazepine, it is generally advisable to check only serum TSH unless there is clinical concern for central hypothyroidism.

This patient has a known diagnosis of celiac disease (Answer B). This autoimmune inflammatory disorder of the small intestine occurs in 2% to 5% of patients with autoimmune thyroid disease and is managed primarily with a gluten-free diet. Although an investigation for occult celiac disease should be considered in patients with autoimmune hypothyroidism who require escalating dosages of levothyroxine, there is no indication that the patient described here is nonadherent to the recommended diet. Similarly, there is no reason to suspect nonadherence to levothyroxine therapy (Answer C). His serum TSH concentration was previously normal on the prescribed dosage, and his carbamazepine level is therapeutic, thus supporting his adherence to medical therapy in general.

Nonthyroidal illness syndrome (Answer D) is not the most likely explanation for the patient's abnormal thyroid function test results. In the setting of nonthyroidal illness, serum T_3 is decreased due to a reduction in 5'-monodeiodinase activity, and T_4 and free T_4 are normal or low. Serum TSH is normal or mildly decreased during the initial phase of a nonthyroidal illness, but it may be mildly elevated during recovery. The patient described here was diagnosed with epilepsy 3 months ago and there is no description a severe intercurrent medical illness.

Weight gain (Answer E) can lead to an increase in levothyroxine dosage requirements; however, a 5-lb (2.3-kg) increase in body weight should have little to no impact on serum TSH. In general, a 10% change in body weight is necessary to affect serum TSH and levothyroxine dosing.

Educational Objective
Describe the effect of certain anticonvulsant drugs (phenobarbital, phenytoin, and carbamazepine) on thyroid hormone metabolism and the consequences for hypothyroidism treatment.

Reference(s)

Burch HB. Drug effects on the thyroid. *N Engl J Med.* 2019;381(8):749-761. PMID: 31433922

Jonklaas J, Bianco AC, Bauer AJ, et al; American Thyroid Association Task Force on Thyroid Hormone Replacement. Guidelines for the treatment of hypothyroidism: prepared by the american thyroid association task force on thyroid hormone replacement. *Thyroid.* 2014;24(12):1670-1751. PMID: 25266247

Surks MI, DeFesi CR. Normal serum free thyroid hormone concentrations in patients treated with phenytoin or carbamazepine: a paradox resolved. *JAMA.* 1996;275(19):1495-1498. PMID: 8622224

42 ANSWER: B) *SDHB* (succinate dehydrogenase subunit B)

This patient had episodic hyperadrenergic symptoms, marked elevations in normetanephrine, and a large adrenal mass that was not lipid rich. Collectively, this confirms the diagnosis of a pheochromocytoma. At least one-third of all pheochromocytomas and paragangliomas are attributed to a known germline (inherited) pathogenic variant. For this reason, it is recommended that all patients with one of these tumors be offered genetic testing. More than a dozen genes that cause inherited pheochromocytoma-paraganglioma syndromes have thus far been identified. In most of these cases, harboring a pathogenic variant not only predisposes the individual to developing pheochromocytoma and/or paraganglioma, but potentially other tumors that may be benign or malignant. In this regard, identifying a pathogenic variant prompts surveillance for tumor syndromes in the patient and also allows for testing of at-risk family members.

This patient's family history of metastatic gastrointestinal stromal tumor should raise concern for a pathogenic variant in one of the succinate dehydrogenase genes (subunits A, B, C, D, or AF2). Pathogenic variants in the *SDHx* genes can predispose an individual to a lifetime risk of developing pheochromocytoma, paraganglioma, renal cell carcinoma, and gastrointestinal stromal tumors. Thus, *SDHB* (Answer B) is the most likely culprit gene in this case.

Pathogenic variants in the *VHL* gene (Answer E) are also common in persons with pheochromocytoma. Individuals with *VHL* pathogenic variants can develop von Hippel–Lindau syndrome, and they have a lifetime risk of developing pheochromocytoma, paraganglioma, renal cell carcinoma, cerebellar hemangioblastomas, neuroendocrine tumors, retinal angiomas, and more.

Pathogenic variants in the *RET* gene (Answer C) cause multiple endocrine neoplasia type 2 in which the hallmark features are medullary thyroid carcinoma and pheochromocytoma. Patients with multiple endocrine neoplasia type 2A can also develop primary hyperparathyroidism, whereas patients with type 2B develop mucosal neuromas, a marfanoid habitus, and intestinal ganglioneuromas.

VHL and *RET* pathogenic variants have reasonably good genotype-phenotype correlations. Knowledge of the specific variant can often allow prediction of the potential phenotype and thus inform how and when to survey patients with imaging and other modalities. In contrast, there is very poor genotype-phenotype correlation with *SDHB* variants (and variants in other *SDHx* genes). Therefore, patients with *SDHx* variants are currently monitored with standardized imaging every 2 to 5 years. For example, patients with *SDHB* variants may be followed with MRI (to avoid radiation) to cover areas from the base of the skull to the pelvis every 2 to 3 years. Evolving research will most likely lead to revision of these surveillance modalities and their recommended frequency.

Pathogenic variants in *TMEM127* (Answer D) and *EPAS1* (Answer A) are very rare causes of pheochromocytoma. Other potential tumors that may be associated with *TMEM127* are not well defined. Pathogenic variants in *EPAS1* may also predispose to paraganglioma and somatostatinomas.

None of the genes listed in the answer choices is known to increase the risk for breast cancer.

Educational Objective

Differentiate among the genes associated with pheochromocytoma and paraganglioma.

Reference(s)

Lenders JW, Duh QY, Eisenhofer G, et al; Endocrine Society. Pheochromocytoma and paraganglioma: an Endocrine Society clinical practice guideline. *J Clin Endocrinol Metab.* 2014;99(6):1915-1942. PMID: 24893135

Neumann HPH, Young WF Jr, Eng C. Pheochromocytoma and paraganglioma. *N Engl J Med.* 2019;381(6);552-565. PMID: 31390501

43

ANSWER: B) Initiate prednisone

This patient has Riedel thyroiditis, a rare form of thyroiditis that is defined by a fibrotic process accompanied by monocellular cell inflammation that extends beyond the thyroid into perithyroidal soft tissue. This is in contrast to other types of inflammatory or infiltrative diseases that do not extend beyond the thyroid capsule. Therefore, the infiltration and inflammation can involve the recurrent laryngeal nerves, parathyroid glands, trachea, esophagus, and other structures close to the thyroid gland. Women in their 30s, 40s, and 50s are more frequently affected. The etiology of Riedel thyroiditis remains unknown. An association between Reidel thyroiditis and autoimmunity has been observed. Riedel thyroiditis can occur in association with Hashimoto thyroiditis and also Graves disease. In addition, it may occur as part of immunoglobulin G4 (IgG4)–related systemic disease, including multifocal systemic sclerosis, retroperitoneal fibrosis, IgG4-related hypophysitis and idiopathic autoimmune pancreatitis.

Patients with Riedel thyroiditis can be asymptomatic, but more often they experience dysphagia, dysphonia, neck pressure, shortness of breath, or hypoparathyroidism. In this setting, thyroid function tests are usually consistent with hypothyroidism, but affected patients can also have normal serum TSH levels. Thyroid ultrasonography demonstrates a diffuse, hypoechoic, hypovascular appearance of the thyroid gland due to extensive fibrosis. In the workup of a thyroid nodule, FNA biopsy is often nondiagnostic, and patients require a core biopsy to confirm the diagnosis. Histologic sections from lesions early in the disease demonstrate intense infiltration of lymphocytes, plasma cells, neutrophils, and eosinophils. Later in the disease process, specimens show infiltration of the thyroid with dense, hyalinized fibrous tissue that contains few lymphocytes, plasma cells, and eosinophils and almost no thyroid follicles. The evidence of storiform fibrosis, presence of obliterative phlebitis, and an IgG4-to-IgG ratio greater than 40% are suggestive of IgG4-related disease. The tissue planes are obliterated, and therefore surgical intervention is usually difficult. Elevation of serum IgG4 can also be seen in patients with IgG4-related disease. However, only about 50% of patients with IgG4-related disease have elevated serum IgG4.

The treatment of Riedel thyroiditis includes managing hypothyroidism if present and decreasing the size of the goiter. Glucocorticoids are the first-line therapy (usually 40 mg daily but higher dosages have been prescribed), and steroid treatment is typically long-term. Recurrence can be seen when steroid dosages are tapered. Tamoxifen is second-line therapy. In some cases, both glucocorticoids and tamoxifen have been used. Rituximab and mycophenolate mofetil have been used in patients with Riedel thyroiditis and systemic fibrosclerosis (IgG4-related disease). Surgery is indicated to relieve tracheal or esophageal compression. The operation should be limited to relieving the obstruction, usually by excising a wedge of thyroid isthmus to relieve tracheal compression. Extensive resection such as total thyroidectomy is not routinely indicated because of the lack of resection planes and risk of injury to adjacent adhering structures, including the parathyroid glands and recurrent laryngeal nerves. Finally, low-dosage radiation therapy has been used in cases refractory to other treatments.

The patient in this vignette has Riedel thyroiditis and should be started on prednisone (Answer B). Total thyroidectomy (Answer A) or isthmusectomy with left lobectomy (Answer D) are not usually pursued due to lack of resection planes and risk of injury to nearby structures. As previously mentioned, isthmusectomy can be performed to relieve compressive symptoms when medical therapy has not been effective. Tamoxifen (Answer C) is usually the second-line agent when prednisone is ineffective, and dosages of 10 to 20 mg twice daily have been used. Before initiating tamoxifen, the patient should be informed of possible adverse effects, including hot flashes, night sweats, increased risk of blood clots, and mood changes. Increasing the levothyroxine dosage (Answer E) would not have an effect on the natural history of Riedel thyroiditis and is not needed given the patient's TSH level.

Educational Objective
Diagnose and manage Riedel thyroiditis.

Reference(s)
Fatourechi MM, Hay ID, McIver B, Sebo TJ, Fatourechi V. Invasive fibrous thyroiditis (Riedel thyroiditis): the Mayo Clinic experience, 1976-2008. *Thyroid.* 2011;21(7):765-772. PMID: 21568724

Deshpande V. IgG4 related disease of the head and neck. *Head Neck Pathol.* 2015;9(1):24-31. PMID: 25804380

44 **ANSWER: D) Treatment-induced neuropathy of diabetes**

In this patient, a vascular cause (Answer A) for the pain is unlikely, as pedal pulses are easily palpable and ambulation does not appear to worsen the discomfort. Neuropathy is the most likely cause. Although distal sensory polyneuropathy is the most common finding in patients with diabetes, other syndromes exist and can overlap. Polyneuropathy (Answer B) often begins with progressive sensory loss that starts in distal extremities and moves proximally. It can be associated with loss of ankle reflexes and motor dysfunction. This patient might very well have longstanding diabetic polyneuropathy, but the recent rapid changes suggest a second superimposed process. Radiculopathy (Answer C) presents either in the lumbar or thoracic area, usually in a contiguous nerve root distribution. It can present with fairly acute pain, and motor weakness pain is usually proximal and unilateral although it can become bilateral. A form of lumbosacral radiculopathy or plexopathy called diabetic amyotrophy presenting with predominant proximal weakness and muscle wasting often occurs in older men and can improve after a few years. This patient's presentation does not fit this pattern.

Treatment-induced neuropathy of diabetes (Answer D), also known as insulin neuritis, is associated with rapid improvement of blood glucose values. Defined as acute onset of neuropathic pain or autonomic dysfunction within 8 weeks of improved glycemic control (hemoglobin A_{1c} reduction >2% within 3 months). It is a small-fiber neuropathy, thought to be due to endoneurial edema and ischemia. A drop of 2% to 3% in hemoglobin A_{1c} in 3 months is associated with a 20% risk of treatment-induced neuropathy. If hemoglobin A_{1c} drops more than 4% in this same timeframe, the risk of treatment-induced neuropathy is greater than 80%. This patient's hemoglobin A_{1c} has decreased from 11.0% to 8.5% in 3 months. The burning pain in her feet is acute in onset, and her symptoms correlate with improvements in glycemic control.

In patients with treatment-induced neuropathy of diabetes, Gibbons and Freeman describe presence of autonomic cardiovascular, gastrointestinal, and genitourinary symptoms and worsened retinopathy in all patients studied. Improvement in painful neuropathy was noted at about 18 months in patients with type 1 diabetes but not in patients with type 2 diabetes.

Diabetic neuropathic cachexia (Answer E) is a term used to describe a presentation in middle-aged or older men on oral hypoglycemic agents. There is severe unintentional weight loss and severe painful peripheral neuropathy. Weight loss in this middle-aged woman was intentional.

Educational Objective
Differentiate among various causes of painful neuropathy in a patient with diabetes mellitus.

Reference(s)
Pop-Busui R, Boulton AJ, Feldman EL, et al. Diabetic neuropathy: a position statement of the American Diabetes Association. *Diabetes Care.* 2017;40(1):136-154. PMID: 27999003

Gibbons CH, Freeman R. Treatment-induced diabetic neuropathy: a reversible painful autonomic neuropathy. *Ann Neurol.* 2010;67(4):534-541. PMID: 20437589

Gibbons CH, Freeman R. Treatment-induced neuropathy of diabetes: an acute, iatrogenic complication of diabetes. *Brain.* 2015;138(Pt 1):43-52. PMID: 25392197

45 **ANSWER: C) *AIP* (aryl hydrocarbon receptor interacting protein)**

This patient's family has clear features of familial isolated pituitary adenoma syndrome (FIPA). The patient has early-onset acromegaly and a large tumor, which is consistent with this syndrome. FIPA is an autosomal dominant disease that is caused by heterozygous germline pathogenic variants in the gene encoding the aryl hydrocarbon receptor interacting protein (*AIP*). *AIP* is probably a tumor suppressor gene. These pathogenic variants cause the development of an adenoma only when the function of the normal allele is lost ("second hit" in the Knudson hypothesis, also known as the 2-hit hypothesis, which stipulates that most genes require 2 pathogenic variants to cause a phenotypic change). Therefore, the disease penetrance is about 15% to 30%, meaning that only 15% to 30% of individuals who have the pathogenic variant will develop a pituitary adenoma in their lifetime. This explains why the patient's father (from whom she inherited the pathogenic variant) does not have evidence of a pituitary adenoma. Each of the patient's children has a 50% chance of having inherited the pathogenic variant. Due to the low disease penetrance, no agreement has been reached on whether AIP genetic testing is warranted in asymptomatic children of an affected parent. Patients with FIPA present with large tumors at an early age (<30 years). The tumors are most often GH secreting, followed by prolactinomas, nonsecreting tumors, ACTH-secreting adenomas, and thyrotropinomas. Different kinds of pituitary adenomas may be present in the same family. The tumors tend to be more aggressive than sporadic adenomas and less responsive to medication.

This family has no history of pancreatic or parathyroid tumors or hypercalcemia suggestive of multiple endocrine neoplasia type 1, so a pathogenic variant in the *MEN1* gene (Answer A) is unlikely (by age 50 years, almost all affected patients have hypercalcemia). *RET* pathogenic variants (Answer B) cause multiple endocrine neoplasia type 2A and 2B, and pituitary adenomas are not part of these syndromes. The *PRKAR1A* gene (Answer D) is associated with Carney complex. Although acromegaly is sometimes part of this syndrome, affected individuals also develop benign cardiac myxomas, skin schwannomas, and skin pigmentation abnormalities (multiple lentigines) and can also develop Cushing syndrome due to primary pigmented nodular hyperplasia. None of these features is present in this family. Pathogenic variants in the *GNAS* gene (Answer E) cause McCune-Albright syndrome. While acromegaly can be part of this syndrome, affected patients often have severe polyostotic fibrous dysplasia. Additionally, McCune-Albright syndrome is never inherited, as it is caused by a somatic (postzygotic) pathogenic variant in the *GNAS* gene that occurs very early in development.

Educational Objective
Describe the genetic causes of familial pituitary adenoma syndromes.

Reference(s)
Beckers A, Aaltonen LA, Daly AF, Karhu A. Familial isolated pituitary adenomas (FIPA) and the pituitary adenoma predisposition due to mutations in the aryl hydrocarbon receptor interacting protein (AIP) gene. *Endocr Rev*. 2013;34(2):239-277. PMID: 23371967

Marques P, Korbonits M. Genetic aspects of pituitary adenomas. *Endocrinol Metab Clin North Am*. 2017;46(2):335-374. PMID: 28476226

46 ANSWER: E) Recommend no change at this time

The patient in this vignette has progressive atherosclerotic cardiovascular disease and is at very high risk for recurrent cardiovascular events. He meets the criteria for further LDL-cholesterol lowering despite already having a low LDL-cholesterol concentration. In the 2018 American Heart Association/American College of Cardiology multisociety guidelines for cholesterol lowering, very high risk is defined by having a history of multiple major atherosclerotic cardiovascular disease events or 1 major event and multiple high-risk conditions. These guidelines recommend addition of a PCSK9 inhibitor in patients at very high risk whose LDL-cholesterol concentration remains at 70 mg/dL or higher (≥1.81 mmol/L) on maximally tolerated statin and ezetimibe therapy. However, there is evidence that in patients at very high risk, a lower LDL-cholesterol goal of less than 55 mg/dL (<1.42 mmol/L) is appropriate and this is recommended in other recent cardiovascular risk modification guidelines. PCSK9 inhibitor monoclonal antibodies such as evolocumab and alirocumab bind to the liver-derived PCSK9 serine protease and prevent LDL-receptor degradation, leading to more available LDL receptors and therefore lower LDL-cholesterol levels in the blood. When a PCSK9 inhibitor is added to high-intensity statin therapy, up to 100% of the PCSK9 is bound by the antibody, resulting in up to a 60% reduction in LDL cholesterol from baseline. A randomized controlled trial of evolocumab vs placebo added to the regimen of individuals with known atherosclerotic cardiovascular disease already receiving statin therapy showed a 15% reduction in cardiovascular events. In this patient's case, LDL-cholesterol levels dropped to the single digits.

Several issues must be considered in such situations. It is worth noting that the LDL cholesterol reported as part of a lipid panel is a calculated value using the Friedewald formula and is generally accurate in patients with serum triglyceride concentrations less than 150 mg/dL (<1.70 mmol/L) and LDL-cholesterol concentrations of at least 70 mg/dL (≥1.70 mmol/L). However, this formula underestimates LDL-cholesterol at concentrations less than 70 mg/dL (<1.70 mmol/L), and in this setting an alternative method of measurement should be done (such as the Martin-Hopkins equation now used by several commercial laboratories or a direct LDL-cholesterol measurement). Long-term effects of such low LDL-cholesterol levels are yet to be determined. There is an ongoing debate on ultra-low LDL-cholesterol levels and safety considerations. Some studies have reported increased incidence of adverse events such as hemorrhagic strokes, dementia, depression, hematuria, and cancers with extremely low LDL cholesterol. However, individuals who have loss-of-function pathogenic variants in the *PCSK9* gene have very low LDL-cholesterol concentrations (~15 mg/dL [0.39 mmol/L]) without any ill effects. The safety of such low LDL-cholesterol levels was first addressed in a post hoc analysis of 10 trials of alirocumab, which suggested that lower on-treatment LDL cholesterol (<50 mg/dL [<1.30 mmol/L]) was associated with lower incidence of major adverse cardiovascular outcomes. Subsequent evaluations of LDL-cholesterol concentrations less than 25 mg/dL (<0.65 mmol/L) and less than 15 mg/dL (<0.39 mmol/L) have not revealed adverse effects in the same study population. In an exploratory analysis of LDL-cholesterol levels attained 4 weeks after initiation of PCSK9 inhibitor therapy with evolocumab, there was a larger relative cardiovascular risk reduction in individuals who attained an LDL-cholesterol concentration less than 10 mg/dL (<0.26 mmol/L), with no significant differences in adverse effects. Such analyses seem to suggest that ultra-low levels of LDL cholesterol are safe and convey additional benefit.

Stopping evolocumab or the statin (Answers A and B) is incorrect, as this would result in increased LDL-cholesterol levels in this patient who is at very high risk. Decreasing the rosuvastatin dosage from 40 mg to 20 mg daily (which is still considered high-intensity statin therapy) would be reasonable, but it was not offered as an answer option. Fenofibrate is a peroxisome proliferator–activated receptor α agonist with triglyceride-lowering effects. Stopping fenofibrate (Answer C) would most likely result in increased triglycerides. PCSK9 inhibitors do not have any significant triglyceride-lowering capability. The fibrate should be continued for now and ongoing need should be reassessed at a later time. Semaglutide (Answer D) is a GLP-1 receptor agonist with cardiovascular benefit used in individuals for treatment of type 2 diabetes. This patient's hemoglobin A_{1c} level is currently optimal.

At this time, no change in the patient's treatment regimen is necessary (Answer E).

Educational Objective
Manage ultra-low LDL-cholesterol levels in a patient on PCSK9 inhibitor therapy.

Reference(s)

Bandyopadhyay D, Quereshi A, Ghosh S, et al. Safety and efficacy of extremely low LDL-cholesterol levels and its prospects in hyperlipidemia management. *J Lipids*. 2018;8598054. PMID: 29850255

Olsson AG, Angelin B, Assmann G, et al. Can LDL cholesterol be too low? Possible risks of extremely low levels. *J Intern Med*. 2017;281(6):534-553. PMID: 28295777

Giugliano RP, Pedersen TR, Park JG, et al; FOURIER Investigators. Clinical efficacy and safety of achieving very low LDL-cholesterol concentrations with the PCSK9 inhibitor evolocumab: a prespecified secondary analysis of the FOURIER trial. *Lancet*. 2017;390(10106):1962-1971. PMID: 28859947

Qamar A, Libby P. Low-density lipoprotein cholesterol after an acute coronary syndrome: how low to go. *Curr Cardiol Rep*. 2019;21(8):77. PMID: 31250329

47 ANSWER: D) Perform neck ultrasonography

Hypercalcemia is a common indication for referral for endocrine consultation. Elevated blood calcium is often present for many years based on retrospective review. Hypercalcemia in outpatients is often due to primary hyperparathyroidism, the most common presentation of which is minimal to no symptoms. When symptomatic, the most frequent symptoms voiced by patients include fatigue, polyuria, polydipsia, cognitive impairment, and bone pain. This patient, however, was previously healthy and presents with a 6-month history of fatigue and polyuria. In addition, he has a palpable neck mass on physical examination and evidence of more pronounced hypercalcemia. This constellation of clinical signs and symptoms should prompt consideration of parathyroid carcinoma. Although parathyroid carcinoma is rare and occurs in only 1% to 2% of patients with hypercalcemia and hyperparathyroidism, preoperative identification and aggressive surgical resection are critical to optimal management given the poor prognosis (<50% 10-year survival).

Parathyroid carcinoma is more common in patients with hereditary hyperparathyroidism, such as multiple endocrine neoplasia type 1, multiple endocrine neoplasia type 2, and *CDC73* pathogenic variants (the latter of which is associated with nonossifying fibromas of the jaw). In the absence of a family history to support a genetic abnormality, additional factors are needed to precipitate consideration of parathyroid carcinoma. Fortunately, specific clinical information can assist in this process. Specifically, the "<3 + <3" rule, based on the fact that 80% to 85% of parathyroid carcinomas present with lesions larger than 3 cm and a serum calcium concentration greater than 3.0 mmol/L (>12 mg/dL), provides a positive predictive value of 99.8% to rule out the presence of parathyroid carcinoma if both criteria are met (ie, size <3.0 cm in maximal diameter and serum calcium adjusted for albumin <12.0 g/dL). In this patient, therefore, accurate determination of tumor size with neck ultrasonography (Answer D) is critical. Although this rule is most useful for excluding the presence of parathyroid carcinoma, only approximately 5% of patients who exceed this rule have malignancy. Nonetheless, given the markedly poor prognosis with incomplete resection of parathyroid carcinoma, application of a more aggressive surgical approach (ie, en bloc resection with ipsilateral hemithyroidectomy and centrocervical lymphadenectomy) is recommended. Referral for minimally invasive parathyroidectomy (Answer A) without extensive surgical resection is not appropriate for this patient. Cinacalcet (Answer C), which is FDA approved for parathyroid carcinoma, may be indicated for this patient if he develops persistent or recurrent disease. However, cinacalcet is not indicated now.

He does have coexisting vitamin D deficiency, which could be contributing to PTH elevation as well. In addition, there is a theoretical risk for postparathyroidectomy hypocalcemia if vitamin D levels are not restored, although this has not been definitively confirmed in studies to date. However, cholecalciferol (Answer B) is not the best next step in this patient's management based on his clinical presentation.

Finally, although renal ultrasonography (Answer E) could be indicated in the preoperative assessment for nephrolithiasis in patients with asymptomatic hyperparathyroidism to determine their candidacy for parathyroidectomy based on current guidelines, such an assessment would not assist in the management of this patient who has already been deemed a surgical candidate.

Educational Objective
Identify risk factors and explain the most prudent clinical approach in a patient with hypercalcemia due to parathyroid carcinoma.

Reference(s)
Schulte KM, Talat N. Diagnosis and management of parathyroid cancer. *Nat Rev Endocrinol.* 2012;8(10):612-622. PMID: 22751344

48 **ANSWER: A) SHBG measurement and free testosterone estimation**
This man had a testosterone concentration drawn without a valid clinical indication. In line with recommendations of the Endocrine Society, testosterone concentrations should be measured to confirm a clinical suspicion of androgen deficiency, which is lacking in this man. Moreover while total testosterone using an accurate and reliable assay is recommended as the initial diagnostic test, the sample should be drawn in the morning in the fasted state. Due to circadian rhythmicity, afternoon testosterone concentrations can be more than 30% lower than morning values, and food intake can acutely reduce testosterone concentrations by a similar percentage (conversely in night-shift workers, testosterone should be measured upon waking in the evening). In this vignette, the patient's total testosterone concentration was still low at 268 ng/dL (9.3 nmol/L) when drawn in the morning while fasting. However, he has no clinical features of androgen deficiency. Of note, gynecomastia is diagnosed by the presence of palpable breast tissue. This man had lipomastia due to obesity, which occurs independent of gonadal status. The LH concentration in the reference range can therefore be considered to be appropriately (rather than inappropriately) normal, and the index of suspicion for organic hypogonadotropic hypogonadism is low. Measuring serum prolactin (Answer C) or performing pituitary-directed MRI (Answer B) is not the best next step. There is no clinical suspicion of hemochromatosis, so iron studies (Answer D) are not indicated. Of note, ferritin may be elevated simply because of the proinflammatory state associated with insulin resistance. There is no clinical suspicion of estradiol excess, and its measurement (Answer E) is not warranted.

This man is centrally obese and has clinical evidence of insulin resistance (ie, acanthosis nigricans), features commonly associated with a low SHBG concentration. In this context, given that total testosterone will reduce in parallel to the reduction in SHBG, documenting a normal free testosterone concentration can be reassuring if trying to confirm a eugonadal status. The Endocrine Society recommends measuring free testosterone using either equilibrium dialysis or estimating it using an accurate formula in men whose total testosterone is near the lower limit of normal or in those who have a condition that alters SHBG concentrations. In clinical practice, gold standard equilibrium dialysis is generally not available, and free testosterone is usually estimated by calculation with a formula that requires SHBG measurement. Measuring SHBG and estimating free testosterone (Answer A) is the best next step. In this man, SHBG was low-normal at 1.1 μg/mL (1.1-6.7 μg/mL) (SI: 10 nmol/L [10-60 nmol/L]), and calculated free testosterone was normal at 11.4 ng/dL (9.0-31.2 ng/dL) (SI: 0.40 nmol/L [0.31-1.04 nmol/L]).

While some uncertainty exists regarding age-dependent reference ranges and optimal methodology for quantifying free testosterone, the European Male Ageing Study, an observational study in community-dwelling middle-aged and older men, has provided epidemiologic proof of principle data to support the clinical usefulness of free testosterone concentrations. In the European Male Ageing Study, men with low total testosterone but normal free testosterone were younger, more obese, and had lower SHBG levels compared with men with low free testosterone. In the men with low total testosterone but normal free testosterone, features of androgen deficiency were lacking. In contrast, men with low free testosterone had clinical evidence of androgen deficiency, even when total testosterone was normal.

In this man, metabolic risk is clinically obvious and should initially be addressed by lifestyle measures, especially weight loss (which, if successful, will lead to an increase in SHBG and total testosterone concentrations).

Educational Objective
Explain how men can have a falsely low total testosterone concentration due to low SHBG, commonly caused by central adiposity and insulin resistance.

Reference(s)
Bhasin S, Brito JP, Cunningham GR, et al. Testosterone therapy in men with hypogonadism: an Endocrine Society clinical practice guideline. *J Clin Endocrinol Metab*. 2018;103(5):1715-1744. PMID: 29562364

Antonio L, Wu FC, O'Neill TW, et al. Low free testosterone is associated with hypogonadal signs and symptoms in men with normal total testosterone. *J Clin Endocrinol Metab*. 2016;101(7):2647-2657. PMID: 26909800

49 ANSWER: D) Refer for genetic testing

This patient has an incidentally detected pituitary abnormality, which is unlikely to be related to her headaches for which the working diagnosis is migraine. There are no clinical features to suggest a previously undiagnosed functioning pituitary adenoma. However, the initial laboratory tests unexpectedly show elevated free thyroid hormone levels without corresponding suppression of TSH. These findings are confirmed on repeated testing and are not explained by assay artifact (ie, laboratory assay interference).

Accordingly, rarer causes of this pattern of thyroid function test results should be considered, including a TSH-secreting pituitary adenoma (thyrotropinoma) or resistance to thyroid hormone (RTH) caused by a loss-of-function pathogenic variant in the human thyroid hormone receptor β gene (*THRB*). The finding of a microadenoma on pituitary imaging might be interpreted as confirmation that the patient has a thyrotropinoma. However, concentrations of both SHBG and α-subunit of pituitary glycoprotein hormones are normal, which is not typical (*see table*). A thyrotropin-releasing hormone (TRH) test (200 mcg intravenously with measurement of serum TSH at baseline, 20 minutes, and 60 minutes) may help to distinguish these disorders but is not available at all centers. The TSH response to TRH is preserved or exaggerated in *THRB*-associated RTH but is attenuated or absent in thyrotropinoma (*see table*).

Table. Discrimination Between Thyrotropinoma and *THRB*-Associated Resistance to Thyroid Hormone

Investigation	Thyrotropinoma	Resistance to thyroid hormone (THRB-associated resistance to thyroid hormone)
Serum SHBG	Increased (but may be normal if there is co-secretion of GH)	Normal
Serum α-subunit	Increased/normal	Normal
Thyrotropin-releasing hormone stimulation test	Absent/attenuated TSH response	Preserved/exaggerated TSH response
Pituitary MRI	Adenoma (although some microadenomas may not be visualized on standard MRI sequences)	Normal (but incidentalomas in 10%-15% as per the general population)

Importantly, the patient has a history of attention-deficit/hyperactivity disorder and recurrent ear infections as a child, exhibits no clinical features of hyperthyroidism, and has a smooth goiter, all of which raise the possibility of previously undiagnosed *THRB*-associated RTH. Even in the absence of a relevant family history or similarly affected relatives, it is appropriate to arrange for genetic testing (Answer D) as the next step in this patient's management.

If she is subsequently confirmed to have *THRB*-associated RTH with a pituitary incidentaloma, surveillance pituitary MRI (Answer A) would be required in due course, but repeated scanning at 3 months (Answer A) would be considered too early (12 months is the normal recommended interval).

If the pattern of initial investigations favored a thyrotropinoma, then a trial of depot somatostatin analogue (Answer C) could be considered and could prove both diagnostic and therapeutic. Thyroid function tests typically normalize in thyrotropinoma but are unaffected in *THRB*-associated RTH.

Although transsphenoidal surgery (Answer E) is the primary treatment option for most thyrotropinomas, it would not be routinely recommended for an incidentally detected nonfunctioning pituitary microadenoma.

In *THRB*-associated RTH, the hypothalamic-pituitary-thyroid axis has an altered set-point, and treatment with antithyroid drugs such as methimazole (Answer B) is best avoided, as the fall in thyroid hormone levels is typically accompanied by a dramatic rebound rise in TSH. This can lead to further thyroid enlargement and possible thyrotroph hyperplasia. Alternative treatment options for those with thyrotoxic symptoms include 3,5,3´-triiodothyroacetic acid (TRIAC), a thyroid hormone analogue that acts centrally to inhibit TSH secretion, thereby reducing thyroid hormone levels, yet is devoid of peripheral thyromimetic activity. TRIAC has been shown to be beneficial in both childhood and adult cases of *THRB*-associated resistance to thyroid hormone, but it is not available at all centers and should only be prescribed under expert supervision. Antithyroid drugs are also generally not preferred in thyrotropinoma, although they may be used in the short term in preparation for surgery if depot somatostatin analogue therapy does not deliver sufficient control of thyrotoxicosis to allow safe anesthesia.

Educational Objective
Plan a systematic approach, combining clinical, laboratory, and radiologic parameters, to ensure reliable discrimination among various causes of hyperthyroxinemia with a nonsuppressed TSH level.

Reference(s)
Gurnell M, Visser T, Beck-Peccoz PB, Chatterjee VKK. Resistance to thyroid hormone. In: Jameson JL, De Groot LJ, eds. *Endocrinology*. 7th ed. Saunders Elsevier. 2015:1649-1665.

Koulouri O, Gurnell M. TSH-secreting pituitary adenomas. In: Huhtaniemi I, Martini L, eds. *Encyclopedia of Endocrine Diseases*. 2nd ed. Academic Press. 2018:261-266.

50 ANSWER: A) Order a basic metabolic panel and measure serum ketones

The correct answer is to obtain a basic metabolic panel and check serum ketones (Answer A). Patients taking SGLT-2 inhibitors are at increased risk of developing euglycemic diabetic ketoacidosis (DKA). Insulin-dependent patients are at highest risk. This patient has type 2 diabetes, but her history of early failure of oral therapy and the need to initiate multiple daily insulin injections is suspicious for latent autoimmune diabetes of adulthood (LADA). Her symptoms are concerning for DKA, but given that her blood glucose values are not considerably elevated, which has historically been observed in patients with DKA, it is possible that neither she nor her health care provider would consider DKA to be the potential etiology of her symptoms.

SGLT-2 inhibitors reduce hyperglycemia via blocking the reabsorption of glucose in the proximal tubule, thereby inducing glucosuria. This occurs independent of insulin action. However, the glucose-lowering efficacy of the SGLT-2 inhibitor is partly offset by a rise in endogenous glucose production, and the plasma glucagon concentration tends to increase, while the plasma insulin concentration decreases. SGLT-2 inhibitors also induce an increase in the levels of ketone bodies. These metabolic changes appear to be what predispose patients receiving an SGLT-2 inhibitor to an increased risk of DKA, particularly a variant called euglycemic DKA. In euglycemic DKA, blood glucose levels may be within the normal reference range, or only mildly to moderately elevated, because hyperglycemia is being attenuated by the glucosuria being induced by the SGLT-2 inhibitor therapy.

Patients who develop DKA while taking an SGLT-2 inhibitor usually have precipitating factors (eg, infection, surgical procedures, decreased oral intake, or initiation of very low-carbohydrate diets [ketogenic or ketogenic-like diets]). While a precipitating factor is usually present, in some instances, precipitating factors or events may not be identified. It is very important that patients are counseled on the potential precipitating factors of DKA while taking an SGLT-2 inhibitor. When SGLT-2 inhibitor therapy is initiated, patients should be educated regarding the symptoms that should prompt an investigation for DKA, and they should also have the ability to check urinary ketones if they feel unwell. If DKA is suspected while taking an SGLT-2 inhibitor, particularly in patients who are insulin-dependent, the "STICH" protocol should be followed:

STop SGLT-2 inhibitor treatment

Insulin administration (dose determined based on discussion with health care provider)

Carbohydrate consumption (generally 30 g or less)

Hydration with water or sugar-free electrolyte drink

A routine dipstick urinalysis (Answer B) would not be sufficient to evaluate this patient's symptoms. It would not assess for ketones, and the urine sample would be expected to demonstrate a very high glucose concentration in a patient receiving an SGLT-2 inhibitor, regardless of whether the patient were in DKA.

Given that her therapy has been stable for the past 2 years, if her symptoms were related to metformin, they should have manifested much earlier during the treatment course. Thus, stopping metformin (Answer E) is incorrect.

Performing esophagogastroduodenoscopy (Answer D) or a gastric-emptying study (Answer C) would not be appropriate at this point in the evaluation. The onset of symptoms is suggestive of an acute process, rather than being related to an underlying gastrointestinal disorder such as gastroparesis or additional esophageal/stomach pathology.

Educational Objective

Diagnose euglycemic diabetic ketoacidosis in a patient receiving an SGLT-2 inhibitor.

Reference(s):

Burke KR, Schumacher CA, Harpe SE. SGLT2 inhibitors: a systematic review of diabetic ketoacidosis and related risk factors in the primary literature. *Pharmacotherapy*. 2017;37(2):187-194. PMID: 27931088

Garg SK, Peters AL, Buse JB, Danne T. Strategy for mitigating DKA risk in patients with type 1 diabetes on adjunctive treatment with SGLT inhibitors: a STICH protocol. *Diabetes Technol Ther*. 2018;20(9):571-575. PMID: 30129772

Ferrannini E, Muscelli E, Frascerra S, et al. Metabolic response to sodium-glucose cotransporter 2 inhibition in type 2 diabetic patients. *J Clin Invest*. 2014;124(2):499-508. PMID: 24463454

Mudaliar S, Polidori D, Zambrowicz B, Henry RR. Sodium-glucose cotransporter inhibitors: effects on renal and intestinal glucose transport: from bench to bedside. *Diabetes Care*. 2015;38(12):2344-2353. PMID: 26604280

Peters AL, Buschur EO, Buse JB, Cohan P, Diner JC, Hirsch IB. Euglycemic diabetic ketoacidosis: a potential complication of treatment with sodium-glucose cotransporter 2 inhibition. *Diabetes Care*. 2015;38(9):1687-1693. PMID: 26078479

Nodzynski T, Lee TC. A rose by any other name: ketoacidosis due to SGLT2 inhibitors reveals latent autoimmune diabetes. *Am J Med*. 2018;131(1):e1-e3. PMID: 28982583

51 ANSWER: B) Liraglutide

Weight-loss medications should be considered in addition to diet, exercise, and behavioral modification to help individuals during their weight-loss journey. The patient described in this vignette is a candidate for pharmacotherapy given that her BMI is greater than 30 kg/m². When selecting the best medication, factors such as adverse effects, comorbidities, contraindications, patient preference, and cost should be considered.

Liraglutide (Answer B) is a long-acting GLP-1 receptor agonist. This medication is administered subcutaneously. The starting dosage is 0.6 mg daily and the dosage is increased by 0.6-mg increments every week until the patient reaches the recommended dosage of 3 mg daily. Liraglutide is contraindicated when patients have a personal or family history of medullary thyroid carcinoma or multiple endocrine neoplasia type 2. It should be used with extreme caution in patients with a history of pancreatitis. The most common adverse effects include nausea, diarrhea, and increased heart rate (>10 beats/min from baseline). Given the options listed, her initial best choice is liraglutide, 3 mg daily.

Naltrexone/bupropion extended-release (Answer A) is a combination pill with an opioid antagonist and a reuptake inhibitor of dopamine and norepinephrine. Each tablet has 8 mg of naltrexone and 90 mg of bupropion and the approved dosage is 2 tablets twice daily. Contraindications to this combination pill include uncontrolled hypertension; opioid use; history of seizures; bulimia or anorexia nervosa; use of monoamine oxidase inhibitors; or abrupt discontinuation of alcohol, benzodiazepines, barbiturates, or anticonvulsant drugs. The most commonly reported adverse effects include headache, sleep disorders, nausea, constipation, and vomiting. This patient's history of a seizure disorder is a contraindication to the use of naltrexone/bupropion, as bupropion lowers the seizure threshold.

Orlistat (Answer C) is an intestinal lipase inhibitor. This medication is taken before each meal, and the recommended dosage ranges from 60 mg to 120 mg 3 times daily. Contraindications to this medication include oxalate nephrolithiasis, cholestasis, and chronic malabsorption syndrome. Adverse effects include steatorrhea, fecal urgency, oily spotting, abdominal pain, and headache. Orlistat is not an appetite suppressant, so other weight-loss medications should be considered first, as this patient is struggling with hunger. Also given her history of Crohn disease, orlistat should not be used as first-line therapy because of its gastrointestinal adverse effects.

Phentermine is a norepinephrine-releasing agent. Phentermine monotherapy (Answer D) was approved by the US FDA in 1959 for short-term treatment (12 weeks) of patients with obesity. This medication is the most prescribed weight-loss medication in the United States. The recommended dosage is 15 to 37.5 mg daily. The most common adverse effects include dry mouth, tachycardia, anxiety, insomnia, and hypertension. This medication is contraindicated for individuals with a history of cardiovascular disease such as this patient, so starting phentermine alone would not be the best option.

Phentermine and topiramate (a GABA receptor modulator) were approved in a combination pill (Answer E) that is available in 4 different doses. The recommended dosage is 7.5 mg of phentermine and 46 mg of topiramate daily, and the maximum dosage is 15 mg of phentermine and 92 mg of topiramate daily. The other 2 doses are used for escalation purposes for 14 days. Contraindications to this combination pill are glaucoma, coronary heart disease, hyperthyroidism, pregnancy, or use during or within 14 days following monoamine oxidase inhibitor therapy. The most common adverse effects include dry mouth, tachycardia, anxiety, insomnia, hypertension, paresthesias, somnolence, and increased risk of developing kidney stones. Given her personal history of ischemic heart disease and glaucoma, phentermine/topiramate is contraindicated.

Educational Objective
Identify candidates for weight-loss medications, bearing in mind their comorbidities.

Reference(s)
Apovian CM, Aronne LJ, Bessesen DH, et al; Endocrine Society. Pharmacological management of obesity: an Endocrine Society clinical practice guideline. *J Clin Endocrinol Metab*. 2015;100(2):342-362. PMID: 25590212

52 ANSWER: E) Perform a 250-mcg cosyntropin-stimulation test

This patient is experiencing recurrent hypoglycemic episodes despite making adjustments to his insulin regimen, and his hemoglobin A_{1c} level suggests very tight glycemic control. In this context, it is clearly appropriate to review his current insulin dosages and insulin-to-carbohydrate ratio. However, he is already taking a total daily insulin dosage (maximum 28 units) that is considerably lower than would be predicted based on body weight and duration of diabetes, especially in the context of reduced exercise. Therefore, simply continuing with further down-titration of either his basal insulin (Answer A) or bolus insulin is unlikely to completely resolve his symptoms. Moreover, the total daily insulin dosage is not consistent with a high insulin-to-carbohydrate ratio. Thus, reducing this ratio (Answer B) is incorrect unless he is consuming very little carbohydrate.

He also reports tiredness, and his laboratory panel shows mild hyponatremia, mild hyperkalemia, and a minor elevation in serum urea nitrogen. ACE inhibitors and angiotensin II receptor blockers could lead to this constellation of features, and there are rare case reports of ramipril being associated with hypoglycemia. However, in the clinical context described here, it is important to consider other possibilities.

The combination of unexplained recurrent hypoglycemia, tiredness, hyponatremia, and hyperkalemia all suggest the possibility of primary adrenal insufficiency, and it is mandatory in this setting to arrange urgent assessment for and/or treatment of possible coexistent Addison disease (Answer E).

One must also consider other potential features of autoimmune polyglandular syndrome type 2; in particular, Graves disease (Answer D) and celiac disease (Answer C), which may both predispose to weight loss and hypoglycemic episodes. However, given the combination of clinical and laboratory features in this case, the most important condition to screen for first is primary adrenal insufficiency.

Educational Objective
Consider other causes for hypoglycemia in a patient with type 1 diabetes mellitus.

Reference(s)

McAulay V, Frier BM. Addison's disease in type 1 diabetes presenting with recurrent hypoglycaemia. *Postgrad Med J.* 2000;76(894):230-232. PMID: 10727569

Chantzichristos D, Persson A, Miftaraj M, Eliasson B, Svensson AM, Johannsson G. Early clinical indicators of Addison disease in adults with type 1 diabetes: a nationwide, observational, cohort study. *J Clin Endocrinol Metab.* 2019;104(4):1148-1157. PMID: 30476180

53 ANSWER: A) Neck ultrasonography in 24 months

The characteristic ultrasonography appearance of the thyroid nodule shown is associated with a very low risk of malignancy. Spongiform or honeycomb thyroid nodules are mixed cystic and solid nodules containing an aggregation of numerous microcystic areas that account for more than 50% of the nodule volume. A systematic review and meta-analysis that included more than 18,000 thyroid nodules from 31 studies found that spongiform appearance was associated with a posttest probability of malignancy of only 2%. This is similar to the false-negative rate associated with benign thyroid cytology.

The 2015 American Thyroid Association (ATA) Guidelines for Thyroid Nodules and Differentiated Thyroid Cancer and the American College of Radiology (ACR) Thyroid Imaging, Reporting, and Data System (TI-RADS) are 2 commonly used systems that delineate the risk of thyroid malignancy based on sonographic findings and dictate the need for thyroid nodule tissue sampling. Because individual features of malignancy tend to occur together in malignant thyroid nodules, the ATA system classifies thyroid nodules into 5 distinct sonographic risk categories based on constellations of features (patterns). Conversely, ACR TI-RADS uses a point-based system that assigns a point value to each thyroid nodule architectural category and the total points determine the TI-RADS level. Recommended management, including size thresholds for FNA biopsy and timing of ultrasonography follow-up, are specified for each ATA pattern and TI-RADS level. Both systems have been prospectively validated in independent studies.

The patient's nodule demonstrates classic spongiform morphology and should be classified as ATA very low suspicion sonographic pattern or TI-RADS level 1 (benign). The estimated risk of malignancy for ATA very low suspicion pattern nodules is less than 3%, and FNA biopsy is considered optional for nodules larger than 2 cm and is not recommended for smaller nodules. FNA biopsy is not recommended according to the ACR for any TI-RADS level 1 nodule.

The ATA Guidelines for Thyroid Nodules and Differentiated Thyroid Cancer advise that if follow-up imaging is to be performed for ATA very low-suspicion pattern nodules, such as the nodule shown, the initial follow-up interval should be at least 2 years (Answer A). Ultrasound-guided FNA biopsy (Answer E) would not be considered given the nodule size smaller than 2 cm.

There is no clinical suspicion for substernal goiter or tracheal compression in this patient and thus no indication to perform neck CT (Answer B). Neck CT is less sensitive and specific than neck ultrasonography in the evaluation of thyroid nodules.

A radioactive iodine uptake and scan (Answer C) is not indicated in the evaluation of thyroid nodules in the absence of low serum TSH.

Serum calcitonin measurement (Answer D) would not be indicated in the evaluation of this thyroid nodule with very low-risk sonographic appearance. Most medullary thyroid carcinomas (>80%) are hypoechoic on ultrasonography. Irregular margins and microcalcifications are both relatively common sonographic findings and can be demonstrated on ultrasonography in at least one-third of cases. Although there are differences in the use of serum calcitonin in the evaluation of thyroid nodules across the globe, routine measurement of serum calcitonin is generally not done in the United States. There is a lack of prospective survival data related to earlier medullary thyroid carcinoma case detection with routine serum calcitonin measurement, unresolved issues of serum calcitonin assay performance, and a lack of availability of pentagastrin stimulation in North America.

Educational Objective

Identify thyroid nodules with a very low likelihood of malignancy based on ultrasonography findings.

Reference(s)

Brito JP, Gionfriddo MR, Al Nofal A, et al. The accuracy of thyroid nodule ultrasound to predict thyroid cancer: systematic review and meta-analysis. *J Clin Endocrinol Metab.* 2014;99(4):1253-1263. PMID: 24276450

Haugen BR, Alexander EK, Bible KC, et al. 2015 American Thyroid Association management guidelines for adult patients with thyroid nodules and differentiated thyroid cancer: the American Thyroid Association Guidelines Task Force on Thyroid Nodules and Differentiated Thyroid Cancer. *Thyroid.* 2016;26(1):1-133. PMID: 26462967

Tessler FN, Middleton WD, Grant EG, et al. ACR thyroid imaging, reporting and data system (TI-RADS): white paper of the ACR TI-RADS committee. *J Am Coll Radiol.* 2017;14(5):587-595. PMID: 28372962

54 ANSWER: D) Amlodipine and chlorthalidone

There is strong evidence that pharmacologic treatment for patients with diabetes who have an initial blood pressure higher than 140/90 mm Hg reduces cardiovascular events and progression of microvascular disease. Interestingly, one meta-analysis suggests that reduction of stroke risk and albuminuria occurs with pharmacologic treatment regardless of whether initial blood pressure is above or below 140/90 mm Hg. Agents that have been shown to reduce cardiovascular events in persons with diabetes include ACE inhibitors, angiotensin-receptor blockers, thiazidelike diuretics, and dihydropyridine calcium-channel blockers.

An important consideration is the initial level of blood pressure. The American Diabetes Association Standards of Clinical Care guidelines emphasize that for patients with an initial blood pressure greater than or equal to 160/100 mm Hg, dual treatment is more likely than monotherapy (Answers A and B) to achieve blood pressure targets, and a 2-drug regimen should be initiated (simultaneously or very quickly in succession, based on one's clinical judgment regarding the risk of hypotension). As monotherapy, ACE inhibitors, thiazidelike diuretics, β-adrenergic blockers, and calcium-channel blockers are associated with systolic/diastolic blood pressure reductions of 12.5/9.5 mm Hg, 15.3/9.8 mm Hg, 14.8/12.2 mm Hg, and 15.3/10.5 mm Hg, respectively. These data demonstrate that single-drug treatment is not likely to achieve a systolic blood pressure less than 140 mm Hg in this patient. Also, in the absence of albuminuria, ACE inhibitors or angiotensin-receptor blockers have not been shown to offer more cardiovascular benefit than calcium-channel blockers or thiazidelike diuretics. Therefore, it would be difficult to choose between Answers A and B.

The combination of ACE inhibitors and angiotensin-receptor blockers (Answer C) has been shown to offer no additional benefit in terms of cardiovascular risk compared with monotherapy with these agents. Further, the risk of hyperkalemia or acute kidney injury is higher with dual ACE inhibitor and angiotensin-receptor blocker treatment, making this a poor choice for this patient.

β-Adrenergic blockers (Answer E) are useful in reducing mortality in patients with angina, prior myocardial infarction, or heart failure. However, as this patient has no history of such conditions, there is no demonstrated benefit of using β-adrenergic blockers in terms of mortality or cardiovascular events.

Since both amlodipine and chlorthalidone (Answer D) reduce cardiovascular events in persons with diabetes, this combination would be most reasonable among the given answer choices.

Educational Objective

Prescribe appropriate antihypertensive pharmacologic treatment for reducing cardiovascular risk based on a patient's blood pressure.

Reference(s)

American Diabetes Association. 10. Cardiovascular disease and risk management: *standards of medical care in diabetes-2020. Diabetes Care.* 2020;43(Suppl 1):S111–S134. PMID: 31862753

Emdin CA, Rahimi K, Neal B, Callender T, Perkovic V, Patel A. Blood pressure lowering in type 2 diabetes: a systematic review and meta-analysis. *JAMA.* 2015;313(6):603-615. PMID: 25668264

Wu J, Kraja AT, Oberman A, et al. A summary of the effects of antihypertensive medications on measured blood pressure. *Am J Hypertens.* 2005;18(7):935-942. PMID: 16053990

55

ANSWER: D) Order ¹²³I whole-body scan with SPECT-CT

This 48-year-old woman has biochemical and clinical findings consistent with hyperthyroidism. However, her thyroid scan demonstrates decreased uptake in her neck. Her serum thyroglobulin remains measurable, which indicates production of thyroid hormone from an ectopic thyroid source. Therefore, one should become suspicious of thyroid tissue in another part of the body producing thyroid hormones that are causing hyperthyroidism. The diagnosis of struma ovarii should be considered in a patient with hyperthyroidism that persists for more than 3 to 6 months who also has measurable serum thyroglobulin, low/absent uptake in the neck, and no goiter. Patients who have been exposed to an iodine load such as intravenous radiographic contrast or amiodarone may have a low radioiodine uptake and decreased tracer uptake in the neck. In the case of intravenous radiographic contrast, the pinhole thyroid scan should be postponed 4 to 6 weeks and a spot urine iodine measurement can be used to document depletion of excess iodine loads. In contrast, amiodarone contains a large amount of iodine with a half-life of approximately 100 days. After stopping amiodarone, it will be longer before a patient is able to undergo a thyroid scan or uptake.

Struma ovarii is a rare form of ovarian teratoma in which greater than 50% of the germ-cell neoplasm is comprised of thyroid tissue. Struma ovarii accounts for less than 1% of all ovarian tumors and approximately 5% of all ovarian teratomas. Struma ovarii commonly occurs in women aged 40 to 60 years. The risk of malignancy is less than 5%. Affected patients commonly have normal thyroid function, but hyperthyroidism can be present at diagnosis in 5% to 8%. The thyroid gland is not typically enlarged. Affected patients usually experience pelvic pain, and the occurrence of ascites has been observed.

Although struma ovarii can be diagnosed by traditional planar ¹²³I or ¹³¹I whole-body scintigraphy, fusion ¹²³I SPECT-CT (Answer D) provides accurate identification and localization of ectopic thyroid tissue in suspected cases of extrathyroidal thyrotoxicosis. Before ordering any scintigraphy imaging, pelvic ultrasonography can document the presence of an ovarian mass. Ovarian resection or unilateral oophorectomy is the primary therapy for benign struma ovarii. For patients with struma ovarii and overt hyperthyroidism, surgery should be postponed until the hyperthyroidism is adequately controlled by β-adrenergic blockers and a thionamide (methimazole) for 4 to 6 weeks before surgery. The methimazole dosage should be chosen according to the severity of hyperthyroidism, as it is in Graves disease.

As this patient has hyperthyroidism with decreased tracer uptake in the both thyroid lobes, thyroid ultrasonography (Answer A) would most likely not provide further information to diagnose the cause of her hyperthyroidism. Methimazole, an antithyroid drug, is usually prescribed to treat Graves disease, hyperthyroidism due to toxic multinodular goiter, or toxic adenoma, and can be used in patients with struma ovarii to control the hyperthyroidism. However, as the diagnosis has not yet been established in this patient, methimazole (Answer B) is not the best option now. Thyroid-stimulating immunoglobulin (Answer C) is usually elevated in patients with Graves disease. In Graves disease, the thyroid scan shows increased uptake in both thyroid lobes, which is the not the case here. Prednisone (Answer E) can be used for patients with subacute thyroiditis, but it is not indicated for this patient.

Educational Objective
Diagnose struma ovarii in a patient with persistent hyperthyroidism.

Reference(s)

Roth LM, Talerman A. The enigma of struma ovarii. *Pathology*. 2007;39(1):139-146. PMID: 17365830

Yoo SC, Chang KH, Lyu MO, Chang SJ, Ryu HS, Kim HS. Clinical characteristics of struma ovarii. *J Gynecol Oncol*. 2008;19(2):135-138. PMID: 19471561

56

ANSWER: E) 2-Hour 75-g oral glucose tolerance test

Current guidelines from the Endocrine Society and European Society for Human Reproduction and the American Society for Reproductive Medicine for the diagnosis of polycystic ovary syndrome follow the Rotterdam International Consensus criteria requiring 2 of 3 of the following criteria: (1) hyperandrogenism—clinical (hirsutism, excessive terminal hair growth, acne, or androgenic alopecia) or biochemical androgen; (2) oligoovulation or anovulation—fewer than 8 to 9 menses per year or frequent bleeding (<21 days) or normal intervals of 25 to 35 days with midluteal progesterone consistent with anovulation; and/or (3) polycystic ovarian morphology—presence of 12 or more follicles 2 to 9 mm in diameter and/or ovarian volume greater than 10 mL in either ovary without a dominant follicle or cyst greater than 1 cm. This young woman has 2 criteria: irregular menses consistent with oligo-anovulation (6 to 8 periods per year) that persisted through adolescence into adulthood and an elevated total testosterone concentration. Other secondary causes have been ruled out. Since polycystic ovary syndrome can be diagnosed with the information given, pelvic ultrasonography (Answer A) is not necessary. Although an elevated LH-to-FSH ratio is also associated with polycystic ovary syndrome, measurement of LH and FSH is not required or sufficient to make the diagnosis without 2 of the 3 criteria.

Antimullerian hormone (Answer B) is associated with antral follicle count and might be particularly helpful in assessing for polycystic ovarian morphology in adolescents when transvaginal ultrasonography might not be easily performed. However, until improved standardization of assays allows for established thresholds and validation on a large scale in population samples of different ages and ethnicities, antimullerian hormone cannot be used as a diagnostic criterion for polycystic ovarian morphology or polycystic ovary syndrome.

Since this patient already has evidence of anovulatory cycles with an intermenstrual interval of 45 to 60 days, measurement of day 21 progesterone (Answer C) is not necessary to document oligoovulatory and anovulatory cycles. It would be useful to document anovulatory cycles if a woman has monthly menses and other possible symptoms of polycystic ovary syndrome.

Screening for nonclassic congenital adrenal hyperplasia is recommended in all women with a possible diagnosis of polycystic ovary syndrome. Screening baseline 17-hydroxyprogesterone is ideally obtained in the early morning (7:30 to 8:00 AM) during the follicular phase if testing can be timed to menses. If the 17-hydroxyprogesterone concentration is greater than 200 ng/dL (>6.1 nmol/L) but less than 1500 ng/dL (<45.5 nmol/L), a high-dose (250-mcg) cosyntropin-stimulation test should be performed. Because this patient has a normal 17-hydroxyprogesterone concentration, she does not require further evaluation for nonclassic congenital adrenal hyperplasia with cosyntropin-stimulation testing (Answer D).

Normal-weight women with polycystic ovary syndrome can have insulin resistance, so guidelines recommend screening for impaired glucose tolerance or type 2 diabetes with a 2-hour 75-g oral glucose tolerance test (Answer E) in all women diagnosed with polycystic ovary syndrome. The presence of a normal hemoglobin A_{1c} level does not exclude the possibility of impaired glucose tolerance, which is more common than impaired fasting glucose in women with polycystic ovary syndrome. Even if a woman with polycystic ovary syndrome does not have prediabetes or type 2 diabetes, metformin can be used to increase the frequency of ovulatory cycles, especially when oral contraceptives cannot be tolerated or might be lead to a higher risk of stroke or venous thrombosis.

Educational Objective
Diagnose polycystic ovary syndrome and recommend appropriate screening for impaired glucose tolerance and type 2 diabetes mellitus.

Reference(s)

Legro RS, Arslanian SA, Ehrmann DA, et al; Endocrine Society. Diagnosis and treatment of polycystic ovary syndrome: an Endocrine Society clinical practice guideline. *J Clin Endocrinol Metab.* 2013;98(12):4565-4592. PMID: 24151290

Teede HJ, Misso ML, Costello MF, et al; International PCOS Network. Recommendations from the international evidence-based guideline for the assessment and management of polycystic ovary syndrome. *Hum Reprod.* 2018;33(9):1602-1618. PMID: 30052961

Abbara A, Eng PC, Phylactou M, et al. Anti-mullerian hormone (AMH) in the diagnosis of menstrual disturbance due to polycystic ovarian syndrome. *Front Endocrinol (Lausanne).* 2019;10:656. PMID: 31616381

Legro RS, Kunselman AR, Dodson WC, Dunaif A. Prevalence and predicators of risk for type 2 diabetes mellitus and impaired glucose tolerance in polycystic ovary syndrome: a prospective, controlled study in 254 affected women. *J Clin Endocrinol Metab.* 1999;84(1):165-169. PMID: 9920077

57 ANSWER: E) Monitor laboratory values for the remainder of her pregnancy

The patient described in this vignette has hypercalcemia and has just started her third trimester of pregnancy. Her hypercalcemia is mild and is associated with a mid-normal PTH level, an elevated 1,25-dihydroxyvitamin D level, and hypercalciuria. In this scenario, one must consider the physiologic changes that occur during normal pregnancy, which include decrease in PTH, increase in calcitriol, and increase in the fractional excretion of calcium. Calcitriol levels begin to increase in the first trimester and may reach more than triple the nonpregnant value by the third trimester. This increase contributes to upregulation of intestinal calcium absorption during pregnancy and to suppression of PTH. Increased production of calcitriol comes almost entirely from maternal kidneys and not the placenta or fetus, although the factors that stimulate renal 1α-hydroxylase during pregnancy are yet to be elucidated. Therefore, the most likely cause of this patient's hypercalcemia remains primary hyperparathyroidism and not extrarenal production of 1,25-dihydroxyvitamin D (which can occur with lymphoma). Hence, referral to oncology for evaluation of possible lymphoma recurrence (Answer D) would not be the most appropriate next step in this patient's management.

Initiating cinacalcet therapy (Answer A) or treating with an intravenous bisphosphonate infusion such as intravenous pamidronate (Answer B) is not indicated in this patient with mild asymptomatic hypercalcemia. Furthermore, there are very limited data regarding the use of cinacalcet in pregnant women, and the US FDA classifies pamidronate as category D (positive evidence of risk in pregnancy).

Given this patient's age, she is a candidate for surgical intervention for primary hyperparathyroidism. The ideal time to operate during pregnancy is the second trimester, and she has just entered her third trimester. In addition, she is asymptomatic with only mild hypercalcemia. Given the inherent potential risks of surgery for the pregnant patient and limited data showing that mild hypercalcemia in gestational primary hyperparathyroidism is generally not associated with an increased risk of obstetric complications, the most appropriate next step would be to monitor her laboratory values during pregnancy (Answer E) and defer parathyroid surgery (Answer C) until after delivery. It is important to note that there may be a risk of transient hypocalcemia in the newborn in pregnant women with primary hyperparathyroidism. In fact, this patient had an uncomplicated delivery, but her baby boy had hypocalcemia for about 2 weeks after birth; his PTH level improved at 2 months and had normalized at his 4-month checkup.

It is interesting to note that this patient's laboratory values 4 months post partum revealed a serum calcium concentration of 10.3 mg/dL (2.6 mmol/L) and a serum intact PTH concentration of 111 pg/mL (111 ng/L). Even though she has no family history of parathyroid disease, it would be prudent to pursue genetic testing to rule out a familial form of primary hyperparathyroidism given her young age and lack of history of radiation exposure.

Educational Objective
Diagnose primary hyperparathyroidism as a cause of hypercalcemia in a pregnant patient and recommend the appropriate management.

Reference(s)
Hirsch D, Kopel V, Nadler V, Levy S, Toledano Y, Tsvetov G. Pregnancy outcomes in women with primary hyperparathyroidism. *J Clin Endocrinol Metab.* 2015;100(5):2115-2122. PMID: 25751112

Horton WB, Stumpf MM, Coppock JD, et al. Gestational primary hyperparathyroidism due to ectopic parathyroid adenoma: case report and literature review. *J Endocr Soc.* 2017;1(9):1150-1155. PMID: 29264569

Kirby BJ, Ma Y, Martin HM, Buckle Favaro KL, Karaplis AC, Kovacs CS. Upregulation of calcitriol during pregnancy and skeletal recovery after lactation do not require parathyroid hormone. *J Bone Miner Res.* 2013;28(9):1987-2000. PMID: 23505097

58   ANSWER: A) Refer to a dietician for lifestyle modification

Women with polycystic ovary syndrome (PCOS) often have a clustering of risk factors for cardiovascular disease. Dyslipidemia is a common occurrence in women with PCOS and is characterized by high triglycerides, low HDL cholesterol, and increased numbers of small, dense LDL-cholesterol particles. These changes are associated with coexisting insulin resistance and are similar to the atherogenic dyslipidemia of metabolic syndrome. Non–HDL-cholesterol levels are often elevated; LDL-cholesterol values vary widely and can be increased in these women. The woman in this vignette has a lipid profile that is often encountered in patients with PCOS. There are no clear guidelines on management of dyslipidemia in PCOS. In addition to obtaining a screening lipid profile at the time of diagnosis, screening for cardiovascular risk factors, such as family history of early cardiovascular disease, cigarette smoking, impaired glucose tolerance/type 2 diabetes, hypertension, obstructive sleep apnea, and abdominal obesity, is important to stratify risk in these women. In this vignette, the patient has dyslipidemia and mild central adiposity but no other traditional risk factors.

Lifestyle modification is recommended as first-line therapy for all women with PCOS. Dietary modification, exercise, smoking cessation, and behavioral techniques (reduction of psychosocial stressors) are used to decrease cardiovascular risk. These modifications cause changes in dyslipidemia, thereby beneficially influencing cardiovascular risk. While optimum lifestyle modifications are not known, most studies have used structured exercise programs with protein-rich hypocaloric diets and, on occasion, psychological support. A recent meta-analysis of lifestyle intervention in women with PCOS showed evidence of improvements in body composition, hyperandrogenism, and insulin resistance without changes in lipid profiles. Overall, data are limited regarding the effects of lifestyle intervention on lipids in women with PCOS, as most studies focus on reproductive outcomes. There are no large randomized controlled trials of exercise therapy in women with PCOS, alone or in combination with dietary intervention. However, it is well established that these interventions improve weight loss and reduce cardiovascular risk factors and diabetes risk in the general population. Therefore, aggressive lifestyle modification with the help of a skilled dietitian (Answer A) is the best first step in managing this woman's dyslipidemia. These efforts can also help improve elevations on liver function tests, as seen in this patient. Combination oral contraceptives commonly used to treat menstrual irregularity in such women can result in triglyceride elevations and should be used with caution and close monitoring of lipids.

Large-scale clinical studies of statins (Answer B) in women with PCOS, either as monotherapy or in combination with other therapies, are very limited. Statins are effective in decreasing total cholesterol and LDL cholesterol in women with PCOS, with no evidence of effect on HDL cholesterol when compared with placebo or oral contraceptive pills. Significant triglyceride reductions have been observed. There is some limited evidence that statins may improve ovarian testosterone levels. There is no clinical trial evidence that statins decrease cardiovascular risk burden in women of childbearing age who have PCOS. Statins are teratogenic and should be used with caution in women of childbearing age and should be used only in women who meet current cardiovascular risk reduction indications. Due to the paucity of data regarding benefit, prescribing a statin for this patient is incorrect.

Fibrates (Answer C) are triglyceride-lowering agents that work by activating peroxisome proliferator–activated receptor α, increasing lipoprotein lipase activity, and increasing catabolism of triglycerides. These agents are particularly effective in individuals with marked hypertriglyceridemia (20%-50% reduction, sometimes up to 70%). They are the recommended first-line agents in patients at risk for triglyceride-induced pancreatitis, but evidence of benefit in primary cardiovascular risk reduction or in PCOS is lacking.

Omega-3 fish oil (Answer D) as concentrated eicosapentaenoic acid and docosahexaenoic acid has modest effects on triglycerides, with reductions up to 50%. Fish oil, when used in high dosages, reduces triglycerides by decreasing VLDL synthesis and increasing catabolism. However, there is no clear evidence of benefit in primary cardiovascular risk reduction or in PCOS, and it is therefore not the best option.

Metformin (Answer E) is an insulin sensitizer widely used in women with PCOS. The effect of metformin on lipid levels in women with PCOS appears to be variable. In some studies, women with PCOS who respond to metformin demonstrate a reduction in total and LDL cholesterol. A Cochrane database review did not find evidence of improved cholesterol or triglyceride levels with metformin therapy. Hence, metformin is not the correct choice for managing dyslipidemia.

Educational Objective
Manage cardiovascular risk in a woman of childbearing age with polycystic ovary syndrome.

Reference(s)

Fauser BC, Tarlatzis BC, Rebar RW, et al. Consensus on women's health aspects of polycystic ovary syndrome (PCOS): the Amsterdam ESHRE/ASRM-Sponsored 3rd PCOS Consensus Workshop Group. *Fertil Steril.* 2012;97(1):28-38. PMID: 22153789

Papadakis G, Kandaraki E, Papalou O, Vryonidou A, Diamanti-Kandarakis E. Is cardiovascular risk in women with PCOS a real risk? Current insights. *Minerva Endocrinol.* 2017;42(4):340-355. PMID: 28146139

Torchen LC. Cardiometabolic risk in PCOS: more than a reproductive disorder. *Curr Diab Rep.* 2017;17(12):137. PMID: 29128916

Legro RS, Arslanian SA, Ehrmann DA, et al; Endocrine Society. Diagnosis and treatment of polycystic ovary syndrome: an Endocrine Society clinical practice guideline. *J Clin Endocrinol Metab.* 2013;98(12):4565-4592. PMID: 24151290

59
ANSWER: B) Ethanol

Determining the cause of hypoglycemia in patients without a history of diabetes mellitus can be difficult. True hypoglycemia must first be established by documenting the Whipple triad and then the etiology must be determined in a timely manner. The Whipple triad includes: (1) symptoms of hypoglycemia, (2) confirmation of a low plasma glucose concentration at the time the patient is symptomatic, and (3) resolution of symptoms after hypoglycemia is treated. Blood glucose assessed using a glucose meter (point-of care) can be suggestive of hypoglycemia but cannot be used for confirmation of true hypoglycemia because the results may be unreliable.

In this vignette, the Whipple triad has been met, as the patient had symptoms of hypoglycemia, the plasma glucose concentration was confirmed to be less than 55 mg/dL (<3.1 mmol/L), and symptoms of hypoglycemia resolved after treatment with D50 and glucagon. The insulin, C-peptide, and proinsulin levels are in the normal range. In a patient with normal renal function, the plasma insulin level should be less than 3.0 µIU/ mL (<20.8 pmol/L) at the time of confirmed hypoglycemia. In a patient with stage 4 chronic kidney disease who does not have diabetes, insulin levels may be nonsuppressed, even during hypoglycemia, due to impaired clearance of insulin. Patients with an insulin-secreting neuroendocrine tumor (Answer A) would be expected to have frankly elevated insulin, C-peptide, and proinsulin values at the time of hypoglycemia, which was not the case in this vignette.

In this patient who has chronic alcohol abuse and has not eaten for more than 18 hours, glycogen stores have been depleted. Therefore, maintenance of normal blood glucose is dependent on gluconeogenesis. During oxidation of ethanol to acetaldehyde, nicotinamide-adenine dinucleotide (NAD) is reduced to NADH. The increased ratio of NADH to NAD prevents oxidation of substrate such as lactate and glutamate to pyruvate and α-ketoglutarate, respectively, essentially inhibiting gluconeogenesis. The main factor in the development of hypoglycemia in this case is the effect of alcohol (Answer B) on prevention of gluconeogenesis by the liver, thereby causing hypoglycemia.

Patients with stage 4 chronic kidney disease (Answer C) may have some impairment of gluconeogenesis by the kidney. However, renal gluconeogenesis is likely at least partially intact, and chronic kidney disease is not the most important factor in the development of hypoglycemia in this patient given the history of chronic alcohol ingestion.

Metoprolol (Answer D) and other β-adrenergic blockers may impair recognition of hypoglycemia but should not cause overt hypoglycemia.

Hypoglycemia has been reported in a subset of patients treated with fluoroquinolone antibiotics. A review by the FDA reported that gatifloxacin had a 10-fold higher risk of causing hypoglycemia or hyperglycemia compared with other quinolones. There have been rare case reports of hypoglycemia occurring in patients treated with ciprofloxacin (Answer E). However, a retrospective study of dysglycemia occurring in patients treated with fluoroquinolones in Veterans Affairs clinics reported that ciprofloxacin had a similar odds ratio to that of azithromycin for causing hypoglycemia. Given this, ciprofloxacin is unlikely to have caused hypoglycemia in this patient.

Educational Objective
Explain how ethanol inhibits gluconeogenesis in the liver and can lead to hypoglycemia and consider this as an etiology of hypoglycemia in a patient without diabetes mellitus.

Reference(s)

Aspinall SL, Good CB, Jiang R, McCarren M, Dong D, Cunningham FE. Severe dysglycemia with the fluoquinolones: a class effect? *Clin Infect Dis.* 2009;49(3):402-408. PMID: 19545207

Service FJ. Diagnostic approach to adults with hypoglycemic disorders. *Endocrinol Metab Clin North Am.* 1999;28(3):519-532. PMID: 10500929

Marks V. Spontaneous hypoglycaemia. *Br Med J.* 1972;1(5797):430-432. PMID: 4333485

60
ANSWER: C) Familial adenomatous polyposis

This patient has autosomal dominant familial adenomatous polyposis (FAP) (Answer C). FAP occurs in association with germline pathogenic variants in the adenomatous polyposis coli gene (*APC*) and is characterized by the development of hundreds of colorectal adenomatous polyps, nearly a 100% lifetime risk of colorectal cancer, and death by the fourth decade of life if untreated. Thyroid cancer has been reported in approximately 1% of patients with FAP, although this most likely represents an underestimate of the true prevalence. A study that used neck ultrasonography to screen patients with FAP for thyroid cancer determined the prevalence to be approximately 7%. Up to 40% of patients with FAP develop the cribriform-morular variant of papillary thyroid carcinoma (CMVPTC), which is an indolent malignancy. CMVPTC has a predilection for females younger than 35 years and may precede colon cancer diagnosis as in the case described. Pathology shows a combination of epithelial and morular components with characteristic nuclear clearing. The finding of CMVPTC in patients without a known diagnosis of FAP should prompt genetic testing to exclude the diagnosis. The prognosis of CMVPTC is generally excellent and spontaneous regressions have been reported. Other extracolonic manifestations of FAP include congenital hypertrophy of retinal pigmentation, gastric and duodenal polyps, epidermoid cysts (as seen in this patient), and desmoid tumors (as described in her brother).

Carney complex (Answer A) is an autosomal dominant multiple endocrine neoplasia syndrome that is associated with pathogenic variants in the protein kinase A type I alpha regulatory subunit gene (*PRKAR1A*). GH excess or acromegaly, Cushing syndrome due to primary pigmented nodular adrenocortical disease, and large-cell calcifying Sertoli-cell tumors in males are common findings. While thyroid nodules are seen in 75% of patients with Carney complex, papillary and follicular thyroid carcinomas are much less common, affecting less than 10% of patients. Nonendocrine manifestations of Carney complex include characteristic pigmented lesions of the skin and mucosa and cardiac myxomas.

PTEN hamartoma tumor syndrome (Cowden syndrome) (Answer B) results from pathogenic variants in the phosphatase and tensin homolog gene (*PTEN*) and is associated with an increased risk of benign thyroid nodules, as well as papillary and follicular thyroid carcinoma. There is also an elevated risk of breast, endometrial, and renal cell carcinoma. Colonic polyps, usually hamartomas, are almost universal. Macrocephaly, learning disabilities, and autism are also characteristic findings in Cowden syndrome.

Hereditary nonpolyposis colorectal cancer (Lynch syndrome) (Answer D) is an autosomal dominant syndrome caused by pathogenic variants in DNA mismatch-repair genes and is the most common hereditary cause of colorectal cancer. In addition to conferring an extremely high risk of colorectal cancer, there is an increased risk of endometrial cancer and other epithelial malignancies. However, no clear association between Lynch syndrome and thyroid cancer has been established.

Medullary thyroid carcinoma, rather than papillary thyroid carcinoma, is seen in the setting of multiple endocrine neoplasia type 2B (Answer E) and multiple endocrine neoplasia type 2A. Both hereditary syndromes are associated with pathogenic variants in the *RET* proto-oncogene.

Note: Image reprinted from Uchino S, Ishikawa H, Miyauchi A, et al. Age-and gender-specific risk of thyroid cancer in patients with familial adenomatous polyposis. *J Clin Endocrinol Metab*. 2016;101(12):4611-4617.

Educational Objective
Diagnose familial adenomatous polyposis in a patient with cribriform-morular variant of papillary thyroid cancer and a family history of tumors associated with familial adenomatous polyposis.

Reference(s)
Feng X, Milas M, O'Malley M, et al. Characteristics of benign and malignant thyroid disease in familial adenomatous polyposis patients and recommendations for disease surveillance. *Thyroid*. 2015;25(3):325-332. PMID: 25585202

Uchino S, Ishikawa H, Miyauchi A, et al. Age-and gender-specific risk of thyroid cancer in patients with familial adenomatous polyposis. *J Clin Endocrinol Metab*. 2016;101(12):4611-4617. PMID: 27623068

61 **ANSWER: B) Immune checkpoint inhibitor therapy–associated orchitis**
This man presents with symptomatic new-onset primary hypogonadism. His serum testosterone concentration before initiation of immune checkpoint inhibitor therapy was normal. Combined treatment with the programmed cell death receptor 1 (PD-1) inhibitor nivolumab and the cytotoxic T lymphocyte-associated antigen 4 (CTLA-4) inhibitor ipilimumab achieved a tumor response, as evidenced by fluorodeoxyglucose-PET. Unfortunately, immunotherapy had to cease because of a fulminant autoimmune response with multiple immune-related autoimmune events, including hepatitis, thyroiditis, and adrenalitis. Given the clinical presentation, immune checkpoint inhibitor therapy–associated orchitis (Answer B) is the most likely cause of his acute-onset primary hypogonadism. Although orchitis due to immune checkpoint inhibitor therapy is less common than other endocrine immune-related autoimmune events such as hypophysitis or thyroiditis, it has been described in several case reports, usually in the context of a fulminant autoimmune response with several other simultaneous immune-related autoimmune events, as in this case.

Orchitis is a rare immune-related autoimmune event because the testis is considered an immuno-privileged organ. The testis is able to tolerate autoantigens from germ cells that appear only after puberty when immunocompetence is already established. Mechanisms include the presence of an immunologic blood-testis barrier, secretion of immunosuppressive factors by testicular macrophages, and an anti-immunogenic repertoire of resident testicular T cells. The massive checkpoint inhibitor treatment–mediated cytotoxic T-cell activation, evidenced by multiple immune-related autoimmune events in this patient, most likely overwhelmed testicular immune defenses. In experimental models of autoimmune orchitis, a cytokine-mediated breakdown of the blood-testis barrier has been demonstrated, allowing inflow of immune cells with subsequent tissue infarction and cellular necrosis. Typically, orchitis is clinically manifested by testicular pain and swelling. While this patient did not recall localizing symptoms during his hospitalization, he was very unwell with marked delirium and was given high-dosage opioids. Interestingly, despite the fact that the female ovary is, compared with the male testis, a less immune-privileged organ, checkpoint inhibitor therapy–associated oophoritis leading to ovarian failure has not been described in the literature to date.

Although glucocorticoid and prolactin excess (Answers A and C) and high-dosage opioids can suppress the male gonadal axis, this suppression occurs at the hypothalamic-pituitary unit, leading to hypogonadotropic hypogonadism (ie, low testosterone with low or inappropriately normal gonadotropin concentrations). The clear-cut elevation of gonadotropins despite exposure to hyperprolactinemia, supraphysiologic glucocorticoids, and opioids denotes primary hypogonadism.

Similarly, severe illness (Answer E) leads to central gonadal axis suppression and can cause temporary hypogonadotropic hypogonadism. Recovery of the hypothalamic-pituitary unit is usually the rate-limiting step in the restoration of eugonadism, especially if the illness is relatively short-lived, and persistent primary hypogonadism is unlikely in the absence of coincidental direct testicular damage. This patient's severe primary hypogonadism persisted on follow-up review 1 month later and long-term testosterone replacement was initiated with resolution of his hypogonadal symptoms.

Thyroid hormone excess stimulates hepatic SHBG production (SHBG concentrations are sometimes measured to help distinguish a TSH-secreting pituitary adenoma from resistance to thyroid hormone), and thyrotoxicosis-associated elevations in SHBG (Answer D) can increase the estradiol-to-testosterone ratio, leading to gynecomastia. While a marked SHBG elevation can lead to a reflex rise in LH by reducing free testosterone, SHBG elevation to such an extent is unusual in the setting of thyrotoxicosis. This patient's thyroid function is currently relatively normal, consistent with recovery from thyroiditis. Moreover, his very low total testosterone is inconsistent with this diagnosis.

Educational Objective
Identify immune checkpoint inhibitor therapy–associated orchitis as a potential cause of primary hypogonadism.

Reference(s)
Quach HT, Robbins CJ, Balko JM, et al. Severe epididymo-orchitis and encephalitis complicating anti-PD-1 therapy. *Oncologist*. 2019;24(7):872-876. PMID: 30936376

Jacobo P, Guazzone VA, Theas MS, Lustig L. Testicular autoimmunity. *Autoimmun Rev*. 2011;10(4):201-204. PMID: 20932942

Brunet-Possenti F, Opsomer MA, Gomez L, Ouzaid I, Descamps V. Immune checkpoint inhibitors-related orchitis. *Ann Oncol*. 2017;28(4):906-907. PMID: 28039179

62 ANSWER: A) Low-carbohydrate

Medical nutrition therapy is a cornerstone of management in persons with diabetes. Data suggest that patients with type 2 diabetes can achieve up to a 2% reduction in hemoglobin A_{1c} levels after 3 to 6 months of medical nutrition therapy guided by a registered dietician. Furthermore, ongoing medical nutrition therapy has been shown to help maintain glycemia. The American Diabetes Association suggests individualized, diabetes-focused medical nutrition therapy. A variety of eating patterns are acceptable for diabetes management. Although long-term trials comparing patterns are not available, there is helpful information from shorter studies.

Low-carbohydrate diets generally imply less than 40% of calories from carbohydrates. As a reference, this equates to less than 200 g of carbohydrates for an individual consuming 2000 calories per day but less than 150 g for those consuming 1500 calories per day. One meta-analysis demonstrated that a low-carbohydrate diet (<45% calories from carbohydrates) was associated with 0.34% lowering of hemoglobin A_{1c} compared with diets with a higher percentage of carbohydrates within the first year of interventions. Further, greater carbohydrate restriction was associated with better glucose lowering. One study of patients with newly diagnosed type 2 diabetes prospectively followed for 4 years suggests that compared with a low-fat diet (Answer C), a Mediterranean diet that was noted to have lower carbohydrate content (<50%) as percentage of calories consumed improves glycemia and reduces the need for medication. Taken together, if the goal is improving glycemic control, patients should be encouraged to substantially reduce overall carbohydrate consumption (Answer A); the greater the carbohydrate reduction, the better the glycemic-lowering effect.

A Paleo eating pattern (Answer B) includes lean meats, fish, fruits, vegetables, nuts, and seeds, similar to what might have been eaten in the Paleolithic era. It limits dairy products, grains, and legumes. The DASH diet (Dietary Approaches to Stop Hypertension) (Answer D) is aimed at reducing hypertension. As such, it emphasizes foods that are lower in sodium and rich in potassium, magnesium, and calcium. DASH diet menus are plentiful in fruits, vegetables, low-fat dairy products, whole grains, nuts, fish, and poultry. Intermittent fasting programs (Answer E) suggest limiting intake of calories to specific hours of the day. Published data regarding the Paleo diet, DASH diet, and intermittent fasting strategies show either no or modest benefit regarding glycemic control. All of these studies are small and of such short duration that it would not be appropriate to recommend these strategies for the sake of glycemic control.

Educational Objective
Make recommendations on the basis of the recent nutrition therapy consensus statement from the American Diabetes Association and data supporting medical nutrition therapy useful in glycemic management.

Reference(s)

Esposito K, Maiorino MI, Ciotola M, et al. Effects of a Mediterranean-style diet on the need for antihyperglycemic drug therapy in patients with newly diagnosed type 2 diabetes: a randomized trial. *Ann Intern Med.* 2009;151(5):306-314. PMID: 19721018

Snorgaard O, Poulsen GM, Andersen HK, Astrup A. Systematic review and meta-analysis of dietary carbohydrate restriction in patients with type 2 diabetes. *BMJ Open Diabetes Res Care.* 2017;5(1):e3000354. PMID: 28316796

Evert AB, Dennison M, Gardner CD, et al. Nutrition therapy for adults with diabetes or prediabetes: a consensus report. *Diabetes Care.* 2019;42(5):731-754. PMID: 31000505

63 ANSWER: B) Very high, as he has other impaired pituitary axes

The pituitary gland is made of several kinds of cells, the most abundant of which are somatotroph cells. In general, but not always, when there is an insult to the gland, GH secretion is affected first, followed by gonadotroph function, and eventually TSH and ACTH secretory capacity. As a result, patients who have hypopituitarism are highly likely to be GH deficient.

In a study by Hartman et al including 817 patients with a history of either adult-onset hypothalamic-pituitary disease or childhood-onset GH deficiency, the probability of GH deficiency (diagnosed with a variety of GH-stimulation tests) increased progressively with the number of other axes that were affected. The proportion of patients in each group with severe GH deficiency was 41%, 67%, 83%, 96%, and 99% for patients with 0, 1, 2, 3, and 4 pituitary hormones deficiencies, respectively. Therefore, because this patient has central hypogonadism (treated) and central hypothyroidism (low free T_4 in the presence of inappropriately normal TSH), his pretest probability of having GH deficiency is about 80% (thus, Answer B is correct and Answers A and D are incorrect). It is not unusual for patients who are GH deficient to have a normal serum IGF-1 level, particularly in males. Indeed, in a study of adults with proven GH deficiency, the serum IGF-1 concentration was normal in 57% of men and 43% of women. In these cases, the only way to prove that the patient is indeed GH deficient is to perform a GH-stimulation test. If this patient had a frankly abnormal age-adjusted serum IGF-1, a stimulation test would not be needed to diagnose GH deficiency.

Although empty sella (Answer C) may be associated with GH deficiency, it is not a good predictor of insufficient GH secretion. The lack of symptoms (Answer D) does not exclude GH deficiency. GH deficiency in adults has important consequences on body composition, cholesterol levels, and bone density, so the diagnosis is not irrelevant because of his age (Answer E).

When interpreting results of GH-stimulation tests, one must remember that in general the GH peak is inversely proportional to BMI. Therefore, the cut-off may need to be adjusted depending on the patient's BMI. Different tests may have different cut-offs, and physicians should be familiar with the performance aspects of the test they use.

Educational Objective
Predict the probability of GH deficiency independently from the serum IGF-1 concentration in patients with hypopituitarism.

Reference(s)

Hartman ML, Crowe BJ, Biller BM, Ho KK, Clemmons DR, Chipman JJ; HyposCCS Advisory Board; U.S. HypoCCS Study Group. Which patients do not require a GH stimulation test for the diagnosis of adult GH deficiency? *J Clin Endocrinol Metab.* 2002;87(2):477-485. PMID: 11836272

Molitch ME, Clemmons DR, Malozowski S, Merriam GR, Vance ML; Endocrine Society. Evaluation and treatment of adult growth hormone deficiency: an Endocrine Society clinical practice guideline. *J Clin Endocrinol Metab.* 2011;96(6):1587-1609. PMID: 21602453

Svensson J, Johannsson G, Bengtsson BA. Insulin-like growth factor-I in growth hormone-deficient adults: relationship to population-based normal values, body composition and insulin tolerance test. *Clin Endocrinol (Oxf).* 1997;46(5):579-586. PMID: 9231054

64 ANSWER: A) Normocalcemic primary hyperparathyroidism

Primary hyperparathyroidism is typically characterized by hypercalcemia in the setting of inappropriately normal or elevated PTH levels. A newer presentation of primary hyperparathyroidism has been described in which serum PTH is elevated but serum calcium is consistently normal. This form of primary hyperparathyroidism, referred to as normocalcemic primary hyperparathyroidism (Answer A), was first formally recognized at the time of the Third International Workshop on the Management of Asymptomatic Primary Hyperparathyroidism in 2008. These patients have no obvious causes for secondary elevations of PTH and seem to have more substantial skeletal involvement than is typical in primary hyperparathyroidism. In making this diagnosis, it is critical to exclude other disorders that are associated with secondary or compensatory elevated PTH with normal calcium concentrations, such as vitamin D deficiency, chronic kidney disease (estimated glomerular filtration rate ≤60 mL/min per 1.73 m^2), medications known to increase PTH (eg, thiazides, bisphosphonates, denosumab, lithium), hypercalciuria, and malabsorption syndromes.

The woman described in this vignette has worsening osteoporosis in the setting of high-normal serum calcium, normal urinary calcium excretion, and elevated serum PTH. In addition, she has a normal vitamin D level and normal kidney function, making normocalcemic primary hyperparathyroidism (Answer A), and not secondary hyperparathyroidism (Answer B), the most likely diagnosis.

Tertiary hyperparathyroidism (Answer C) specifically refers to the development of autonomous parathyroid function and excessive PTH secretion after longstanding secondary hyperparathyroidism, resulting in hypercalcemia, which is not the case here. It typically occurs in patients with end-stage renal disease and after kidney transplant.

Familial hypocalciuric hypercalcemia (FHH) (Answer D) is a rare condition inherited in an autosomal dominant pattern, and it results from loss-of-function pathogenic variants in the calcium-sensing receptor gene (*CASR*). This makes the parathyroid glands less sensitive to calcium and also leads to an increase in tubular calcium reabsorption in the kidney, resulting in hypercalcemia and hypocalciuria. In patients with FHH, serum PTH concentrations are typically inappropriately normal or high in the presence of mild hypercalcemia, which again is not the case here. The major feature that distinguishes FHH from primary hyperparathyroidism is low urinary calcium excretion, with the calcium-to-creatinine clearance ratio typically less than 0.01. Individuals with FHH usually present in childhood and there is often a family history of asymptomatic hypercalcemia.

Finally, pseudohypoparathyroidism refers to a group of heterogeneous disorders defined by targeted organ (kidney and bone) unresponsiveness to PTH. Pseudohypoparathyroidism type 1a (Answer E) is an autosomal dominant disease caused by a loss-of-function pathogenic variant in the *GNAS* gene, and it requires maternal transmission of the variant. Patients with pseudohypoparathyroidism type 1a exhibit PTH resistance characterized by hypocalcemia, high-normal to high serum phosphate levels, and low serum 1,25-dihydroxyvitamin D levels despite significantly elevated serum PTH levels, which is not consistent with this patient's presentation. Affected patients also manifest Albright hereditary osteodystrophy, which is characterized by round facies, short stature, obesity, short fourth metacarpal bones, subcutaneous calcifications, and developmental delay.

Educational Objective
Recognize normocalcemic primary hyperparathyroidism as a form of primary hyperparathyroidism.

Reference(s)

Lowe H, McMahon DJ, Rubin MR, Bilezikian JP, Silverberg SJ. Normocalcemic primary hyperparathyroidism: further characterization of a new clinical phenotype. *J Clin Endocrinol Metab*. 2007;92(8):3001-3005. PMID: 17536001

Bilezikian JP, Khan AA, Potts JT Jr; Third International Workshop on the Management of Asymptomatic Primary Hyperthyroidism. Guidelines for the management of asymptomatic primary hyperparathyroidism: summary statement from the third international workshop. *J Clin Endocrinol Metab*. 2009;94(2):335-339. PMID: 19193908

Bilezikian JP, Silverberg SJ. Normocalcemic primary hyperparathyroidism. *Arq Bras Endocrinol Metabol*. 2010;54(2):106-109. PMID: 20485897

Cusano NE, Silverberg SJ, Bilezikian JP. Normocalcemic primary hyperparathyroidism. *J Clin Densitom*. 2013;16(1):33-39. PMID: 23374739

Cusano NE, Cipriani C, Bilezikian JP. Management of normocalcemic primary hyperparathyroidism. *Best Pract Res Clin Endocrinol Metab*. 2018;32(6):837-845. PMID: 30665550

65 ANSWER: E) Reassurance and no further testing

Recommendations for the evaluation and follow-up of incidentally discovered adrenal masses have evolved. The 2 key questions to ask when evaluating an incidentally discovered adrenal mass are: (1) could it be malignant? and (2) does it overproduce adrenal hormones?

This patient has a small, round, lipid-rich mass. An attenuation value less than 10 Hounsfield units on unenhanced CT is indicative of a lipid-rich entity, which is very reassuring for a benign adenoma. Lipid-rich consistency can similarly be demonstrated when a contrast protocol CT demonstrates absolute washout of 60% or more on delayed imaging. Similarly, lipid-rich characteristics can be assessed on MRI using in- and out-of-phase imaging. Although benign adenomas can still secrete excess hormones, they do not need to be radiographically surveilled prospectively when the initial imaging is this reassuring (thus, Answer E is correct).

The strongest evidence for this approach comes from a large meta-analysis and systematic review published in *Annals of Internal Medicine* in 2019 (Elhassan et al). After including more than 4000 patients with adrenal tumors followed in 32 studies, the authors made a number of important conclusions:

- Lipid-rich and benign-appearing adrenal tumors rarely exhibit meaningful growth over time; the mean growth was only 2 mm over 4 years and only 2.5% of masses grew more than 1 cm.
- There were no instances where a benign-appearing adrenal mass transformed into a malignancy.
- The initial hormone profile rarely changed; tumors that had mild hypercortisolism maintained this profile and only 4% of tumors developed new cortisol excess over time.

The findings of this study provide strong evidence to support recent recommendations from the European Society of Endocrinology, the European Network for the Study of Adrenal Tumors, and the American Association of Clinical Endocrinologists Adrenal Disease Network. These recommendations state that when an incidentally discovered adrenal mass exhibits a lipid-rich and reassuring appearance, no further radiographic imaging (Answer D) or surveillance is necessary. Further, if the initial cortisol profiling indicates nonfunctional status (ie, cortisol <1.8 μg/dL [<49.7 nmol/L] after 1 mg of dexamethasone), repeated biochemical testing is not indicated. One could consider retesting for hypercortisolism if there is substantial change in a patient's weight, glycemic status, blood pressure, or bone density in subsequent years; however, the likelihood of detecting a new clinically significant abnormality is very low.

Testing for hypercortisolism with a 1-mg dexamethasone-suppression test is recommended for every incidentally discovered adrenal mass because the prevalence of an abnormal finding (>1.8 μg/dL [>49.7 nmol/L]) may be 5% to 10%. Testing for aldosterone and renin (Answer A) is indicated when a patient with an adrenal mass also has hypertension and/or hypokalemia, which this patient does not. Although older guidelines underscored the importance of measuring metanephrines to assess all, or most, adrenal tumors, we have now learned that the probability of a pheochromocytoma is essentially zero among adrenal masses with a lipid-rich appearance. Therefore, testing for metanephrines (Answer C) is not necessary in these situations and may have a much higher false-positive rate when compared with a true-positive value. Measurement of adrenal androgens (Answer B) can be helpful in patients who exhibit clinical signs of hyperandrogenism, or when there is concern that the adrenal mass may be a primary adrenal carcinoma. However, this patient has neither indication.

Educational Objective

Evaluate and manage incidentally discovered adrenal masses.

Reference(s)

Elhassan YS, Alahdab F, Prete A, et al. Natural history of adrenal incidentalomas with and without mild autonomous cortisol excess. *Ann Intern Med.* 2019;171(2):107-116. PMID: 31234202

Fassnacht M, Arlt W, Bancos I, et al. Management of adrenal incidentalomas: European Society of Endocrinology clinical practice guideline. *Eur J Endocrinol.* 2016;175(2):G1-G34. PMID: 27390021

Vaidya A, Hamrahian A, Bancos I, Fleseriu M, Ghayee HK. The evaluation of incidentally discovered adrenal masses. *Endocr Pract.* 2019;25(2):178-192. PMID: 30817193

66 ANSWER: C) Recommend massage, warm compresses, oral hydration, and nonsteroidal antiinflammatory drugs as needed for pain

This patient is experiencing acute sialadenitis of the submandibular glands following radioactive iodine therapy. The parotid, submandibular, and sublingual glands all contain the sodium-iodide symporter and are able to concentrate iodine to as high as 7 to 700 times the plasma levels. The salivary glands can thus receive a significant radiation dose as a consequence of radioactive iodine therapy for thyroid cancer, leading to salivary gland dysfunction. The parotid glands are most commonly affected. The reported frequency of salivary gland adverse effects after radioactive iodine varies widely, ranging from 5% to 86%. Long-term salivary gland dysfunction is uncommon, occurring in approximately 5% of patients. Risk factors for sialadenitis following radioactive iodine include higher administered activity of ^{131}I, female sex, history of sialadenitis, and concomitant Sjogren syndrome.

Acute sialadenitis classically presents with swollen and painful salivary glands, but it can be asymptomatic, with patients presenting with xerostomia many months later. Acute salivary gland signs and symptoms often resolve spontaneously within hours to several days without any specific treatment. The development of xerostomia predisposes patients to dental caries.

Conservative measures, including massage, warm compresses, oral hydration, and nonsteroidal antiinflammatory drugs as needed for pain (Answer C), are often recommended in the initial management of sialadenitis following radioactive iodine therapy unless symptoms are severe, although the efficacy of nonsteroidal antiinflammatory drugs is unproven. Sialogogic agents (eg, sour candies) can also be considered, but evidence of benefit is lacking. Avoidance of anticholinergic medications is generally recommended. In the setting of severe pain or swelling, oral glucocorticoid therapy (eg, methylprednisolone) should be considered. Sialendoscopy has been shown to be an effective treatment option for the management of radioactive iodine-associated sialadenitis that is refractory to conservative therapy. Signs and symptoms of suppurative sialadenitis include pain, purulent salivary return, foul taste, and fever. This diagnosis should prompt an urgent referral to a dentist, oral surgeon, or otolaryngologist and the initiation of antibiotic therapy. The patient's clinical presentation is not consistent with suppurative sialadenitis; initiating amoxicillin-clavulanate twice daily (Answer A) is not indicated.

There is no evidence that the patient has persistent thyroid cancer. The palpable mass in right zone 1B is a swollen submandibular gland. Lymph node metastasis to neck zone 1 is exceedingly uncommon in thyroid cancer, and the patient's stimulated thyroglobulin and posttherapy whole-body scan are reassuring and indicative of an excellent response to therapy. Increasing the levothyroxine dosage to achieve a serum TSH value less than 0.1 mIU/L (Answer B), performing FNA biopsy (Answer D) of the right zone 1 mass, or administering radioactive iodine therapy again with a higher administered activity of ^{131}I (Answer E) would be inappropriate. Additional radioactive iodine therapy would most likely exacerbate the patient's ongoing salivary gland dysfunction and would put her at unnecessary risk for additional complications.

Educational Objective

Manage the most common complication of radioactive iodine therapy—sialadenitis.

Reference(s)

Bhayani MK, Acharya V, Kongkiatkamon S, et al. Sialendoscopy for patients with radioiodine-induced sialadenitis and xerostomia. *Thyroid.* 2015;25(7):834-838. PMID: 25860842

Hollingsworth B, Senter L, Zhang X, et al. Risk factors of 131I-induced salivary gland damage in thyroid cancer patients. *J Clin Endocrinol Metab.* 2016;101(11):4085-4093. PMID: 27533304

Mandel SJ, Mandel L. Radioactive iodine and the salivary glands. *Thyroid.* 2003;13(3):265-271. PMID: 12729475

67 ANSWER: D) Liraglutide

Despite numerous attempts by the patient to increase exercise and reduce caloric intake, he admits that he always relapses to his old dietary and sedentary habits. His BMI remains greater than 30 kg/m². Among many other potential interventions (bariatric surgery referral, individual exercise prescription, continued nutrition counseling, etc), he is a candidate for antiobesity therapy. Liraglutide (Answer D) is a GLP-1 receptor agonist indicated as an adjunct to a reduced-calorie diet and increased physical activity for chronic weight management in adult patients with an initial BMI of:

- ≥30 kg/m² (obesity)
- ≥27 kg/m² (overweight) in the presence of at least 1 weight-related comorbid condition (eg, hypertension, type 2 diabetes, or dyslipidemia)

The recommended liraglutide dosage for the management of obesity is 3 mg daily. It is initiated at 0.6 mg daily for 1 week and then increased at weekly intervals as tolerated until a dosage of 3 mg daily is reached. The cost of antiobesity medications such as liraglutide may serve as a barrier to use in many instances, as in general, insurance coverage for these therapies is limited.

The primary intent of using liraglutide therapy in this patient is weight loss. However, results from the SCALE Obesity and Prediabetes 3-year extension trial showed that individuals who took liraglutide, 3 mg once daily, for 3 years, in addition to making healthy lifestyle changes to diet and exercise, were 79% less likely to be diagnosed with type 2 diabetes in that timeframe than individuals who changed their diet and exercise alone (placebo group). By week 160, 26 of 1472 participants (2%) in the liraglutide group vs 46 of 738 participants (6%) in the placebo group were diagnosed with diabetes while on treatment. The mean time from randomization to diagnosis was 99 weeks (SD 47) for the 26 participants in the liraglutide group vs 87 weeks (SD 47) for the 46 participants in the placebo group. Accordingly, among the treatment options offered in this case, liraglutide (Answer D) would be the best option.

The Diabetes Prevention Program demonstrated a reduced risk of developing type 2 diabetes in patients with impaired glucose tolerance who received metformin therapy or lifestyle intervention (lifestyle intervention decreased the incidence of type 2 diabetes by 58% compared with 31% in the metformin-treated group). Metformin in this case would have been a great choice had it been a potential answer option.

While some early reports suggested that there may be links between vitamin D levels and type 2 diabetes, in a randomized controlled clinical trial of patients at high risk for type 2 diabetes not selected for vitamin D insufficiency, vitamin D_3 supplementation (Answer A) at a dose of 4000 IU per day did not result in a significantly lower risk of diabetes when compared with placebo.

Pioglitazone (Answer B) (and other thiazolidinediones) have demonstrated an ability to reduce the risk of progressing from prediabetes to type 2 diabetes. However, this patient's 30 pack-year history of cigarette smoking and employment in the rubber manufacturing industry, both risk factors for developing bladder cancer, do not make pioglitazone a good option in this case. Recognition of risk factors that would preclude use of any medical therapy is very important; it is critical that the risks and benefits of any medical therapy are thoroughly reviewed before they are initiated. Lastly, pioglitazone may also potentiate further weight gain, which would be undesirable in this patient.

While Yassin et al recently reported that long-term testosterone therapy (Answer C) prevents progression from prediabetes to type 2 diabetes in men with hypogonadism and improves glycemia, lipids, and metabolic and anthropometric parameters, it is important to note that this was an observational study, not a randomized controlled trial. In addition, this patient has obstructive sleep apnea with reported nonadherence to CPAP therapy (supported by his slightly elevated hematocrit noted on laboratory assessment, which is indicative of hypoxia). In this setting, testosterone replacement therapy would not be advised. His fatigue would best be addressed by attempts to improve his adherence to CPAP therapy and engagement in a lifestyle modification program to assist him in losing weight, which may also improve his state of hypogonadism. Lastly, generally speaking, testosterone therapy usually does not result in weight loss, which is one of the primary goals in this patient.

Angiotensin-receptor blocker therapy (Answer E) has been reported to reduce the risk of developing new-onset type 2 diabetes, but in this patient with normal blood pressure, it is not indicated.

Educational Objective

Differentiate among interventions that have been reported to reduce the risk of progression to type 2 diabetes in at-risk patients.

Reference(s)

Bhasin S, Brito JP, Cunningham GR, et al. Testosterone therapy in men with hypogonadism: an Endocrine Society clinical practice guideline. *J Clin Endocrinol Metab.* 2018;103(5):1715-1744. PMID: 29562364

Knowler WC, Barrett-Connor E, Fowler SE, et al; Diabetes Prevention Program Research Group. Reduction in the incidence of type 2 diabetes with lifestyle intervention or metformin. *N Engl J Med.* 2002;346(6):393-403. PMID: 11832527

Yassin A, Haider A, Haider KS, et al. Testosterone therapy in men with hypogonadism prevents progression from prediabetes to type 2 diabetes: eight-year data from a registry study. *Diabetes Care.* 2019;42(6):1104-1111. PMID: 30862651

Kernan WN, Viscoli CM, Furie KL, et al; Iris Trial Investigators. Pioglitazone after ischemic stroke or transient ischemic attack. *N Engl J Med* 2016;374(14):1321-1331. PMID: 26886418

U.S. Food and Drug Administration. FDA Drug Safety Communication: Updated FDA review concludes that use of type 2 diabetes medicine pioglitazone may be linked to an increased risk of bladder cancer. Available at: https://www.fda.gov/drugs/drug-safety-and-availability/fda-drug-safety-communication-updated-fda-review-concludes-use-type-2-diabetes-medicine-pioglitazone. Accessed for verification December 2019.

Letašiová S, Medveďová A, Šovčíková A, et al. Bladder cancer, a review of the environmental risk factors. *Environ Health.* 2012;11(Suppl 1):S11. PMID: 22759493

Gillespie EL, White CM, Kardas M, Lindberg M, Coleman CI. The impact of ACE inhibitors and angiotensin II type 1 receptor blockers on the development of new-onset type 2 diabetes. *Diabetes Care.* 2005;28(9):2261-2266. PMID: 16123505

le Roux CW, Astrup A, Fujioka K, et al; SCALE Obesity Prediabetes NN8022-1839 Study Group. 3 years of liraglutide versus placebo for type 2 diabetes risk reduction and weight management in individuals with prediabetes: a randomised, double-blind trial. *Lancet.* 2017;389(10077):1399-1409. PMID: 28237263

Pittas AG, Dawson-Hughes B, Sheehan P, et al. Vitamin D supplementation and prevention of type 2 diabetes. *N Engl J Med.* 2019;381(6):520-530. PMID: 31173679

68 ANSWER: C) [131]I whole-body scan with SPECT-CT

Differentiated thyroid carcinoma (DTC) accounts for most thyroid cancers and usually has a good prognosis. In rare cases, it can present with distant metastasis at the time of diagnosis. Among DTC, papillary thyroid carcinoma is the most common (85%), followed by follicular thyroid carcinoma (12%). Papillary thyroid carcinoma can spread to cervical lymph nodes, but follicular thyroid carcinoma typically spreads via hematogenous dissemination to distant sites and usually does not spread to cervical lymph nodes. Distant metastases occur in 10% to 15% of patients with follicular thyroid carcinoma. Common sites of distant metastases are the lungs and bone. Other sites such as the liver, brain, skin, and adrenal glands can harbor distant metastases, but these are less common. When metastasis to the adrenal glands occurs, it can be unilateral, solitary, and often asymptomatic.

Staging after thyroidectomy provides prognostic information. TNM classification (tumor, node, metastasis) predicts disease-specific mortality, and the American Thyroid Association risk of recurrence staging system predicts recurrence risk. Important prognostic features include stage, age, tumor characteristics, and presence of distant metastases. The treatment of follicular thyroid carcinoma consists of surgery, followed by radioiodine treatment in patients at high risk and selected patients at intermediate risk, and thyroid hormone suppressive therapy. In the case of persistent disease after suppressive thyroid hormone therapy and radioiodine treatment with no further evidence of radioactive iodine–avid disease, external beam radiation therapy can be considered. Additionally, tyrosine kinase inhibitors may be indicated for persistent/progressive non–iodine-avid disease despite other mentioned treatments.

The patient in this vignette recently underwent total thyroidectomy for an FNA-proven follicular neoplasm. The final pathology revealed an invasive follicular thyroid carcinoma. Due to hematuria 4 weeks later, abdominal CT was performed, which showed a 2.6-cm heterogeneous mass in the right adrenal gland. Further evaluation for pheochromocytoma, aldosteronism, and Cushing syndrome was unremarkable. As this adrenal nodule is not producing hormones, and it is heterogeneous, it could be either adrenal carcinoma (although the size is small for a typical adrenal carcinoma) or metastasis from follicular thyroid carcinoma. The imaging characteristics on abdominal CT rule out the possibility of a benign adrenal mass. Low unenhanced CT attenuation values (≤10 Hounsfield units) suggest that the likelihood of a benign adenoma is close to 100%. If the unenhanced CT attenuation is greater than 10 Hounsfield units, the contrast washout should be measured in the adrenal lesion. An absolute contrast medium washout greater than 50% after 10 minutes following contrast administration is consistent with a benign adenoma. The patient in this vignette has a 2.6-cm heterogeneous right adrenal mass with a precontrast attenuation value of 20 Hounsfield units and less than 50% contrast washout at 10 minutes. All these findings suggest that the adrenal mass is not benign. Although adrenal metastases from differentiated thyroid cancer are uncommon, this possibility should be included in the differential diagnosis of a patient with follicular thyroid cancer and an adrenal gland lesion. This patient should have measurement of serum TSH (>30 mIU/L), thyroglobulin, and thyroglobulin antibodies and undergo a radioactive iodine whole-body scan (Answer C) to check for distant metastases and to determine whether the right adrenal lesion concentrates radioactive iodine.

FNA biopsy of the adrenal mass (Answer A) is not recommended because of the potential risk of seeding adrenal cancer, but it might be indicated in distinguishing between an adrenal tumor and a metastatic tumor. Right adrenalectomy (Answer D) is not yet indicated, as there is not enough information about the adrenal mass. If the ^{131}I whole-body scan with SPECT-CT shows uptake in the right adrenal gland, right adrenalectomy should be considered followed by radioiodine treatment. In the case of non–iodine-avid metastases, tyrosine kinase inhibitors can be considered. The patient has follicular thyroid carcinoma and this does not usually metastasize to cervical lymph nodes. Therefore, neck ultrasonography (Answer B) is not the best answer. Chest CT (Answer E) is also not necessary, as the ^{131}I whole-body scan with SPECT-CT can provide further information about the presence or absence of lung metastasis.

Educational Objective
Identify different sites of metastasis from thyroid cancer, including the adrenal glands.

Reference(s)

Grebe SK, Hay ID. Follicular thyroid cancer. *Endocrinol Metab Clin North Am*. 1995;24(4):761-801. PMID: 8608779

Haugen BR, Alexander EK, Bible KC, et al. 2015 American Thyroid Association management guidelines for adult patients with thyroid nodules and differentiated thyroid cancer: the American Thyroid Association Guidelines Task Force on Thyroid Nodules and Differentiated Thyroid Cancer. *Thyroid*. 2016;26(1):1-133. PMID: 26462967

Ranade R, Thapa P, Basu S. Adrenal metastasis from differentiated thyroid carcinoma documented on post-therapy (131)I scan: a case based discussion. *World J Radiol*. 2014;6(3):56-61. PMID: 24765241

69 ANSWER: C) Progesterone test for withdrawal bleed

Although an adult endocrinologist might not be the first to evaluate an adolescent with primary amenorrhea, they might need to pursue additional testing to confirm a diagnosis if an adolescent did not have a complete evaluation. Combined oral contraceptives would restore estrogen deficiency, but they would not exclude the possibility of secondary hypogonadism. The key question that changes the nature of the evaluation is whether the patient has evidence of delayed puberty vs stalled puberty, growth failure, and estrogen deficiency, which would lead to additional testing. This patient did have evidence of some pubertal development, with thelarche occurring at age 11 years. Adolescents with thelarche followed by delayed development of secondary sex characteristics and primary amenorrhea within 4 years of thelarche are considered to have stalled puberty. Further evaluation is more likely when an adolescent with delayed puberty also demonstrates growth failure and an evaluation for GH deficiency is initiated. Secondary hypogonadism or hypogonadotrophic hypogonadism can be caused by constitutional delay of growth and puberty, which is the most common cause of delayed puberty. The diagnosis of isolated GnRH deficiency or idiopathic hypogonadotropic hypogonadism is typically a diagnosis of exclusion. Although there can be associated anosmia or hyposmia in Kallmann syndrome and other rare phenotypic associations of midline defects, hearing loss, unilateral renal agenesis or skeletal defects, absent or stalled puberty development can both occur. Although constitutional delay of growth is usually diagnosed by spontaneous progression through puberty, this might also occur in isolated GnRH deficiency, which is not exclusively diagnosed by associated pathogenic variants. Although isolated GnRH deficiency might be suspected more with known family history of isolated GnRH deficiency or pathogenic variants, congenital delay of growth and puberty can be familial as well or be seen at higher rates in families with isolated GnRH deficiency. Isolated GnRH deficiency is often diagnosed if puberty has not progressed by age 18.

The patient's estradiol concentrations are not in the ideal confirmatory estrogen-sufficient range (100-200 pg/mL [367.1-734.2 pmol/L]). Therefore, the best next step would be to prescribe progesterone for 10 days (Answer C) to see if there is enough endogenous estrogen present to develop an endometrial lining and result in a menstrual period after about 2 weeks of completing the progesterone treatment.

Antimullerian hormone (Answer D) is associated with antral follicle count and could be particularly helpful in assessing for polycystic ovarian morphology in adolescents when transvaginal ultrasonography might not be easily performed. However, until improved standardization of assays allows for established thresholds and validation on a large scale in population samples of different ages and ethnicities, antimullerian hormone cannot be used as a diagnostic criterion for polycystic ovarian morphology or polycystic ovary syndrome. Although it might be low in secondary hypogonadism, there is insufficient evidence to suggest that it can be used to differentiate primary ovarian insufficiency or secondary hypogonadism from anovulatory amenorrhea.

If the patient does not have a withdrawal bleed after progesterone, pituitary MRI (Answer B) would be reasonable, but it would not be necessary if she has a withdrawal bleed.

If she did not have clinically significant recurrent cystic acne in an androgenetic pattern, more detailed testing for androgen excess with measurement of androstenedione and free testosterone (Answer A) might be considered.

Even though polycystic ovary syndrome is commonly associated with obesity, a lean or normal BMI, as in this patient, does not exclude the diagnosis. Before diagnosing polycystic ovary syndrome, measuring 17-hydroxyprogesterone (Answer E) would be recommended. However, the more important step is to exclude secondary hypogonadism in this patient, so the progesterone withdrawal test is the best recommendation now.

Educational Objective
Diagnose polycystic ovary syndrome in a woman with primary amenorrhea.

Reference(s)
Legro RS, Arslanian SA, Ehrmann DA, et al; Endocrine Society. Diagnosis and treatment of polycystic ovary syndrome: an Endocrine Society clinical practice guideline. *J Clin Endocrinol Metab.* 2013;98(12):4565-4592. PMID: 24151290

Iwase A, Nakamura T, Osuka S, Takikawa S, Goto M, Kikkawa F. Anti-mullerian hormone as a marker of ovarian reserve: what have we learned, and what should we know? *Reprod Med Biol.* 2015;15(3):127-136. PMID: 29259429

Abbara A, Eng PC, Phylactou M, et al. Anti-mullerian hormone (AMH) in the diagnosis of menstrual disturbance due to polycystic ovarian syndrome. *Front Endocrinol (Lausanne).* 2019;10:656. PMID: 31616381

70   ANSWER: D) Measure serum 24,25-dihydroxyvitamin D

In patients who present with hypercalcemia, the initial clinical question is to define whether the condition is PTH dependent or independent. This patient's PTH concentration is below 20 pg/mL (<20 ng/L), which would be considered a PTH-independent process. Having established this, it is important to know that the differential diagnosis for PTH-independent hypercalcemia is relatively broad. Causes of PTH-independent hypercalcemia can generally be stratified into those with or without excessive 1,25-dihydroxyvitamin D production. This patient has elevated serum calcitriol with hypercalciuria, the latter of which is generally defined as calcium excretion of more than 4 mg/kg per day. In addition, there is evidence that the hypercalciuria is longstanding and chronic based on the presence of nephrocalcinosis. Finally, a family history of nephrolithiasis and osteoporosis in her father is consistent with an inherited disorder of vitamin D metabolism. Given her constellation of signs and symptoms, this patient most likely has a pathogenic variant in the *CYP24A1* gene, resulting in diminished catabolism of calcitriol to the inert compound 24,25-dihydroxyvitamin D. While this disorder can be confirmed by genetic testing, the initial recommended screening test is measurement of the ratio of serum 25-hydroxyvitamin D to 24,25-dihydroxyvitamin D. A ratio greater than 99 reliably identifies patients who are candidates for genetic testing of the *CYP24A1* gene. Thus, measuring 24,25-dihydroxyvitamin D (Answer D) is the best next step. While there is no definitive therapy for this disease, treatment with P450 enzyme inhibitors such as fluconazole have been shown to benefit patients by reducing 1,25-dihydroxyvitamin D levels and improving hypercalcemia and hypercalciuria.

Although granulomatous disease is not an uncommon cause of PTH-independent hypercalcemia, this patient has no pertinent symptoms (cough, fever, weight loss) or chest x-ray findings, making a diagnosis of tuberculosis-induced hypercalcemia extremely unlikely. Thus, a test for tuberculosis (Answer E) is not needed.

The negative chest x-ray findings and the patient's ethnicity render a diagnosis of sarcoidosis very unlikely. Furthermore, measuring serum angiotensin-converting enzyme (Answer A) is not an established diagnostic test for sarcoidosis.

Malignant disorders such as multiple myeloma can also cause PTH-independent hypercalcemia, although this would not result in elevated serum calcitriol. Her young age and normal total protein-to-albumin ratio (<2) are inconsistent with paraprotein-related hypercalcemia, and protein electrophoresis (Answer B) is not needed. Other malignancies such as lymphoma can also cause PTH-independent hypercalcemia with concomitant elevation of serum 1,25-dihydroxyvitamin D, although the patient's age and lack of constitutional symptoms make this very unlikely.

Finally, although vitamin A toxicity is a rare cause of PTH-independent hypercalcemia, it is due to retinoid-induced osteoclast activation and is not associated with altered calcitriol production or catabolism. Thus, measuring vitamin A (Answer C) is incorrect.

Educational Objective
Recommend appropriate management for hypercalcemia and nephrocalcinosis in a patient with a pathogenic variant in the *CYP24A1* gene.

Reference(s)
Ketha H, Kumar R, Singh RJ. LC-MS/MS for identifying patients with CYP24A1 mutations. *Clin Chem.* 2016;62(1):236-242. PMID: 26585929

Tebben PJ, Milliner DS, Horst RL, et al. Hypercalcemia, hypercalciuria, and elevated calcitriol concentrations with autosomal dominant transmission due to CYP24A1 mutations: effects of ketoconazole therapy. *J Clin Endocrinol Metab.* 2012;97(3):E423-E427. PMID: 22337913

71 ANSWER: E) Insufficient data to make a diagnosis
Determining the etiology of diabetes mellitus can be challenging. It is critical to determine whether a patient has type 1 diabetes, type 2 diabetes, or another form of diabetes, as the correct diagnosis will lead to treatment with the appropriate antihyperglycemic medication.

Given that more than 90% of patients with diabetes in industrialized countries have type 2 diabetes (Answer C), this is certainly a possible diagnosis in this patient. However, there are clues that she may have an atypical form of diabetes. She has a history of gestational diabetes treated with insulin. The insulin was stopped at the time of delivery and she had no antihyperglycemic treatment until she presented in mild diabetic ketoacidosis 8 months later. She was appropriately started on insulin and now has reasonable glycemic control on basal insulin alone. Even though she presented in mild diabetic ketoacidosis, this is unlikely to represent type 1 diabetes (Answer A), as her C-peptide concentration was in the normal range at the most recent clinic visit.

Latent autoimmune diabetes in adults (LADA) (Answer B) is a heterogeneous disorder that may affect up to 10% of all patients with diabetes, and it shares genetic and clinical features of both type 1 and type 2 diabetes. Patients with LADA are generally 30 years or older at the time of diagnosis, have detectable C-peptide levels, and have elevated autoimmune diabetes markers (eg, glutamic acid decarboxylase antibodies, islet-cell antibodies, insulinoma-associated antigen 2 antibodies, and/or zinc transporter 8 antibodies). Patients with LADA tend to progress more rapidly to insulin treatment than patients with typical type 2 diabetes. The patient in this vignette may have LADA, as her C-peptide level was in the normal range at the time of diabetes diagnosis. However, autoimmune markers have not been obtained. Therefore, LADA cannot be diagnosed until further testing is completed.

Given the history and examination findings, this patient could also have a monogenic form of diabetes (maturity-onset diabetes of the young [MODY]) (Answer D). Patients with MODY are usually normal weight or overweight, are usually diagnosed in the second or third decade of life, have an autosomal dominant mode of transmission, have detectable C-peptide levels, do not require insulin treatment initially, and lack autoimmune diabetes markers. Patients with MODY are often misdiagnosed as having either type 1 or type 2 diabetes. However, she presented in mild diabetic ketoacidosis and this would not favor a diagnosis of monogenic diabetes. Autoimmune markers should be assessed and would be undetectable if the patient had MODY. Therefore, MODY cannot be diagnosed at this time.

The vignette contains insufficient data to make a diagnosis (Answer E). Measuring glutamic acid decarboxylase antibodies (or other autoimmune markers) would help to differentiate the type of diabetes this patient has and may be important in the treatment of other family members with diabetes.

Educational Objective
Determine the etiology of diabetes based on the medical and family history, physical examination, and laboratory data.

Reference(s)
Cervin C, Lyssenko V, Bakhtadze E, et al. Genetic similarities between latent autoimmune diabetes in adults, type 1 diabetes, and type 2 diabetes. *Diabetes.* 2008;57(5):1433-1437. PMID: 18310307

Thanabalasingham G, Owen KR. Diagnosis and management of maturity onset diabetes of the young (MODY). *BMJ.* 2011;343:d6044. PMID: 22012810

72 ANSWER: C) Measurement of plasma metanephrines

A new adrenal mass in this patient with a recent history of lymphoma is concerning for recurrence of lymphoma in the adrenal gland. However, the adrenal mass could also represent a coincident primary adrenal neoplasm. This patient's subsequent management will depend on how well these entities can be distinguished.

The radiographic characteristics of an adrenal mass are critical in evaluating whether the mass is benign or potentially malignant. Reassuring features that are suggestive of a benign adrenal mass include small size (generally <4 cm), round and uniform shape, homogenous appearance, and high lipid content (such as low attenuation on unenhanced CT [<10 Hounsfield units] or loss of signal on out-of-phase sequencing on MRI), and high contrast washout on delayed contrast CT imaging (>60% absolute washout and >40% relative washout).

Features that raise concern for a malignant process include larger size (generally >4 cm), irregular shape or contours, heterogeneous content, calcifications, low lipid content on CT or MRI, poor washout on delayed contrast CT imaging, and fluorodeoxyglucose avidity on PET scan.

A benign pheochromocytoma or a malignant adrenocortical carcinoma usually displays poor lipid content, poor washout on delayed contrast CT imaging, and fluorodeoxyglucose avidity. Pheochromocytomas almost never exhibit an unenhanced CT attenuation value less than 10 Hounsfield units.

The best way to ascertain the origins of the adrenal mass is to review the findings on histopathology. The specimen can be obtained either by biopsy or surgery (Answers A, B, and E); however, a pheochromocytoma must be excluded before proceeding with either option. Biopsy of a pheochromocytoma is not advised given the risk of precipitating a catecholamine crisis. Therefore, the best step now is to measure plasma metanephrines (Answer C) to evaluate for a pheochromocytoma. The absence of hallmark hyperadrenergic symptoms and signs does not exclude the diagnosis of a pheochromocytoma. Resumption of lymphoma-directed chemotherapy (Answer D) can be considered; however, a tissue diagnosis to confirm lymphoma, and/or metanephrines and other hormonal evaluation to exclude a primary adrenal tumor, are warranted before proceeding with chemotherapy.

In this case, the patient's plasma metanephrines were markedly elevated, and pheochromocytoma was diagnosed. He was ultimately found to have a pathogenic variant in the *SDHD* gene. The patient's lymphoma and pheochromocytoma were incidental issues, as there is currently no known connection between the 2 conditions.

Educational Objective
Evaluate and manage incidentally discovered adrenal masses and list indications for biopsy of an adrenal mass.

Reference(s)
Lenders JW, Duh QY, Eisenhofer G, et al; Endocrine Society. Pheochromocytoma and paraganglioma: an Endocrine Society clinical practice guideline. *J Clin Endocrinol Metab.* 2014;99(6):1915-1942. PMID: 24893135

73 ANSWER: E) Cholestatic liver disease

In the setting of cholestatic liver disease (Answer E), a unique abnormal lipoprotein is often present that has similar density to that of LDL, but it does not have its surface protein signature, apolipoprotein B. This lipoprotein contains only phospholipid and unesterified cholesterol and is referred to as lipoprotein X. In cholestasis there is impaired bile flow; it is believed that these lipoprotein-like lipoprotein X particles are due to reflux of biliary lipoproteins into the systemic circulation. Lipoprotein X elevation is common in cholestatic liver diseases, occurring in up to 45% of cases. Extreme cholesterol elevations can occur with resultant artifactual abnormalities in electrolytes (hyponatremia) and hyperviscosity. Apolipoprotein B levels are typically low. Xanthomas can occur in the palms. However, such significant elevations in cholesterol are often reflective of significant liver dysfunction, as lipoprotein X can only be cleared by hepatocytes. Hypercholesterolemia will resolve only after liver dysfunction resolves. Plasma exchange can be used as a temporizing measure to decrease cholesterol levels. In end-stage liver disease, liver transplant results in complete reversal of the lipid abnormalities. LDL apheresis, which physically removes LDL particles (by virtue of the presence of apolipoprotein B on LDL) from the blood, will not clear lipoprotein X because it lacks apolipoprotein B on its surface. Lipoprotein X is not thought to be an atherogenic lipoprotein. Diagnosis of lipoprotein X is usually made clinically, although the presence or absence of these particles can be measured using agarose gel electrophoresis (a send-out test not widely available). Resolution of cholestasis will result in the disappearance of these particles and often involves liver transplant.

This patient has very high cholesterol and triglyceride levels in the setting of severe cholestatic liver disease. Homozygous familial hypercholesterolemia (Answer A) is a rare, life-threatening genetic disorder resulting from pathogenic variants in the gene encoding the LDL receptor, which result in lack of LDL receptors. It is characterized by extremely high plasma cholesterol levels greater than 500 mg/dL (>12.95 mmol/L). The incidence is approximately 1 in 1 million, and affected individuals present at a very young age with tendon xanthomas and accelerated, progressive, premature coronary disease before age 20 years. The patient in this vignette has no clinical findings suggestive of homozygous familial hypercholesterolemia.

Familial forms of hypertriglyceridemia (Answer B) can result in very high triglyceride levels (>2000 mg/dL [>22.60 mmol/L]), but cholesterol levels are seldom as high as those seen in this patient.

Hepatic lipase deficiency (Answer C) is an extremely rare autosomal recessive disorder caused by pathogenic variants in the gene encoding the enzyme hepatic lipase. Hepatic lipase is synthesized in hepatocytes and breaks down phospholipids and triglycerides of circulating lipoproteins. Hepatic lipase removes triglycerides from intermediate-density lipoproteins and converts these to LDL particles. Individuals with hepatic lipase deficiency have abnormally high levels of HDL cholesterol and very low numbers of LDL particles. This patient's lipid panel is not consistent with hepatic lipase deficiency.

Ursodiol (Answer D) is a water-soluble bile acid derived from cholesterol and is used in patients with cholestatic liver disease. Administration increases concentration of endogenous ursodiol in the bile-acid pool and can replace toxic bile acids in cholestasis. Ursodiol has no known direct effects on lipids.

Educational Objective
Explain the effect of cholestatic liver disease on lipoprotein metabolism and lipoprotein X.

Reference(s)
Heinl RE, Tennant HM, Ricketts JC, et al. Lipoprotein-X disease in the setting of severe cholestatic hepatobiliary autoimmune disease. *J Clin Lipidol.* 2017;11(1):282-286. PMID: 28391896

Fellin R, Manzato E. Lipoprotein-X fifty years after its original discovery. *Nutr Metab Cardiovasc Dis.* 2019;29(1):4-8. PMID: 30503707

74 ANSWER: D) Trimethoprim-sulfamethoxazole

Several case reports have demonstrated an association between trimethoprim-sulfamethoxazole (Answer D) and hypoglycemia, particularly with higher dosages in the setting of renal failure, in which case the hypoglycemia may be prolonged and last several hours despite dextrose infusion. Studies suggest that this is due to inappropriate insulin secretion with documentation of elevated C-peptide levels. Therefore, evaluating C-peptide levels after the dose would be appropriate. It is postulated that this may be caused by sulfonamides acting at the sulfonylurea receptor, although this is not proven. In this patient, there was a temporal association between the dose of trimethoprim-sulfamethoxazole and the occurrence of hypoglycemia, highlighting the importance of reviewing the medication record. When dosed intravenously, it is advised that the dose be given over 3 to 4 divided doses. It is possible that this high dose, given once every 24 hours, accounted for the patient's hypoglycemia.

Primary adrenal insufficiency (Answer E) is a reasonable consideration in this patient. Early in the history of HIV/AIDS, gross abnormalities in adrenal pathology were not uncommonly found at autopsy. However, with the use of highly active antiretroviral therapy, glucocorticoid deficiency is now rare. Moreover, the absence of hypotension, hyponatremia, and hyperkalemia makes this a less likely consideration.

Malnutrition (Answer C) can predispose to hypoglycemia because of poor glycogen stores, but it is unlikely to be the sole factor in patients who have hypoglycemia in the hospitalized setting. In this patient, hypoglycemia did not develop until hospital day 5, suggesting an additional factor is at play.

Iron (Answer A) and fluconazole (Answer B) are not associated with hypoglycemia.

Educational Objective
Identify high-dosage trimethoprim-sulfamethoxazole as a cause of hypoglycemia.

Reference(s)
Service FJ. Hypoglycemic disorders. *N Engl J Med.* 1995;332(17):1144-1152. PMID: 7700289

75

ANSWER: C) Perform whole-body bone scan

The patient described in this vignette has severe osteoporosis in the setting of end-stage liver disease and elevated bone-specific alkaline phosphatase. While starting teriparatide (Answer E), an osteoanabolic agent used in the treatment of osteoporosis, may be an appealing option to treat his severe osteoporosis, especially given the low bone turnover typically seen in patients with end-stage liver disease, it is important to remember that teriparatide has a black box warning for osteosarcoma. Its use remains limited to 2 years in a lifetime, even though postmarketing surveillance has shown that the incidence of osteosarcoma in teriparatide-treated patients worldwide does not exceed epidemiologic expectations. Contraindications to its use include history of skeletal irradiation, Paget disease of bone, or unexplained elevation in alkaline phosphatase. This patient has a mildly elevated bone-specific alkaline phosphatase concentration, which requires further evaluation before starting teriparatide therapy. There are several different etiologies of elevated alkaline phosphatase of bone origin, including Paget disease of bone, metastatic cancer to bone, hyperparathyroidism, osteomalacia, and recent fracture. A baseline radionuclide bone scan should be performed in all patients with suspected Paget disease to document the extent and locations of skeletal involvement; this should be followed by plain radiographs of the suspicious regions of the skeleton to confirm the

RT Anterior LT   LT Posterior RT

Bone scan.

diagnosis. Therefore, performing a whole-body bone scan (Answer C) is the best next step. This patient's whole-body bone scan showed focal abnormal increased radiotracer uptake involving the right frontal bone (*see images*). Bone biopsy of this skull lesion showed a region of disorganized hyperostotic bone most consistent with the osteosclerotic stage of Paget disease of bone.

Serum protein electrophoresis (Answer A) to test for possible multiple myeloma is unlikely to be diagnostic in this normocalcemic patient with normal kidney function. While measuring 24-hour urinary calcium excretion (Answer B) is helpful in identifying hypocalciuria or hypercalciuria as a cause of secondary osteoporosis, this would not be the best next step in the evaluation of a patient with elevated bone-specific alkaline phosphatase. Similarly, starting alendronate (Answer D) to treat his osteoporosis would not be the most appropriate next step in such a scenario. It would also be important to consider the possibility of esophageal varices in such a patient before initiating an oral bisphosphonate, which could cause esophageal irritation. For Paget disease of bone, the recommended course of therapy with oral alendronate is 40 mg once daily for 6 months. Alternatives include oral risedronate, 30 mg daily for 2 months, or intravenous zoledronic acid given in a dose of 5 mg as an intravenous infusion.

Educational Objective

Evaluate for Paget disease of bone in a patient with elevated bone-specific alkaline phosphatase.

Reference(s)

Singer FR, Bone HG 3rd, Hosking DJ, et al; Endocrine Society. Paget's disease of bone: an Endocrine Society clinical practice guideline. *J Clin Endocrinol Metab*. 2014;99(12):4408-4422. PMID: 25406796

76

ANSWER: A) Obtain 2 bedtime salivary cortisol measurements

The diagnosis of mild Cushing syndrome is challenging, as many symptoms such as weight gain, hypertension, and depression are very common in the general population. Additionally, signs that are best to discriminate (easy bruising, facial plethora, proximal muscle weakness, and purplish striae) do not appear until hypercortisolism is quite severe. Therefore, the clinician must rely heavily on biochemical evaluation. The 3 tests that can be used are 24-hour urinary free cortisol measurement, dexamethasone-suppression test, and late-night salivary cortisol measurement. The 2008 Endocrine Society guidelines recommend initial use of 1 test with high diagnostic accuracy (urinary free cortisol, late-night salivary cortisol, 1-mg overnight or 2-mg 48-hour dexamethasone-suppression test) and recommend that patients

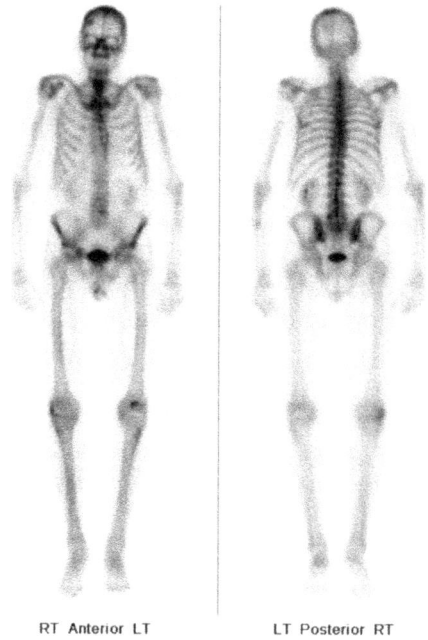

who have an abnormal result undergo a second test—either one of the above, a serum late-night cortisol measurement (not practical) or a dexamethasone–corticotropin-releasing hormone test.

This patient has seemingly failed 1 screening test (the serum cortisol was >1.8 µg/dL [>49.7 nmol/L]) and has a urinary free cortisol value in the upper normal range (not uncommon in mild Cushing syndrome). However, she is on an oral contraceptive pill. Oral estrogens increase cortisol-binding globulin levels, thereby increasing measurement of total serum cortisol. As such, any test that relies on serum cortisol measurement can be affected by oral estrogens, which may cause false positivity by artificially increasing the cortisol level. This is also an issue in interpreting serum cortisol during workup of adrenal insufficiency. Therefore, any test that relies on serum cortisol measurement should not be used in women taking oral estrogen therapy. In this case, the dexamethasone-suppression test (despite dexamethasone reaching an appropriate suppressive level) is not reliable, and other tests must be used to confirm or exclude hypercortisolism. Salivary cortisol (Answer A) correlates with free serum cortisol and is therefore reliable in women on oral estrogen. Another possibility would be to stop the oral contraceptive for 4 to 6 weeks and perform another dexamethasone-suppression test, but this was not offered as an answer option. This patient's bedtime salivary cortisol levels were normal, and ultimately Cushing syndrome was ruled out by repeating dexamethasone-suppression testing after stopping the oral contraceptive pills.

Performing pituitary-directed MRI (Answer C) would not yet be indicated, and it could unveil a common nonfunctioning microadenoma. Measuring plasma ACTH (Answer B) would be indicated after hypercortisolemia is confirmed and thus the diagnosis of Cushing syndrome is established to distinguish between ACTH-dependent and ACTH-independent Cushing syndrome. Repeating the dexamethasone-suppression test with 2 mg (Answer D) is not needed, as dexamethasone reached an appropriately suppressed level with 1 mg and this patient's serum cortisol would most likely not suppress to below 1.8 µg/dL even after 2 mg of dexamethasone. Measuring 24-hour urinary free cortisol after stopping the oral contraceptive (Answer E) would not be helpful, as urinary free cortisol measurement is not affected by changes in cortisol-binding globulin.

Educational Objective
Explain how oral estrogen can cause false positivity in dexamethasone-suppression testing during the workup of possible hypercortisolism.

Reference(s)
Nieman LK, Biller BM, Findling JW, et al. The diagnosis of Cushing's syndrome: an Endocrine Society clinical practice guideline. *J Clin Endocrinol Metab.* 2008;93(5):1526-1540. PMID: 18334580

Qureshi AC, Bahri A, Breen LA, et al. The influence of the route of oestrogen administration on serum levels of cortisol-binding globulin and total cortisol. *Clin Endocrinol (Oxf).* 2007;66(5):632-635. PMID: 17492949

77 ANSWER: A) Reassess continuous glucose monitoring data over a different interval before making recommendations

Continuous glucose monitoring (CGM) systems are increasingly used in the management of diabetes. As a result, there is a need for standardization of data gathering, presentation, and targets for different patient populations. This case highlights the need to review the data gathered before clinical decisions are made (Answer A).

To ensure accurate interpretation of the data gathered, the following information should be documented:

1. Number of days CGM is worn
2. Percentage of time CGM is active
3. Mean glucose value
4. Glycemic variability (often given as standard deviation)
5. Glucose management indicator (if duration of sampling is long enough this reflects hemoglobin A_{1c} reading)
6. Percentage of time spent above range level 2 (>250 mg/dL [>13.9 mmol/L]) and level 1 (180-250 mg/dL [10.0-13.9 mmol/L])
7. Percentage of time spent in the range of 70 to 180 mg/dL (3.9-10.0 mmol/L)
8. Percentage of time spent below range level 1 (54-69 mg/dL [3.0-3.8 mmol/L]) and level 2 (<54 mg/dL [<3.0 mmol/L])

In this vignette, a 90-day tracing is shown; however, the patient used CGM for only 16 of these 90 days. The 16 days of data gathering could have been scattered over the 90 days or could have been every day over the past 2 weeks. Given this uncertainty, making changes to insulin pump settings is inadvisable. A 2- to 4-week tracing from the app should be obtained to get a better sense of CGM use and the most recent trends in glycemia. If the patient had been using the device more than 70% of the time over the course of 14 or 30 days, then the tracing could be more reliably used for clinical decision making.

A recent consensus statement was published that describes possible "ideal" targets for blood glucose when using CGM. Data on long-term implications of achieving these targets are still not available, but data are slowly accruing in this regard. There are 3 sets of targets described: for most patients with type 1 and type 2 diabetes, for older patients who have time-in-range goals and glucose ranges adjusted, and for pregnant women with type 1 diabetes who need glucose ranges adjusted.

Table. Glycemic Targets for the General Population, Older Patients, and Pregnant Women Using CGM

| Population | Time spent in range | | Time spent above range | | Time spent below range | |
	Percentage of time	Blood glucose range	Percentage of time	Blood glucose range	Percentage of time	Blood glucose range
Patients with type 1 or type 2 diabetes	>70%	70-180 mg/dL (SI: 3.9-10.0 mmol/L)	<25%	>180 mg/dL (SI: >10.0 mmol/L)	<4%/<1%	<70 mg/dL/<54 mg/dL (SI: <3.9 mmol/L/<30 mmol/L)
Older patients	>50%	70-180 mg/dL (SI: 3.9-10.0 mmol/L)	<10%	>250 mg/dL (SI: >13.9 mmol/L)	<1%	<70 mg/dL (SI: <3.9 mmol/L)
Patients with type 1 diabetes who are pregnant	>70%	63-140 mg/dL (SI: 3.5-7.8 mmol/L)	<25%	>140 mg/dL (SI: >7.8 mmol/L)	<4%/<1%	<63 mg/dL/<54 mg/dL (SI: <3.5 mmol/L/<3.0 mmol/L)

The goal for this patient is to increase the time spent in the goal range without inducing hypoglycemia (goal is to keep the time spent <70 mg/dL [<3.9 mmol/L] to less than 4% of the time).

Given the limited data available from the tracing provided, changing insulin rates or ratios would be inadvisable at this time. Although her overnight blood glucose values are high, increasing the overnight basal rate from 0.6 to 0.8 units per hour (Answer B) would be a 33% increase, which is too aggressive. Raising all basal intervals (Answer C) is not required, especially since she seems to have a drop in blood glucose in the 7 AM to 9 AM timeframe.

Increasing the insulin-to-carbohydrate ratio (Answer D) also seems premature. She does have an increase in blood glucose after breakfast (which is following lower blood glucose values with exercise), so she might not be accurately counting carbohydrates.

Finally, there is no indication of wide blood glucose fluctuations, no suggestion that the patient is unable to use pump/CGM, and no evidence of device malfunction. Switching her regimen to multiple daily insulin injections (Answer E) is therefore incorrect. This patient should be referred to a nutritionist to review dietary intake, counseled on appropriate use of CGM, and given tips on insulin pump therapy, such as changing pump sites at least every 3 days.

Educational Objective
Evaluate data from continuous glucose monitoring in the management of patients with diabetes mellitus.

Reference(s)

Battelino T, Danne T, Bergenstal RM, et al. Clinical targets for continuous glucose monitoring data interpretation: recommendations from the International Consensus on Time in Range. *Diabetes Care*. 2019;42(8):1593-1603. PMID: 31177185

Xing D, Kollman C, Beck RW, et al; Juvenile Diabetes Research Foundation Continuous Glucose Monitoring Study Group. Optimal sampling intervals to assess long-term glycemic control using continuous glucose monitoring. *Diabetes Technol Ther*. 2011;13(3):351-358. PMID: 21299401

Riddlesworth TD, Beck RW, Gal RL, et al. Optimal sampling duration for continuous glucose monitoring to determine long-term glycemic control. *Diabetes Technol Ther*. 2018;20(4):314-316. PMID: 29565197

78 ANSWER: D) Thyroglobulin measurement by radioimmunoassay

The patient's surgical pathology did not demonstrate any high-risk features, but she was found to have persistently elevated serum thyroglobulin postoperatively. Postoperative imaging, including neck ultrasonography and diagnostic radioactive iodine (^{123}I) whole-body scan, was performed and was negative. Because of the persistent thyroglobulinemia, she was treated with radioactive iodine therapy (100 mCi ^{131}I), but again the posttherapy whole-body scan did not show evidence of persistent locoregional disease or distant metastasis. Subsequent neck and chest CT imaging was also negative. Notably, there was no significant change in the patient's serum thyroglobulin concentration with TSH stimulation or after completion of ^{131}I therapy. The clear mismatch between the serum thyroglobulin results and the clinical and radiographic findings suggests that the persistently elevated serum thyroglobulin result is most likely spurious.

Heterophile antibodies are weak, polyspecific antibodies against animal antigens that are capable of causing positive or negative interference in common laboratory tests. Spurious TSH, thyroglobulin, hCG, and PTH values due to interference from heterophile antibodies have all been described. The most common type of heterophile antibodies are human antimouse antibodies (HAMA). Although HAMA were first described in laboratory workers with mouse exposure, they may occur in up to 10% of the general population. HAMA interference in thyroglobulin testing occurs at a frequency of 0.4% to 3.0%. This is most common with noncompetitive immunometric assays that use murine monoclonal antibodies. Conversely, HAMA interference is not seen with radioimmunoassays or assays that use liquid chromatography–tandem mass spectrometry. Thus, thyroglobulin measurement by radioimmunoassay (Answer D) could be performed to confirm HAMA interference in this patient and yield an accurate determination of her serum thyroglobulin concentration.

Performing additional diagnostic testing, including bone scintigraphy (Answer A), diagnostic radioactive iodine (^{123}I) whole-body scan (Answer B), and PET-CT whole-body imaging (Answer E), would not be appropriate in this patient who had low-risk thyroid cancer and extensive prior imaging to exclude metastasis. Before considering additional diagnostic imaging, it is imperative to first exclude an artifactual cause of persistent thyroglobulinemia. Exploratory central neck dissection (Answer C) is also not indicated in this patient with negative neck imaging, and it would put the patient at unnecessary risk for recurrent laryngeal nerve injury and postsurgical hypoparathyroidism.

Educational Objective
Identify human antimouse antibodies (HAMA) interference in a patient with low-risk thyroid cancer and persistent thyroglobulinemia.

Reference(s)

Giovanella L, Keller F, Ceriani L, Tozzoli R. Heterophile antibodies may falsely increase or decrease thyroglobulin measurement in patients with differentiated thyroid carcinoma. *Clin Chem Lab Med.* 2009;47(8):952-954. PMID: 19589101

Preissner CM, O'Kane DJ, Singh RJ, Morris JC, Grebe SK. Phantoms in the assay tube: heterophile antibody interferences in serum thyroglobulin assays. *J Clin Endocrinol Metab.* 2003;88(7):3069-3074. PMID: 12843145

Verburg FA, Waschle K, Reiners C, Giovanella L, Lentjes EG. Heterophile antibodies rarely influence the measurement of thyroglobulin and thyroglobulin antibodies in differentiated thyroid cancer patients. *Horm Metab Res.* 2010;42(10):736-739. PMID: 20486066

79 ANSWER: C) Increase the basal rate at 7 AM and change the insulin-to-carbohydrate ratio to 1 to 8 at 6:30 PM

Regular assessment of hemoglobin A_{1c} and glucose monitoring data is critical for the management of patients with diabetes on insulin treatment, as demonstrated in the Diabetes Control and Complications Trial (DCCT). The hemoglobin A_{1c} goal should be individualized for each patient, but, in general, a goal of 7.0% or less (≤53 mmol/mol) is reasonable for many patients with type 1 diabetes. Glycemic targets are usually set higher for those patients with hypoglycemia unawareness or advanced complications and for older adults.

Self-monitoring of blood glucose allows for appropriate adjustments in insulin doses. Traditionally, this consisted of home glucose monitoring with a glucose meter. Studies have shown that more frequent glucose monitoring generally leads to improved glycemic control. Increasing numbers of patients are using continuous glucose monitoring (CGM) to augment fingerstick glucose data. CGM uses a subcutaneous sensor that samples glucose continuously from the interstitial fluid and sends the data to a receiver. Most real-time glucose sensors give an integrated glucose level every 5 minutes around the clock. Alarms can be set for both hypoglycemia and hyperglycemia. The immediate feedback of glucose data allows for timely intervention to treat glucose excursions. CGM is particularly helpful in patients with hypoglycemia unawareness. Several randomized controlled trials in adults have demonstrated improvement in glycemic control and a significant reduction in hypoglycemia in patients with type 1 diabetes treated with either multidose subcutaneous insulin or with insulin pumps. The most up-to-date systems combine an insulin pump and CGM that communicates with the pump, as in this vignette.

This patient has longstanding type 1 diabetes and is being treated with an insulin pump and CGM. He has hypoglycemia unawareness, so an appropriate hemoglobin A_{1c} target is in the range of 7.5% to 8.0% (58-64 mmol/mol).

Reviewing the CGM tracing, there is an increase in glucose levels starting at about 3 AM, which may be due to the dawn phenomenon. Increasing the basal insulin rate from 3 to 7 AM is appropriate, but additional changes should be made. The glucose levels remain elevated from 7:30 AM to 1 PM. The glucose values trend down after the noon meal and are lower until about 6 PM. The glucose levels trend upward until about 10:30 PM, then trend down toward midnight. Changing the insulin-to-carbohydrate ratio to 1 unit per 8 g carbohydrate at 7:30 AM (Answers D and E) would be inadequate to maintain improved glucose control from 7 AM to 1 PM. Increasing the basal rate from 7:30 AM to 1 PM is appropriate, but the insulin-to-carbohydrate ratio must be modified at 6:30 PM to counteract hyperglycemia after the evening meal (thus, Answer C is correct and Answer A is incorrect). Increasing the basal insulin rate at 1 PM (Answer B) would most likely increase the risk of hypoglycemia during the afternoon.

Educational Objective
Analyze glucose monitoring data and make adjustments in the insulin regimen to improve glycemic control and minimize the risk of hypoglycemia.

Reference(s)
Diabetes Control and Complications Trial Research Group, Nathan DM, Genuth S, et al. The effect of intensive treatment of diabetes on the development and progression of long-term complications in insulin-dependent diabetes mellitus. *N Engl J Med.* 1993;329(14):977-986. PMID: 8366922

American Diabetes Association. 7. Diabetes technology: standards of medical care in diabetes-2020. *Diabetes Care.* 2020;43(Suppl 1):S77-S88. PMID: 31862750

80 **ANSWER: D) Referral to sleep medicine**
The patient's symptoms and physical examination findings should prompt an evaluation for obstructive sleep apnea (OSA) (Answer D). OSA is a common sleeping disorder characterized by episodes of partial or complete obstruction of the upper airway during sleep. This leads to awakening, which causes sleep fragmentation, sympathetic activation, and desaturation. The prevalence of OSA in the general population ranges from 9% to 38%, and the prevalence is higher in men, obese individuals, and older individuals. Weight gain leading to obesity is a major risk factor for developing OSA. OSA is associated with hypertension, atrial fibrillation, cardiovascular events, pulmonary hypertension, and chronic heart failure.

Symptoms of OSA include snoring, witnessed episodes of apnea, gasping or choking while sleeping, nocturia, daytime fatigue, insomnia, impaired concentration, unrefreshing sleep, recurrent awakening from sleep, morning headaches, irritability, and decreased libido. Associated physical examination findings include neck circumference greater than 16.5 in (42 cm) in men and greater than 14.5 in (37 cm) in women, retrognathia or micrognathia, enlarged tonsils, high arched hard palate, macroglossia, and septal deviation.

Screening questionnaires such as STOP-BANG and the Epworth Sleepiness scale can be used to detect individuals at high risk for OSA. Diagnosis requires overnight polysomnography, which detects episodes of apnea (cessation of airflow for at least 10 seconds despite ongoing inspiratory effort) or hypopnea (more than 50% airflow reduction or reduction in airflow, which leads to desaturation or reduction in airflow with electrocochleographic evidence of awakening). Several parameters are measured during polysomnography, including pulse oximetry, electroencephalography, electro-oculography, nasal and oral air flow measures, chest wall movements, electromyography, and electrocardiography.

The apnea-hypopnea index represents the average number of disordered breathing events per hour of sleep. OSA syndrome is diagnosed when a patient has an apnea-hypopnea index of 15 or more regardless of symptoms, or 5 or more with associated symptoms. Classification of OSA severity is based on the apnea-hypopnea index: patients with mild OSA have an index of 5 to 14, patients with moderate disease have an index of 15 to 29, and patients with severe OSA have an index of 30 or higher.

Treatment of OSA includes weight loss, avoidance of alcohol and sedatives before bedtime, and a continuous positive airway pressure device. The positive pressures prevent the collapse of the upper airway during sleep. There is no evidence to recommend pharmacologic treatments. Surgical interventions on the upper airway are a treatment option.

OSA is a risk factor for insulin resistance and development of type 2 diabetes. This patient has prediabetes. Measuring fasting insulin (Answer B) would not provide additional information to guide his management.

He has no physical findings suggestive of cortisol excess. Therefore, a 24-hour urine collection for cortisol (Answer C) is not needed.

Although this patient has a high cardiovascular risk, he does not present with new-onset chest pain, dyspnea, murmur, or any other symptom or physical examination finding that would prompt one to order echocardiography (Answer E).

This patient's physical examination findings are not consistent with acromegaly, so measuring IGF-1 (Answer A) is not indicated.

Educational Objective
Identify obese patients who should be screened for obstructive sleep apnea.

Reference(s)
Park JG, Ramar K, Olson EJ. Updates on definition, consequences, and management of obstructive sleep apnea. *Mayo Clin Proc.* 2011;86(6):549-554. PMID: 21628617

Senaratna CV, Perret JL, Lodge CJ, et al. Prevalence of obstructive sleep apnea in the general population: a systematic review. *Sleep Med Rev.* 2017;34:70-81. PMID: 27568340

Mannarino MR, Di Filippo F, Pirro M. Obstructive sleep apnea syndrome. *Eur J Intern Med.* 2012;23(7):586-593. PMID: 22939801

81 ANSWER: B) Deoxycorticosterone-producing adrenal tumor

Assuming satisfactory medication adherence, this patient has refractory hypertension (blood pressure not controlled on ≥3 antihypertensive agents). He also has evidence of fluid retention (bilateral lower limb swelling) without other signs of cardiac failure. His recent-onset nocturia is most likely secondary to hypokalemia with consequent nephrogenic diabetes insipidus. Importantly, although he has numerous clinical and laboratory features of mineralocorticoid excess, both his plasma renin activity and plasma aldosterone concentration are suppressed.

Accordingly, the picture is not consistent with a state of secondary aldosteronism, in which there is activation of the renin-angiotensin-aldosterone system, as would be seen in renal artery stenosis (Answer A).

The undetectable aldosterone level also rules out glucocorticoid-remediable aldosteronism (ie, familial hyperaldosteronism type I) (Answer C) due to a chimeric duplication where the 5′-promoter region of the *CYP11B1* gene (encoding 11β-hydroxylase, which is regulated by ACTH) is fused to the coding sequences of *CYP11B2* (encoding aldosterone synthase), leading to ACTH-dependent aldosterone production. Glucocorticoid-remediable aldosteronism also typically presents at a younger age with early-onset/severe hypertension and is inherited in an autosomal dominant manner.

Several conditions can give rise to a state of actual or apparent mineralocorticoid excess, which is independent of aldosterone, including:
- Rarer subtypes of congenital adrenal hyperplasia (eg, 11β-hydroxylase deficiency and 17α-hydroxylase deficiency resulting in excess 11-deoxycorticosterone production)
- Syndrome of apparent mineralocorticoid excess—inherited (autosomal recessive) or acquired (eg, due to excess licorice or carbenoxolone ingestion) with reduced renal 11β-hydroxysteroid dehydrogenase type 2 activity, leading to reduced conversion of cortisol to (inactive) cortisone and consequent activation of the mineralocorticoid receptor by cortisol
- Cushing syndrome; glucocorticoid resistance
- 11-Deoxycorticosterone-producing adrenal tumor
- Liddle syndrome in which there is constitutive activation of the renal epithelial sodium channel due to an activating pathogenic variant in the *SCNN1B* gene, resulting in impaired degradation by the ubiquitin proteasome

In the absence of a history of excess ingestion of licorice containing glycyrrhizic acid causing acquired apparent mineralocorticoid excess, both inherited apparent mineralocorticoid excess (Answer E) and Liddle syndrome (Answer D) are effectively ruled out by the patient's age at presentation and his history of normal blood pressure until age 55 years.

Therefore, given the severity and refractoriness of the hypertension with profound hypokalemia, it is important to investigate for an alternative source of mineralocorticoid excess such as production of 11-deoxycorticosterone by an adrenocortical tumor (Answer B).

Educational Objective
Identify aldosterone-independent causes of mineralocorticoid excess.

Reference(s)
Athimulam S, Lazik N, Bancos I. Low-renin hypertension. *Endocrinol Metab Clin North Am.* 2019;48(4):701-715. PMID: 31655771

Marques P, Tufton N, Bhattacharya S, Caulfield M, Akker SA. Hypertension due to a deoxycorticosterone-secreting adrenal tumour diagnosed during pregnancy. *Endocrinol Diabetes Metab Case Rep.* 2019;18-0164. PMID: 31051469

82 ANSWER: E) Perform thyroid ultrasonography again after delivery

This woman in her second trimester of pregnancy has a 1.5-cm left spongiform thyroid nodule. The prevalence of thyroid nodules during pregnancy in areas of mild to moderate iodine deficiency has been reported to be between 3% and 21%. The frequency of thyroid cancer in pregnant women with thyroid nodules ranges between 12% and 43% in published retrospective studies in the United States and Canada.

The evaluation of a thyroid nodule is the same during pregnancy as it is in nonpregnant women. A thorough family history of benign or malignant thyroid disease should be obtained, as well as a personal history of radiation exposure to the head and neck. Thyroid ultrasonography should be performed, and serum TSH should be measured. Total T_4 increases by week 7 of gestation and reaches a peak by approximately week 16 of gestation. These concentrations then remain high until delivery. Total T_4 range is 50% higher than the nonpregnant range if there is no total T_4 pregnancy reference range. Other imaging studies such as radioactive iodine uptake and radionuclide scintigraphy are contraindicated during pregnancy. However, FNA biopsy can be safely done during pregnancy, and the indications for performing FNA biopsy are the same in pregnant and nonpregnant patients. The decision to perform FNA biopsy of a thyroid nodule during pregnancy should be based on the sonographic pattern, as outlined in the 2015 American Thyroid Association thyroid nodule guidelines. These current guidelines indicate different FNA size cutoffs based on 5 sonographic patterns and their associated risk stratification for thyroid cancer. However, in the absence of worrisome characteristics, the nodule growth, or the appearance of a cervical lymph node during pregnancy, FNA biopsy can be postponed until after delivery. FNA biopsy can be safely performed in any trimester during pregnancy, but if thyroid surgery is indicated, it is only recommended to be performed during the second trimester. When FNA biopsy shows indeterminate cytology results, including follicular neoplasm, atypia of undetermined significance, or follicular lesion of undetermined significance, pregnant women can be followed and further evaluation can be postponed until after delivery. On the basis of the 2017 guidelines of the American Thyroid Association for the diagnosis and management of thyroid disease during pregnancy and in the postpartum period, molecular testing is not recommended during pregnancy, as no validation studies have been performed in pregnant women.

In this vignette, the nodule looks spongiform and is only 1.5 cm in longest dimension. Therefore, this nodule does not meet the criteria for FNA biopsy (Answer D) at this time. FNA biopsy of a spongiform nodule can be performed when it is larger than 2 cm. For a spongiform nodule, the estimated risk of malignancy is 3%. As this patient is pregnant and euthyroid according to her TSH value, a thyroid scan (Answer C) should not be done. Based on the ultrasound characteristics, this nodule does not harbor any worrisome characteristics, so thyroidectomy (Answer A) is not indicated now. There is no evidence that levothyroxine suppression therapy (Answer B) would decrease the size of the nodule during pregnancy. The best approach for this patient is to perform thyroid ultrasonography again after delivery (Answer E). This could determine whether the nodule has increased in size or whether it harbors any worrisome characteristics that should prompt FNA biopsy.

Educational Objective
Manage thyroid nodules in pregnant women.

Reference(s)

Alexander EK, Pearce EN, Brent GA, et al. 2017 guidelines of the American Thyroid Association for the diagnosis and management of thyroid disease during pregnancy and the postpartum. *Thyroid.* 2017;27(3):315-389. PMID: 28056690

Haugen BR, Alexander EK, Bible KC, et al. 2015 American Thyroid Association management guidelines for adult patients with thyroid nodules and differentiated thyroid cancer: the American Thyroid Association Guidelines Task Force on Thyroid Nodules and Differentiated Thyroid Cancer. *Thyroid.* 2016;26(1):1-133. PMID: 26462967

83 ANSWER: B) Discontinue clomiphene and prescribe insulin

This patient has newly diagnosed diabetes and by definition is "pregestational." Pregestational diabetes carries increased risk for fetal and neonatal complications, as well as maternal complications. Fetal and neonatal complications include congenital malformations, prematurity, intrauterine growth restriction, macrosomia, increased perinatal mortality, and possibly long-term sequelae. Hyperglycemia is strongly associated with all of these complications. Multiple lines of largely observational data have shown that the risk of these complications dramatically increases with worsening glycemic control. The risks of congenital malformations in 1 study of 7 cohorts are shown (*see table*).

Hemoglobin A_{1c}	Risk of congenital malformations
5.5% (37 mmol/mol)	2%
6.2% (44 mmol/mol)	2.7%
7.6% (60 mmol/mol)	4%
14% (130 mmol/mol)	20%

Similarly, data from the north of England show that the risk of perinatal mortality starts to increase at hemoglobin A_{1c} levels greater than 6.6% (>49 mmol/mol).

For these reasons, most experts suggest that preconception hemoglobin A_{1c} should be targeted to less than 6.5% (<48 mmol/mol) or as close to normal without associated hypoglycemia. Additionally, some clinicians use the following preconception glycemic targets for fingerstick blood glucose measurements to help guide treatment: 80 to 110 mg/dL (4.4-6.1 mmol/L) in the fasting state and less than 155 mg/dL (<8.6 mmol/L) 2 hours after a meal. (Note that these targets are different from those advised *during* pregnancy.) To this end, patients contemplating pregnancy should spend approximately 6 months optimizing glycemic control. Given this information, the patient should be advised to cease efforts at conception, so continuing clomiphene (Answers A and D) would not be appropriate.

In general, experts suggest the use of the following insulins, which have a good safety profile: insulin detemir, NPH insulin, insulin aspart, and insulin lispro. Further, American Diabetes Association guidelines suggest that patients who are on oral medications to manage diabetes stop these medications before pregnancy and start insulin treatment. While observational data from small studies suggest that insulin glargine is safe, there is the theoretical risk of macrosomia because glargine has higher mitogenic potential. This patient should stop clomiphene and begin insulin (Answer B).

In gestational diabetes, there are limited data that metformin or sulfonylureas used during the third trimester may be safe, as organogenesis is complete, but long-term data on fetal outcomes in those with preexisting diabetes are completely lacking. Regarding metformin, observational data indicate that women with preexisting type 2 diabetes who are well managed on metformin may have generally good outcomes with maintenance of metformin treatment. There are almost no data establishing the safety of GLP-1 receptor agonists in pregestational diabetes mellitus. Therefore, prescription of a sulfonylurea (Answers D and E) or GLP-1 receptor agonist (Answer C) is not the best choice in this setting.

For this particular patient, in reality, her elevated preconception hemoglobin A_{1c} was not recognized and diabetes was not identified till the 20th week of pregnancy during a screening oral glucose tolerance test. The patient's baby was born with congenital heart disease despite good glucose control in the second half of pregnancy.

Educational Objective
Explain risks for complications in women with pregestational diabetes and the thresholds at which these risks occur.

Reference(s)

Tennant PW, Glinianaia SV, Bilous RW, Rankin J, Belle R. Pre-existing diabetes, maternal glycated haemoglobin, and the risks of fetal and infant death: a population-based study. *Diabetologia*. 2014;57(2):285-294. PMID: 24292565

Guerin A, Nisenbaum R, Ray JG. Use of maternal GHb concentration to estimate the risk of congenital anomalies in the offspring of women with prepregnancy diabetes. *Diabetes Care*. 2007;30(7):1920-1925. PMID: 17446531

84 ANSWER: C) Primary hyperparathyroidism

The choice of a specific antifracture therapy for a patient with diagnosed osteoporosis is dependent on several factors, the most important being the degree of osteoporosis based on bone density and fracture risk. Given this patient's DXA results and her absolute fracture risk by FRAX calculation, she is deemed to be at high risk of fracture and, as such, is a candidate for anabolic therapy. This approach is intuitively more attractive as well, based on existing clinical trial data showing abrogation of bone mineral density increases in patients who were treated with a bisphosphonate before anabolic therapy. It is, however, equally important to identify and treat underlying secondary causes of osteoporosis that could complement, but also complicate, a prescribed treatment regimen. On the basis of the pretreatment biochemical and DXA data, this patient has concurrent primary hyperparathyroidism (Answer C). The presence of an elevated serum calcium concentration when corrected for albumin (10.5 mg/dL [2.6 mmol/L], based on the calculation [$calcium_{corrected} = calcium_{actual} - (albumin_{actual} - albumin_{mid-normal}) \times 0.8$]), and an intact PTH concentration in the upper normal range are consistent with autonomous parathyroid disease. If available, measurement of ionized calcium would also be advisable, as this is a more sensitive means of detecting hypercalcemia than measuring serum calcium. Finally, the patient's pattern of bone mineral density deficit, with greater deficit at the cortical-rich proximal one-third radius, is consistent with the presence of underlying primary hyperparathyroidism. Following the initiation of teriparatide, this patient developed hypercalcemia in the context of autonomous parathyroid function. Upon cessation of teriparatide, the patient's calcium returned to baseline.

Although she did have measured hypercalcemia, based on elevated calcium adjusted for albumin, before starting teriparatide, the PTH level was borderline high and not frankly suppressed (ie, serum PTH <20 pg/mL [<20 ng/L]). This result is inconsistent with PTH-independent hypercalcemia and rules out the presence of sarcoidosis (Answer A) and multiple myeloma (Answer D), in which PTH is invariably suppressed. Renal cell carcinoma (Answer E) can be associated with hypercalcemia as well, although it is due to the overproduction of PTHrP. As such, PTH levels are concomitantly suppressed in this disorder. Finally, the patient's PTH and serum calcium levels could be consistent with the presence of familial hypocalciuric hypercalcemia (Answer B). Her 24-hour urinary calcium and calculated fractional excretion of calcium are, however, inconsistent with this diagnosis, as values are typically less than 100 mg daily and less than 0.01, respectively, in patients with familial hypocalciuric hypercalcemia.

Educational Objective
Explain the importance of ruling out primary hyperparathyroidism before starting PTH analogue therapy in a patient with osteoporosis.

Reference(s)

Nordenström E, Katzman P, Bergenfelz A. Biochemical diagnosis of primary hyperparathyroidism: analysis of the sensitivity of total and ionized calcium in combination with PTH. *Clin Biochem*. 2011;44(10-11):849-852. PMID: 21515248

85 ANSWER: A) Administer zoledronic acid infusion

This man has clinical osteoporosis and requires adequate secondary fracture prevention. The Endocrine Society guidelines on male osteoporosis recommend that men with high fracture risk, such as the man in this vignette, should receive osteoporotic drug therapy with proven antifracture benefit, regardless of whether testosterone treatment is considered. Zoledronic acid (Answer A) has proven antifracture benefit in men and there is some evidence of reduced mortality after hip fracture with its use. It is a good choice for this patient; his renal function is normal and his vitamin D level is adequate. While the optimal timing of zoledronic acid treatment is not clear, based on randomized controlled trial protocols demonstrating antifracture benefit, it is recommended that zoledronic acid treatment be given 2 to 12 weeks after the fracture.

While he reports symptoms that could be consistent with androgen deficiency, these are very nonspecific and might be related to his chronic alcoholism. Indeed, he has signs of alcoholic liver disease and his liver function test results are suggestive of alcoholic hepatitis. Low muscle bulk can be due to chronic alcoholism and associated malnutrition (suggested by his low BMI). His testicular size is in the low-normal range. Definitive clinical evidence of androgen deficiency is lacking. While his gonadal studies suggest hypogonadotropic hypogonadism, the stress associated with an acute fracture can suppress the gonadal axis acutely, and this is most likely aggravated by the gonadal axis suppressive effects of opioids. In one longitudinal study, the average acute fracture-associated decrease in serum testosterone was almost 50%. In the subgroup of men requiring hospitalization, serum testosterone was not uncommonly near the castrate range. Therefore, although serum testosterone measurement is an important component of secondary osteoporosis screening in men, it should not be ordered in the acute setting. Indeed, this patient's total testosterone concentration, when remeasured 3 months later, increased to 271 ng/dL (9.4 nmol/L).

Similarly, this patient's modest increase in prolactin was due to the acute fracture-associated stress compounded by the well-described prolactin-stimulatory effects of opioids, and it subsequently normalized. Therefore, a pituitary-directed MRI (Answer E) is not necessary. MRI would only be indicated if hormonal abnormalities had persisted with recovery, especially if there were features of a pituitary mass effect or evidence of involvement of other pituitary axes.

Given that the patient does not have established hypogonadism, testosterone treatment (Answers B and D) is not indicated. Even if there were a clinical indication for testosterone replacement, combined testosterone and osteoporotic drug therapy would have been necessary, as there are no fracture data for testosterone treatment. The Endocrine Society guidelines emphasize that men with high fracture risk need osteoporotic drug treatment with proven antifracture effect, regardless of whether they receive testosterone treatment.

An aromatase inhibitor such as anastrozole (Answer C) is sometimes prescribed off-label by some practitioners for the treatment of functional hypogonadism, with the expectation that by decreasing serum estradiol and its central negative feedback on the hypothalamic pituitary unit, LH and subsequently serum testosterone increase. Aromatase inhibitors are not approved for treatment of male hypogonadism, and there is no convincing evidence of clinical benefit. Moreover, by decreasing estradiol production, aromatase inhibitors have been shown to reduce bone density in men and would be detrimental in this situation.

Educational Objective
Prescribe osteoporotic drug therapy as first-line treatment in a man at high fracture risk, even in the context of hypogonadism.

Reference(s)
Watts NB, Adler RA, Bilezikian JP, Drake MT, Eastell R, Orwoll ES, Finkelstein JS; Endocrine Society. Osteoporosis in men: an Endocrine Society clinical practice guideline. *J Clin Endocrinol Metab.* 2012;97(6):1802-1822. PMID: 22675062

Cheung AS, Baqar S, Sia R, et al. Testosterone levels increase in association with recovery from acute fracture in men. *Osteoporos Int.* 2014;25(8):2027-2033. PMID: 24803329

86 **ANSWER: D) Increase the dosages of calcium to 4 g daily and calcitriol to 2 mcg daily**
The patient described in this vignette has permanent postsurgical hypoparathyroidism treated with calcium, active vitamin D supplementation, and recombinant human PTH (rhPTH) (1-84). The US FDA approved rhPTH (1-84) in 2015 for the management of chronic hypoparathyroidism not well controlled with conventional therapy, as an adjunct to calcium and vitamin D. Based on the prescribing information, it is required to confirm that 25-hydroxyvitamin D stores are sufficient and that the serum calcium concentration is above 7.5 mg/dL (>1.9 mmol/L) before starting rhPTH (1-84) therapy. In September 2019, a recall was issued on all doses of rhPTH (1-84) after observation of visible rubber particles in the drug solution originating from the cartridge needle puncturing the rubber septum of the cartridge each time an injection was done.

Abrupt discontinuation of rhPTH (1-84) can cause a sharp decrease in blood calcium levels, akin to hungry bone syndrome. In response to the recall, the Endocrine Society and the American Society for Bone Mineral Research (ASBMR) issued a joint statement to provide guidance for clinicians treating such patients, since many of these patients transiently require higher dosages of calcium/calcitriol than they did before starting rhPTH (1-84).

The recommendation is to increase the amount of calcium to the pre-rhPTH (1-84) dosage and to increase the amount of calcitriol to double (or triple) the pre-rhPTH (1-84) dosage about 12 hours after the last injection of rhPTH (1-84). Therefore, in this patient who now has symptomatic hypocalcemia since stopping rhPTH (1-84) the day prior, increasing calcium to 4 g daily and calcitriol to 2 mcg daily (Answer D) is correct. Recommending no changes to her current medications (Answer A) is incorrect. Increasing the calcium dosage to 4 g daily (Answer B) or increasing the calcitriol dosage to 1 mcg daily (Answer C) would not be adequate. Furthermore, increasing the calcitriol dosage can also be associated with worsening hyperphosphatemia because active vitamin D therapy increases intestinal phosphate absorption.

While teriparatide (PTH 1-34) is not FDA approved for the treatment of hypoparathyroidism, it has been studied in this setting and shown to be effective. However, teriparatide's effect to raise the serum calcium concentration is shorter-lived than that of rhPTH (1-84), and injections twice daily or even 3 times daily are typically necessary. Therefore, starting once-daily teriparatide injections (Answer E) would not be the most appropriate next step in the management of this patient's hypocalcemia.

Since patients may have individual differences in their calcium/calcitriol requirements and since it is not possible to predict how long the transient increase in these requirements will last after stopping rhPTH (1-84), it is recommended to check serum calcium levels frequently and adjust the dosage of calcium and calcitriol accordingly for each patient. Once the serum calcium level is at goal (mildly low to low-normal range), it is important to check for hypercalciuria (defined as a 24-hour urinary calcium excretion >300 mg). Patients with chronic hypoparathyroidism excrete more calcium than normal persons at the same serum calcium concentration due to the lack of the effect of PTH at the kidney level. Worsening hypercalciuria could contribute to the development of kidney stones or other kidney disease.

Educational Objective
Recognize the transient increase in calcium/calcitriol requirements when stopping rhPTH (1-84) therapy in a hypoparathyroid patient presenting with hypocalcemia and recommend the most appropriate therapeutic intervention.

Reference(s)
Mannstadt M, Clarke BL, Vokes T, et al. Efficacy and safety of recombinant human parathyroid hormone (1-84) in hypoparathyroidism (REPLACE): a double-blind, placebo-controlled, randomised, phase 3 study [published correction appears in *Lancet Diabetes Endocrinol.* 2014;2(1):e3]. *Lancet Diabetes Endocrinol.* 2013;1(4):275-283. PMID: 24622413

Bilezikian JP, Brandi ML, Cusano NE, et al. Management of hypoparathyroidism: present and future. *J Clin Endocrinol Metab.* 2016;101(6):2313-2324. PMID: 26938200

Marcucci G, Della Pepa G, Brandi ML. Drug safety evaluation of parathyroid hormone for hypocalcemia in patients with hypoparathyroidism. *Expert Opin Drug Saf.* 2017;16(5):617-625. PMID: 28332412

Endocrine Society. Endocrine Society, ASBMR Issue Joint Statement on Natpara Recall. Available at: https://endocrinenews.endocrine.org/endocrine-society-asbmr-issue-joint-statement-on-natpara-recall/. Accessed for verification January 2020

Winer KK. Advances in the treatment of hypoparathyroidism with PTH 1-34. *Bone.* 2019;120:535-541. PMID: 30243992

87 ANSWER: B) Clindamycin

Patients with diabetes are at increased risk for lower-extremity wounds that can lead to amputation. Risk factors for lower-extremity wounds are decreased sensation, which increases the risk of injury, vascular compromise to the extremity that can delay healing, neuropathy, and development of foot deformities leading to abnormal pressure points and skin breakdown. This patient with a history of Charcot foot and ulcers is at particularly high risk for recurrent lower-extremity ulcers.

Wounds can be colonized with microorganisms and often do not have to be treated with antibiotics. However, assessing for infection and treating early with antibiotics are essential for limb preservation in patients with high-risk wounds. All patients with a new wound should have a probe-to-bone test and plain x-ray to assess for osteomyelitis.

The Infectious Disease Society of America released guidelines in 2012 on the assessment of diabetic foot infections. When a patient with diabetes presents with a wound, both wound characteristics and vascular characteristics must be assessed. A wound is thought to be infected rather than colonized if there is evidence of inflammation and/or purulence. At least 2 of the following features must be present to diagnose infection: swelling, erythema, pain, increased warmth, or purulence.

If a wound is infected, the next step is to determine severity. It is considered mild if the skin findings are less than 2 cm from the wound and limited to the subcutaneous space. If the findings extend beyond 2 cm, there is lymphatic streaking, or there is involvement beyond the subcutaneous tissue, the infection is considered moderate. Finally, if there are systemic inflammatory response signs, the infection is considered severe (temperature >100.4°F [>38°C] or <96.8°F [<36°C]; heart rate >90 beats/min; respiratory rate >20 breaths/min; Po_2 <32 mm Hg; white blood cell count >12,000/μL, <4000/μL, or >10% bands). This classification is useful in determining the need for hospitalization. Hospitalization was determined to be necessary in 4% of patients with mild infection, 46% of patients with moderate infection, and 71% of patients with severe infection (cited in the guideline). Mild infections can usually be treated with oral antibiotics, while severe infections require admission to the hospital for intravenous antibiotics. Management of moderate infections requires coordination between the patient and provider, and decision making must take into account the patient's social situation and ability to adhere to recommendations such as off-loading weight from the leg with the wound.

This patient has a wound with erythema, streaking up her leg, and purulent drainage, suggesting the wound is infected. The erythema is less than 2 cm from the wound. Probe-to-bone test and x-ray are negative, so she most likely does not have osteomyelitis. Because she has an infected wound, she needs antibiotic therapy, and topic antimicrobial therapy (Answer C) is insufficient. Hyperbaric oxygen therapy (Answer D) may be effective in short-term improvement of a chronic diabetic wound but would not be the first choice in the treatment of an infected wound. Offering no treatment for an ulcer with purulent drainage (Answer E) would be incorrect.

The next consideration is which microorganisms to cover. Most wounds have polymicrobial infection with gram-positive cocci. Given this patient's history of methicillin-resistant *Staphylococcus aureus* infection, the recommendation would be to extend her coverage to include this bacteria. Clindamycin (Answer B) is the most appropriate antibiotic in this scenario. Cephalexin (Answer A) would be appropriate for a mild infection for simple gram-positive coverage. It does not cover methicillin-resistant *Staphylococcus aureus*.

Educational Objective
Manage a diabetic foot infection.

Reference(s)
Lipsky BA, Berendt AR, Cornia PB, et al; Infectious Diseases of America. 2012 Infectious Disease Society of America clinical practice guideline for the diagnosis and treatment of diabetic foot infections. *Clin Infect Dis*. 2012;54(12):e132-e173. PMID: 22619242

88 ANSWER: E) Adiponectin

The relationship between body fat and metabolic disease is dependent on fat distribution. Visceral adipose tissue is stored within the abdominal cavity around internal organs, and its accumulation is linked to chronic inflammation and metabolic disorders. A waist circumference measurement is a good estimator of the amount of visceral adipose tissue. A waist circumference greater than 40 in (>102 cm) in men and greater than 35 in (>88 cm) in women is a risk factor for cardiovascular and metabolic disease.

Traditionally, adipose tissue was considered an energy storage organ, but adipocytes are now recognized to be metabolically active. Adipocytes release adipokines that are involved in regulation of appetite, inflammation, immune response, and glucose metabolism, among other functions. Adipose tissue from obese individuals undergoes hyperplasia, hypertrophy, and infiltration of inflammatory cells. These changes are associated with changes in secretion of adipokines, with upregulation in the expression of proinflammatory adipokines.

Adipokines secreted by visceral adipose tissue that have a role in metabolic disease include resistin, adiponectin, tumor necrosis factor α, interleukin-6, visfatin, serum amyloid A-3, and plasminogen activator inhibitor-1.

Adiponectin (Answer E) is secreted by adipose tissue, and its levels decrease with increasing adiposity. Adiponectin expression is suppressed by proinflammatory cytokines, which explains why its levels are lower in obese individuals. Adiponectin is an insulin-sensitizing, anti-inflammatory, antiapoptotic adipokine. In skeletal muscle, it increases basal and insulin-stimulated glucose uptake via translocation of GLUT-4 to the cell membrane, increases fatty acid uptake and oxidation, and increases mitochondrial mass and oxidative capacity. In the liver, adiponectin also has insulin-sensitizing effects and its levels negatively correlate with tumor necrosis factor α. In the cardiac muscle, it has cardiac remodeling, vasodilating, antiinflammatory, and antiatherogenic effects. Of the options listed in the vignette, adiponectin is the most likely adipokine to be decreased in this patient.

Leptin (Answer A) is an anorexigenic hormone that binds to its receptor in the hypothalamus. Leptin is secreted by adipocytes, and its concentration correlates with the amount of adipose tissue. Since leptin levels are proportional to body fat, obesity is associated with high levels. Obese individuals appear to resist the hypothalamic action of leptin because the body should be able to recognize the excess adipose tissue and decrease food intake and increase energy expenditure to get rid of excess fat. Leptin also has a role in the regulation of the immune response.

Adipocyte secretion of tumor necrosis factor α (Answer B) is increased in obese individuals. Its concentration is correlated with the amount of adipose tissue and the severity of insulin resistance. Tumor necrosis factor α acts locally, inducing adipocyte insulin resistance by deactivating the insulin receptor. Also, it is involved in atherosclerosis by increasing cell adhesion molecules in vascular smooth muscle, altering endothelium-dependent vasodilation, and increasing endothelial cell apoptosis.

Resistin (Answer C) causes insulin resistance by binding to insulin receptors on adipocytes, liver, and muscle. Its level increases in the presence of obesity, and it may have a role in the development of type 2 diabetes. Resistin is an inflammatory marker, and its gene expression is regulated by proinflammatory agents. Resistin also promotes endothelial dysfunction and calcification of coronary arteries.

Plasminogen activator inhibitor-1 (Answer D) is the strongest fibrinolysis inhibitor, and it is involved in insulin resistance and energy balance. An increase in the circulating plasminogen activator inhibitor-1 concentration is observed in individuals with abdominal obesity. Plasminogen activator inhibitor-1 is a proinflammatory agent that promotes the expression of resistin. An increased level of plasminogen activator inhibitor-1 is considered to be a major risk factor for cardiovascular disease.

Educational Objective
Describe the role of different adipokines in obese individuals and recognize that adiponectin is low in the setting of obesity.

Reference(s)
Dutheil F, Gordon BA, Naughton G, et al. Cardiovascular risk of adipokines: a review. *J Int Med Res*. 2018;46(6):2082-2095. PMID: 28974138

Kelesidis T, Kelesidis I, Chou S, Mantzoros CS. Narrative review: the role of leptin in human physiology: emerging clinical applications. *Ann Intern Med*. 2010;152(2):93-100. PMID: 20083828

Nakamura K, Fuster JJ, Walsh K. Adipokines: a link between obesity and cardiovascular disease. *J Cardiol*. 2014;63(4):250-259. PMID: 24355497

89 ANSWER: B) Langerhans cell histiocytosis
This patient has a multisystem disorder, with evidence of endocrine, pulmonary, and skeletal involvement. The results from the water-deprivation test are consistent with central diabetes insipidus, and the pituitary MRI demonstrates focal thickening of the infundibulum. Anterior pituitary function is reasonably well preserved, although dynamic testing would be required to exclude more widespread partial hypopituitarism. Mild hyperprolactinemia is consistent with stalk disconnection syndrome.

Langerhans cell histiocytosis (Answer B) should be considered in the differential diagnosis of any patient with apparently isolated central diabetes insipidus. An estimated 10% to 15% of such patients have Langerhans cell histiocytosis. Pulmonary involvement is seen in approximately 10% of affected patients and is more frequent in adult-onset disease, where cigarette smoking is a key etiologic factor. High-resolution CT of the chest showing a combination of multiple cysts and nodules, with a mid-to-upper zone predominance and interstitial thickening in a young smoker is highly suggestive of Langerhans cell histiocytosis. Bone involvement occurs in most affected patients, and it can be associated with localized pain. Radiologic studies demonstrate lytic lesions that are typically "hot" on radionuclide bone scans. Langerhans cell histiocytosis would therefore account for all of the presenting features in this man.

Sarcoidosis (Answer D) is a multisystem granulomatous disorder that most frequently involves the lungs, although up to 30% of patients present with extrathoracic manifestations (skin, eyes, reticuloendothelial system, musculoskeletal system, cardiac, renal, and central nervous system). Hypothalamic and/or pituitary involvement is rare, but when present it is usually associated with anterior pituitary dysfunction; contrast-enhanced MRI of the brain may reveal more extensive changes with meningeal and/or parenchymal involvement. High-resolution CT of the chest commonly reveals hilar and mediastinal lymphadenopathy, with parenchymal lung changes that mainly affect the mid and upper zones. Therefore, although sarcoidosis is a diagnosis to consider in this case, the clinical and radiologic features are not typical.

Similarly, the findings on cross-sectional imaging of the chest are not classic for pulmonary tuberculosis (Answer E), where patchy or poorly defined consolidation in the upper lobes may progress to cavitation, often with associated lymphadenopathy. Pituitary gland and skeletal involvement are recognized manifestations of mycobacterial infection, but the former is relatively rare, and it would be unusual for a patient with no relevant medical history to present with disseminated tuberculosis.

Lymphangitis carcinomatosis (Answer C) is the term used to denote diffuse infiltration and obstruction of the parenchymal lymphatic system by tumor cells (usually adenocarcinoma) and is most commonly seen in the lungs. High-resolution CT of the chest typically demonstrates interlobular septal thickening and reticulonodular changes. Disseminated malignancy with vertebral and pituitary metastases is possible, but given the patient's young age, relatively short history of symptoms, and no notable medical history, this would be less likely.

The clinical features and radiologic findings in this case would represent a very unusual presentation of Hodgkin lymphoma (Answer A), so this is not the most likely diagnosis.

Educational Objective
Identify the potential causes of central diabetes insipidus in the context of multisystem disease.

Reference(s)
Langrand C, Bihan H, Raverot G, et al. Hypothalamic-pituitary sarcoidosis: a multicenter study of 24 patients. *Q J Med.* 2012;105(10):981-995. PMID: 22753675

Sagna Y, Courtillot C, Drabo JY, et al. Endocrine manifestations in a cohort of 63 adulthood and childhood onset patients with Langerhans cell histiocytosis. *Eur J Endocrinol.* 2019;181(3):275-285. PMID: 31269469

90   ANSWER: D) Start canagliflozin

The sodium-glucose cotransporter 2 (SGLT-2) protein, mainly expressed in the proximal convoluted tubules of the kidney, normally mediates reabsorption of about 90% of filtered glucose. SGLT-2 inhibitors promote the renal loss of glucose by inhibition of the SGLT-2 receptors and have favorable effects on lowering plasma glucose levels and improving renal hemodynamics and cardiovascular outcomes.

Canagliflozin (Answer D) has been approved for treatment of type 2 diabetes and is used as a second- or third-line option to treat hyperglycemia. Canagliflozin improved cardiovascular outcomes in the CANVAS trial, which was a randomized controlled trial of 10,142 participants with type 2 diabetes and elevated cardiovascular risk (65.6% of the patients had documented cardiovascular disease). Patients were randomly assigned to either 100 or 300 mg daily of canagliflozin vs placebo as add-on treatment to other antihyperglycemic medications and were followed for a mean of 188.2 weeks. The primary outcome was a composite of cardiovascular death, nonfatal heart attack, or nonfatal stroke, which was significantly reduced in the patients treated with canagliflozin (hazard ratio, 0.86; 95% CI, 0.75-0.97; $P < .001$). There was an increased risk for lower-extremity amputation in this trial, which was an unexpected finding (hazard ratio, 1.97; 95% CI, 1.41-2.75). Of affected patients, 71% had amputation of the toe or metatarsal. The patients at highest risk for amputation had a previous amputation, peripheral vascular disease, or peripheral neuropathy. The increased risk for amputation in the CANVAS trial has not been found in large randomized controlled trials of other SGLT-1 inhibitors, such as empagliflozin or dapagliflozin, nor was this reported in the CREDENCE trial with canagliflozin.

A second large randomized controlled trial (CREDENCE trial) included 4401 patients with type 2 diabetes who had chronic kidney disease and albuminuria and were treated with renin-angiotensin-aldosterone blockade and diuretics at baseline. Participants were randomly assigned to 100 mg daily of canagliflozin vs placebo and followed for a median of 2.62 years. The primary outcome was a composite of development of end-stage kidney disease (dialysis, transplant, or sustained estimated glomerular filtration rate <15 mL/min per 1.73 m^2), a doubling of serum creatinine, or death of renal or cardiovascular causes, which was significantly reduced in the patients treated with canagliflozin (hazard ratio, 0.70; 95% CI, 0.59-0.82; $P = .00001$). Secondary outcomes included a lower risk of cardiovascular death, myocardial infarction, or stroke (hazard ratio, 0.80; 95% CI, 0.67-0.95; $P = 0.01$) and hospitalization for heart failure (hazard ratio, 0.61; 95% CI, 0.47-0.80; $P < .001$) in the patients treated with canagliflozin. The slope in the decline in estimated glomerular filtration rate was also reduced in patients in the trial's active treatment arm.

Other potential adverse effects of SGLT-2 inhibitors include an increased risk of urinary tract and yeast infections. There is an increased risk of hypotension, particularly in patients treated with moderate or large doses of diuretics and in elderly patients due to potential volume depletion. SGLT-2 inhibitors have been reported to decrease bone density over time in some, but not all, randomized controlled trials and should be used with caution in patients with low bone mass or osteoporosis. The dosage of SGLT-2 inhibitor must be reduced if the estimated glomerular filtration rate is between 45 and 60 mL/min per 1.73 m^2. The recommendation is to avoid use of these medications if the initial estimated glomerular filtration rate is less than 45 mL/min per 1.73 m^2. Finally, a small subset of patients treated with SGLT-2 inhibitors develop "euglycemic ketoacidosis." These patients have biochemical evidence of metabolic acidosis but usually have glucose readings in the range of 100 to 250 mg/dL (5.6-13.9 mmol/L). This unusual form of ketoacidosis can be difficult to recognize. Affected patients should be hospitalized and treated with intravenous fluids and intravenous insulin per protocol until the acidosis has corrected.

The patient in this vignette has suboptimally controlled type 2 diabetes, microalbuminuria, and coronary atherosclerosis with mild systolic dysfunction. Addition of an SGLT-2 inhibitor or GLP-1 receptor agonist with proven efficacy in reducing cardiovascular and renal events is warranted. Of the possible treatment options, canagliflozin (Answer D) is best. Canagliflozin should lower this patient's risk of cardiovascular events and improve renal outcomes. Other SGLT-2 inhibitors such as empagliflozin and dapagliflozin have also been shown to reduce adverse cardiovascular and renal outcomes in large randomized controlled trials but were not listed as treatment options.

The GLP-1 receptor agonists liraglutide, dulaglutide, and semaglutide have been shown to reduce cardiovascular events in patients with type 2 diabetes and increased cardiovascular risk. However, they were not listed as possible treatments in this case. These medications should preferentially be used in patients with atherosclerotic coronary artery disease with retained left ventricular function. Extended-release exenatide (Answer A) and lixisenatide (Answer C) have not been shown to reduce cardiovascular events in large randomized controlled trials and would not be the best treatments in this case.

In a secondary prevention trial (IRIS trial), pioglitazone (Answer E) was demonstrated to reduce the risk of stroke or transient ischemic attack in patients with insulin resistance (but without overt diabetes) who had increased cardiovascular risk. However, the presence of systolic dysfunction in this patient should preclude the use of a thiazolidinedione such as pioglitazone.

Increasing all insulin doses by 10% (Answer B) is a treatment option and it may improve this patient's glycemic control. However, increasing the amount of insulin will most likely not reduce adverse cardiovascular or renal outcomes in this patient and may lead to additional weight gain and fluid retention.

If the patient is prescribed canagliflozin, his blood pressure should be monitored closely and a chemistry panel should be obtained 1 to 3 weeks later to ensure that renal function is stable.

Educational Objective
Determine when SGLT-2 inhibitors are indicated in a patient with type 2 diabetes mellitus, coronary artery disease, and diabetic nephropathy.

Reference(s)
Neal B, Perkovic V, Mahaffey KW, et al; CANAS Program Collaborative Group. Canagliflozin and cardiovascular and renal events in type 2 diabetes. *N Engl J Med*. 2017;377(7):644-657. PMID: 28605608

Perkovic V, Jardine MJ, Neal B, et al; CREDENCE Trial Investigators. Canagliflozin and renal outcomes in type 2 diabetes and nephropathy. *N Engl J Med*. 2019;380(24):2295-2306. PMID: 30990260

Fadini GP, Avogaro A. SGLT2 inhibitors and amputations in the US FDA Adverse Event Reporting System. *Lancet Diabetes Endocrinol*. 2017;5(9):680-681. PMID: 28733172

Peters AL, Buschur EO, Buse JB, Cohan P, Diner JC, Hirsch IB. Euglycemic diabetic ketoacidosis: a potential complication of treatment with sodium-glucose cotransporter 2 inhibition. *Diabetes Care*. 2015;38(9):1687-1693. PMID: 26078479

Kernan WN, Viscoli CM, Furie KL, et al; IRIS Trial Investigators. Pioglitazone after ischemic stroke or transient ischemic attack. *New Engl J Med*. 2016;374(14):1321-1331. PMID: 26886418

91

ANSWER: B) Diffuse sclerosing variant of papillary thyroid carcinoma

This young woman with a history of multiple autoimmune disorders, including autoimmune thyroid disease, has experienced recent enlargement of the right thyroid lobe with associated tenderness. Thyroid ultrasonography shows heterogeneous parenchymal echotexture, which is characteristic of autoimmune thyroid disease. However, the presence of diffuse microcalcifications throughout the right thyroid lobe is not characteristic of Hashimoto thyroiditis. Abnormal-appearing lymph nodes containing microcalcifications in the ipsilateral neck are also described. Together these findings are concerning for thyroid malignancy and are highly characteristic of the diffuse sclerosing variant of papillary thyroid carcinoma (DSVPTC) (Answer B).

Diffuse sclerosing variant accounts for only 6% of PTC, and it is typically seen in young women. It is more aggressive than classic PTC, with lymph node metastases occurring in approximately 80% of patients, extrathyroidal extension in 50%, and structural recurrences in close to one-third. Typical sonographic findings include hyperechogenicity, thyroidal enlargement, and the presence of numerous microcalcifications throughout the gland in the absence of a discrete nodule. Pathologically, DSVPTC is characterized by abundant psammoma bodies, squamoid metaplasia, fibrosis, calcification, and lymphocytic infiltration.

Microcalcifications also commonly occur in classic PTC (Answer A). However, they are seen in the setting of a suspicious thyroid nodule rather than an infiltrative malignancy.

Both metastatic nonthyroidal malignancy and thyroid lymphoma should be included in the differential diagnosis of a rapidly enlarging thyroid mass. However, neither is associated with the presence of diffuse microcalcifications throughout the thyroid gland. Thyroid lymphoma (Answer E) is more common in patients with Hashimoto thyroiditis, affecting approximately 0.5%. Nearly all are of the nonHodgkin type. Thyroid lymphoma is characteristically hypoechoic and pseudocystic in appearance on ultrasonography (although solid, it can appear cystic) and can be nodular or diffuse. Enhancement of posterior echoes is a distinguishing finding.

This patient has a history of abnormal pap smears with high-risk human papillomavirus. However, thyroid metastasis from squamous-cell carcinoma of the cervix (Answer C) has not been reported in patients without a known diagnosis of metastatic cervical cancer. Among nonthyroidal solid malignancies, renal-cell carcinoma is most likely to metastasize to the thyroid gland.

Although subacute thyroiditis (Answer D) is often associated with asymmetric thyroid enlargement, pain, and tenderness, this is usually associated with fever and thyrotoxicosis and is preceded by a viral illness. Evanescent, ill-defined, hypoechoic nodular areas can be seen on ultrasonography in the setting of subacute thyroiditis; however, microcalcifications and highly suspicious cervical lymphadenopathy do not occur.

Educational Objective

Recognize the characteristic ultrasonography appearance of the diffuse sclerosing variant of papillary thyroid cancer.

Reference(s)

Vuong HG, Kondo T, Pham TQ, et al. Prognostic significance of diffuse sclerosing variant papillary thyroid carcinoma: a systematic review and meta-analysis. *Eur J Endocrinol.* 2017;176(4):433-441. PMID: 28183787

Chereau N, Giudicelli X, Pattou F, et al. Diffuse sclerosing variant of papillary thyroid carcinoma is associated with aggressive histopathological features and a poor outcome: results of a large multicentric study. *J Clin Endocrinol Metab.* 2016;101(12):4603-4610. PMID: 27626975

92

ANSWER: C) Measure macroprolactin

Hyperprolactinemia is a common abnormality, and its evaluation must be thoughtful, as elevated prolactin can be due to many different causes. One cause is pregnancy, which in this case has been ruled out. Another cause is drugs, mostly antidopaminergic psychiatric medications or promotility agents such as metoclopramide or domperidone. Other causes include prolactin-secreting pituitary adenomas or sellar masses that cause elevated prolactin due to stalk compression (the stalk effect). An increasingly recognized cause of elevated serum prolactin is macroprolactinemia. In this condition, prolactin binds to immunoglobulins creating an antigen-antibody complex of higher molecular mass than prolactin (>150 kDa). Prolactin antibodies may compete with prolactin molecules for receptor binding, resulting in low bioactivity. The term *macroprolactinemia* is generally used when the concentration of macroprolactin exceeds 60% of the total serum prolactin concentration as determined by measurement of prolactin before and after polyethylene glycol precipitation. Polyethylene glycol removes the prolactin molecules that are bound to proteins, and prolactin is then measured again in the remaining serum.

This allows a measurement of real, or "monomeric," serum prolactin. Hyperprolactinemia occurs in this condition because macroprolactin is not cleared readily from the circulation due to its binding to immunoglobulins. The overall prevalence of macroprolactinemia in patients with hyperprolactinemia is 10% to 30%. Interestingly, the symptoms of hyperprolactinemia (irregular periods, erectile dysfunction) seem to be equally prevalent in patients with macroprolactinemia and in patients with real hyperprolactinemia.

Macroprolactinemia is a benign clinical condition, and no pharmacologic treatment or diagnostic investigations are necessary. However, macroprolactinemia occasionally occurs in the presence of prolactin-secreting pituitary adenomas, and this could be determined by documenting an elevated level of monomeric prolactin after the protein-bound prolactin is removed by polyethylene glycol. Macroprolactin should be measured in this patient before additional testing is done (Answer C).

Performing a pituitary-directed MRI (Answer A) would not be appropriate in this case before proof of real hyperprolactinemia is documented. Although 10% to 15% of GH-secreting adenomas cosecrete prolactin, measuring a random GH concentration (Answer B) is rarely useful, particularly in this patient who has a normal serum IGF-1 value. While primary hypothyroidism is a cause of hyperprolactinemia (due to increased secretion of hypothalamic thyrotropin-releasing hormone), this has been ruled out by the normal TSH measurement. Therefore, measuring free T_4 (Answer D) is not necessary. Finally, sertraline and other selective serotonin reuptake inhibitors are occasionally associated with hyperprolactinemia, but this is generally mild and very rarely causes an elevation above 100 ng/mL (>4.3 nmol/L). Thus, measuring prolactin after stopping sertraline (Answer E) is incorrect.

Educational Objective
Guide the evaluation for macroprolactinemia.

Reference(s)
Kasum M, Pavičić-Baldani D, Stanić P, et al. Importance of macroprolactinemia in hyperprolactinemia. *Eur J Obstet Gynecol Reprod Biol*. 2014;183:28-32. PMID: 25461348

McKenna TJ. Should macroprolactin be measured in all hyperprolactinaemic sera? *Clin Endocrinol (Oxf)*. 2009;71(4):466-469. PMID: 19320649

Glezer A, Bronstein MD. Approach to the patient with persistent hyperprolactinemia and negative sellar imaging. *J Clin Endocrinol Metab*. 2012;97(7):2211-2216. PMID: 22774208

Park YM. Serum prolactin levels in patients with major depressive disorder receiving selective serotonin-reuptake inhibitor monotherapy for 3 months: a prospective study. *Psychiatry Investig*. 2017;14(3):368-371. PMID: 28539956

93 ANSWER: E) Provide reassurance and do not change current therapy

This woman has nonclassic 21-hydroxylase deficiency without evidence of adrenal insufficiency. A basal morning follicular-phase 17-hydroxyprogesterone concentration greater than 1500 ng/dL (>45.5 nmol/L) in an adult woman confirms the diagnosis. In settings when the 17-hydroxyprogesterone concentration is 200 to 1500 ng/dL (6.1-45.5 nmol/L), a cosyntropin-stimulation test can be performed and the diagnosis can made if levels rise above 1500 ng/dL (>45.5 nmol/L).

Although she was treated with nocturnal dexamethasone for many years, the risk-to-benefit value of this treatment strategy is debatable. Hyperandrogenism (hirsutism and acne) and oligomenorrhea in adult women with nonclassic 21-hydroxylase deficiency should be preferentially treated with estrogen-containing oral contraceptives because they can effectively normalize menses, increase SHBG, and lower androgens. If needed, antiandrogens such as spironolactone can be used in addition. Glucocorticoid therapy should be reserved for women who cannot tolerate oral contraceptives or who do not respond to oral contraceptives and antiandrogens. In contrast, glucocorticoids are first-line therapy in classic 21-hydroxylase deficiency.

Although glucocorticoids are especially effective at lowering androgens, they are associated with a higher risk of adverse effects, particularly with nocturnal dosing and long-acting glucocorticoids such as dexamethasone (as was observed with this patient's weight gain). Glucocorticoids can be considered in women with nonclassic 21-hydroxylase deficiency when oral contraceptives and antiandrogens are insufficient or not tolerated, or for infertility and anovulation. If glucocorticoids are used for infertility, dexamethasone should be avoided because it crosses the placenta, and glucocorticoids should be stopped when fertility is no longer sought, with a transition to oral contraceptives and/or antiandrogens, if possible.

This patient has mild nonclassic 21-hydroxylase deficiency. Although she stopped taking dexamethasone 2 years ago, she has no evidence of adrenal insufficiency. She has mild hirsutism and normal menses while on an estrogen-containing oral contraceptive. Therefore, there is no strong indication to initiate glucocorticoids (Answers A, B, C, and D) and expose her to unnecessary risk. The best course of action is to provide reassurance and continue the same therapy (Answer E). If needed, an antiandrogen could be considered in the future.

Educational Objective
Manage nonclassic congenital adrenal hyperplasia in a woman.

Reference(s)
Speiser PW, Arlt W, Auchus RJ, et al. Congenital adrenal hyperplasia due to steroid 21-hydroxylase deficiency: an Endocrine Society clinical practice guideline. *J Clin Endocrinol Metab.* 2018;103(11):4043-4088. PMID: 30272171

94 ANSWER: B) Increase the levothyroxine dosage to 125 mcg daily

This patient had preexisting hypothyroidism before becoming pregnant and is on thyroid hormone replacement therapy. In general, pregnancy affects thyroid gland size and its function. The thyroid gland increases in size during pregnancy and the degree of the size change depends on the patient's iodine status. The size increases more in iodine-deficient areas (20%-40%) and increases less in iodine-replete areas (10%). Production of T_4 and T_3 increases by almost 50%. The daily iodine requirement also increases by 50% during pregnancy. These physiologic changes become challenging for pregnant women with a diagnosis of hypothyroidism. Approximately 50% to 85% of pregnant women with preexisting hypothyroidism need more levothyroxine during pregnancy. Factors responsible for this increased requirement include weight gain, increased T_4 pool size, elevated serum thyroxine-binding globulin concentrations, increased clearance of T_4 due to placental deiodinase activity, transfer of T_4 to the fetus, and reduced gastrointestinal absorption due to iron intake by daily ingestion of prenatal vitamin. Therefore, hypothyroid women of reproductive age on levothyroxine therapy should be counseled regarding the likelihood of increased demand for levothyroxine during pregnancy. They should also be counseled to contact their caregiver immediately upon a confirmed pregnancy to adjust thyroid hormone replacement therapy. In hypothyroid women who become pregnant, the levothyroxine dosage should be increased by 25% to 30%. This is typically accomplished by switching from once-daily dosing to a total of 9 doses per week (double the daily dose 2 days each week), or by prescribing a new daily dose that is increased by 25% to 30% (thus, Answer B is correct and Answers A and C are incorrect). After this change, further dosage adjustment should be made to target a TSH in the lower half of the trimester-specific reference range. When this is not available, it is reasonable to target maternal TSH concentrations below 2.5 mU/L. Once the TSH level is within the desired range, it should be monitored every trimester. Dosage requirements can increase by as much as 50% during pregnancy, and the increase occurs as early as the fifth week of gestation. In a prospective study, the median onset of the dosage adjustment occurred at 8 weeks' gestation with a plateau at 16 weeks' gestation. However, some women required an adjustment in levothyroxine dosage as early as the fifth week of gestation. Following delivery, the levothyroxine dosage should be reduced to the prepregnancy dosage followed by measurement of serum TSH 4 to 6 weeks later.

T_4 delivery is very important for the development of fetal brain. Pregnant women taking either desiccated thyroid or a regimen combining T_3 and T_4 are most likely at risk for having insufficient transfer of maternal T_4 to the fetal brain. The fetal central nervous system is relatively impermeable to T_3 and this is the reason to avoid the use of exogenous T_3 during pregnancy. In addition, most fetal T_3 present in the central nervous system during pregnancy is derived from maternal T_4. Liothyronine treatment (Answers D and E) should not be considered in the management of pregnant women with hypothyroidism.

Educational Objective
Manage hypothyroidism in a pregnant woman with preexisting hypothyroidism.

Reference(s)

Alexander EK, Pearce EN, Brent GA, et al. 2017 guidelines of the American Thyroid Association for the diagnosis and management of thyroid disease during pregnancy and the postpartum. *Thyroid.* 2017;27(3):315-389. PMID: 28056690

Alexander EK, Marqusee E, Lawrence J, Jarolim P, Fischer GA, Larsen PR. Timing and magnitude of increases in levothyroxine requirements during pregnancy in women with hypothyroidism. *N Engl J Med.* 2004;351(3):241-249. PMID: 15254282

95 ANSWER: C) Idiopathic hirsutism

Although this patient meets criteria for hirsutism with a modified Ferriman-Gallwey score of 8 or higher, she does not have polycystic ovary syndrome (Answer A) as defined by Rotterdam criteria: clinical examination findings of moderate hirsutism (Ferriman-Gallwey score ≥8) or androgenetic acne or alopecia or biochemical results of elevated androgens above the reference range. Her ovulatory status was normal in the past based on regular menses and no difficulty conceiving. Pelvic ultrasonography did not reveal enlarged ovarian volume greater than 10 mL (the left ovary is excluded due to the presence of a cyst >1 cm) or multiple follicles smaller than 1 cm (Rotterdam criteria ≥12; 2018 International American Society for Reproductive Medicine/European Society for Human Reproduction and Embryology guideline [with improved transducer frequency ≥8 MHz] ≥20 follicles for women older than 20 years).

She does not have clinical findings of Cushing syndrome on examination, so screening for Cushing syndrome or a pituitary or adrenal tumor is not necessary. The DHEA-S concentration greater than 50 μg/dL (>1.36 μmol/L) also argues against Cushing syndrome. In the evaluation for mild autonomous cortisol secretion, a DHEA-S value lower than 50 μg/dL (<1.36 μmol/L) might increase suspicion for autonomous cortisol secretion from the adrenal glands or an adrenal adenoma (Answer B) due to suppression of ACTH and subsequent decreased DHEA-S concentrations.

Although this woman's symptoms began in pregnancy, luteoma (Answer D) is a cause of gestational hirsutism or virilization that would improve after pregnancy. While deepening of the voice or clitoromegaly would not necessarily resolve after pregnancy in the setting of luteoma, terminal hair growth should not continue to worsen after pregnancy. Luteomas are not tumors but represent hyperplastic masses of large lutein cells that spontaneously resolve within a few weeks after delivery.

Ovarian hyperthecosis (Answer E) is a nonneoplastic condition of androgen excess more common in postmenopausal women, although it can also occur before menopause. The clinical presentation is usually characterized by more severe hirsutism or even virilization (deepening of the voice, frontal balding, clitoromegaly) with a more recent onset, rapid progression, and higher total testosterone concentrations above 150 ng/dL (>5.2 nmol/L). With this woman's presentation of mild hirsutism and normal total testosterone, this diagnosis is far less likely.

Because this woman does not have any other cause of hirsutism, she would be classified as having idiopathic hirsutism (Answer C); that is, hirsutism not caused by another hyperandrogenic endocrine disorder. Hyperinsulinemia is thought to drive excess androgen production by the ovary in polycystic ovary syndrome, and idiopathic hirsutism might also be caused by hyperinsulinemia in obesity, type 2 diabetes, and insulin resistance. She has increased risk from family history and ethnicity. Weight gain and increased insulin resistance during pregnancy could explain why she started developing hirsutism during pregnancy.

Educational Objective

Evaluate hirsutism and diagnose or exclude polycystic ovary syndrome.

Reference(s)

Legro RS, Arslanian SA, Ehrmann DA, et al; Endocrine Society. Diagnosis and treatment of polycystic ovary syndrome: an Endocrine Society clinical practice guideline. *J Clin Endocrinol Metab.* 2013;98(12):4565-4592. PMID: 24151290

Teede HJ, Misso ML, Costello MF, et al; International PCOS Network. Recommendations from the international evidence-based guideline for the assessment and management of polycystic ovary syndrome. *Fertil Steril.* 2018;110(3):364-379. PMID: 30033227

Escobar-Morreale HF, Carmina E, Dewailly D, et al. Epidemiology, diagnosis and management of hirsutism: a consensus statement by the Androgen Excess and Polycystic Ovary Syndrome Society. *Hum Reprod Update.* 2012;18(2):146-170. PMID: 22064667

Martin KA, Anderson RR, Chang RJ, et al. Evaluation and treatment of hirsutism in premenopausal women: an Endocrine Society clinical practice guideline. *J Clin Endocrinol Metab.* 2018;103(4):1-25. PMID: 29522147

96

ANSWER: B) Perform serum protein electrophoresis

This patient presents with very low HDL cholesterol, which has recently developed given documentation of normal HDL cholesterol 2 years ago. Low HDL cholesterol is a commonly observed lipid abnormality, especially in individuals with diabetes or coronary heart disease. Low HDL cholesterol is defined as an HDL-cholesterol concentration less than 40 mg/dL (<1.04 mmol/L) in men and less than 50 mg/dL (<1.30 mmol/L) in women. Patients exhibiting extremely low HDL cholesterol, defined as levels below 20 mg/dL (<0.52 mmol/L), often have hypertriglyceridemia (triglycerides >500 mg/dL [>5.65 mmol/L]). An HDL-cholesterol concentration less than 20 mg/dL (<0.52 mmol/L) (<5th percentile for normal range) in the absence of hypertriglyceridemia is uncommon and suggests abnormal HDL-cholesterol metabolic pathways. Very low HDL cholesterol in the absence of significant hypertriglyceridemia generally results from impaired HDL synthesis.

In the absence of elevated triglycerides, isolated very low HDL cholesterol can be observed due to primary (genetic) or secondary causes. Primary low HDL cholesterol results from rare monogenic disorders, including apolipoprotein A-1 deficiency, Tangier disease, and lecithin cholesterol acyltransferase deficiency. Affected individuals have very low HDL-cholesterol levels (<10 mg/dL [<0.26 mmol/L]) on all lipid measurements. The patient in this vignette has no evidence of a primary genetic HDL disorder since he had a normal HDL-cholesterol concentration 2 years ago.

Secondary reasons for very low HDL cholesterol can result from artifactual causes due to certain drugs, malignancy, or laboratory interference with the HDL assay. Use of androgenic anabolic steroids results in a profound drop in HDL cholesterol through activation of clearance pathways. Androgenic anabolic steroids used for catabolic diseases such as malignancy and AIDS (or used recreationally) may result in extremely low HDL-cholesterol levels. HDL-cholesterol levels decline within days of initiating these agents and normalize after 1 to 3 months of steroid withdrawal. Androgens exert their HDL-lowering effects by accelerating the breakdown of HDL. Occasionally, individuals who are treated with fibrates demonstrate a paradoxical response with dramatic reductions in HDL cholesterol below 20 mg/dL (<0.52 mmol/L). The prevalence and reason for this idiosyncratic response remain unknown. A sudden, dramatic decline in HDL cholesterol may precede overt clinical manifestations of a hematologic malignancy. Extremely low HDL-cholesterol levels have been reported in the setting of lymphoma. The mechanism underlying HDL-cholesterol suppression remains unknown and the suppression resolves with treatment. Assay interference occurs when there is paraproteinemia due to immunoproliferative disorders, with resultant interference in the HDL assay reagents. Measurement by other methods such as ultracentrifugation reveals normal lipid levels. Treatment of the underlying disorder (such as multiple myeloma) normalizes the extremely low HDL cholesterol observed with direct assays.

This patient has experienced a recent drop in HDL-cholesterol levels. Serum protein electrophoresis (Answer B) should be performed to rule out assay interference. This man was found to have a monoclonal spike on serum protein electrophoresis, and he was referred to hematology. A bone marrow biopsy confirmed monoclonal gammopathy due to plasma-cell myeloma. Low HDL cholesterol was believed to be due to interference of paraproteins in the HDL assay used on the autoanalyzer. Sample reanalysis using a different technique revealed an HDL-cholesterol concentration of 43 mg/dL (1.11 mmol/L), similar to values noted previously.

Apolipoprotein A-1 is the structural protein of HDL, and its levels are low when HDL-cholesterol levels are low. Measurement of apolipoprotein A-1 (Answer A) would not add diagnostic value to this patient's evaluation. There is no clinical evidence that he is taking anabolic steroids. Therefore, testosterone measurement (Answer C) is not the best option. HDL efflux capacity (Answer D) is assessed with a functional assay and is not widely available commercially. It would not add diagnostic value in this situation. Lipoprotein (a) (Answer E) is a modified LDL-like particle with structural similarity to plasminogen. Circulating lipoprotein (a) levels are primarily determined by genetics. High lipoprotein (a) levels contribute to atherogenic risk and can be considered a risk-enhancing factor. However, lipoprotein (a) has no known effect on HDL-cholesterol levels, and its measurement in this individual is unlikely to add information that can aid in his management.

Educational Objective

Identify malignancy as a cause of very low HDL cholesterol.

Reference(s)

Rader DJ, deGoma EM. Approach to the patient with extremely low HDL-cholesterol. *J Clin Endocrinol Metab.* 2012;97(10):3399-3407. PMID: 23043194

Goldberg RB, Mendez AJ. Severe acquired (secondary) high-density lipoprotein deficiency. *J Clin Lipidol.* 2007;1(1):41-56. PMID: 21291667

97

ANSWER: B) Hypophosphatasia

On first pass, this patient's "calcium disorder" appears to be due to calcific periarthritis, a condition that involves calcium deposition within tendons and ligaments surrounding joints. The condition typically affects middle-aged adults, is more common in females than in males, and may or may not be associated with antecedent overuse or trauma. The disease has been associated with diabetes mellitus and thyroid disorders, although most affected patients have no specific predisposing risk factors. Genetic disorders of mineral metabolism, however, may also predispose to the disorder, which is likely the case for this patient. She has a constellation of previous metatarsal fractures, family history of a femoral fracture in her mother while on bisphosphonate therapy, and a low alkaline phosphatase level. These findings are most consistent with a diagnosis of hypophosphatasia (Answer B). Hypophosphatasia is due to pathogenic variants in the gene encoding tissue nonspecific alkaline phosphatase (*ALPL*) that result in elevated levels of the substrate molecule pyrophosphate, leading to impaired mineralization and osteomalacia with low-trauma fractures in adults. As such, bisphosphonates, which are often prescribed for low bone density in older women with suspected osteoporosis and can worsen underlying osteomalacia, are contraindicated in patients with hypophosphatasia. In addition, disturbances in pyrophosphate metabolism also result in extraarticular calcification in some patients, causing calcific periarthritis, chondrocalcinosis, or diffuse idiopathic skeletal hyperostosis. The prevalence of hypophosphatasia was historically thought to be low, although a more recent study suggests that the frequency of a dominant allele may be as high as 1 in 6370 in a European population. While there is an FDA-approved therapy for hypophosphatasia (asfotase alfa) in children and in adults with pediatric onset disease, there is no evidence to date that treatment improves the extraarticular consequences of the disease.

Disturbances in phosphorus metabolism, specifically hyperphosphatemia, caused by reduction in FGF-23, a physiologically regulated phosphaturic hormone, can also lead to a disorder of periarticular calcification called tumoral calcinosis (Answer A). Tumoral calcinosis can be due to pathogenic variants in the FGF-23 gene (*FGF23*) or the α-Klotho gene (*KL*), the gene product of which, alpha Klotho, is the obligatory cofactor for FGF-23 action. More recently, pathogenic variants in *GALNT3*, the gene encoding a glycosyltransferase that is thought to prevent the degradation of FGF-23, as well as autoantibodies to FGF-23, have also been described as a cause of tumoral calcinosis. This patient's phosphate level, however, is normal, ruling out tumoral calcinosis as a potential etiology for her calcific periarthritis.

Although pseudogout in the setting of hyperparathyroidism can also be confused with calcific periarthritis, this patient has no evidence for either primary or secondary hyperparathyroidism (Answer C) based on her laboratory values.

Infectious arthritis (Answer E) can potentially mimic the clinical presentation of calcific periarthritis, although this patient's normal white blood cell count and absence of fever make this diagnosis much less likely.

Tumor-induced osteomalacia (Answer D) with mandatorily associated hypophosphatemia is due to overproduction of FGF-23, resulting in bone pain, muscle weakness, and stress or insufficiency fractures. Consistent with a contradistinctive physiology to tumoral calcinosis, however, tumor-induced osteomalacia is not associated with periarticular calcific disease.

Educational Objective
Identify nonskeletal manifestations (calcific periarthritis) in a patient with hypophosphatasia.

Reference(s)
McKiernan FE, Berg RL, Fuehrer J. Clinical and radiographic findings in adults with persistent hypophosphatasemia. *J Bone Miner Res*. 2014;29(7):1651-1660. PMID: 24443354

Guañabens N, Mumm S, Möller I, et al. Calcific periarthritis as the only clinical manifestation of hypophosphatasia in middle-aged sisters. *J Bone Miner Res*. 2014;29(4):929-934. PMID: 24123110

98

ANSWER: A) Continue methimazole at the current dosage

The prevalence of overt hyperthyroidism in pregnancy is 0.9% in the first trimester and 0.65% in the second trimester. Hypertension, heart failure, and thyroid storm are potential maternal complications. Adverse pregnancy outcomes can also include intrauterine growth restriction, placental abruption, preterm labor and birth, low birthweight, and stillbirth. Subclinical hyperthyroidism has not been associated with poor maternal or fetal/neonatal outcomes.

Gestational thyrotoxicosis is the most common cause of thyrotoxicosis during pregnancy. The glycoprotein hormones including TSH and hCG possess a common α subunit and a unique β subunit, which confers their specificity. Because of the considerable homology between TSH and hCG, hCG can bind to and activate the TSH receptor during pregnancy, leading to increased thyroid hormone synthesis and secretion. Gestational thyrotoxicosis occurs concurrently with hyperemesis gravidarum in approximately 50% of cases. Biochemical resolution of gestational thyrotoxicosis usually occurs by 19 weeks' gestation.

Graves disease is the second most common cause of hyperthyroidism in pregnancy, affecting up to 1% of women before pregnancy and 0.2% during pregnancy. Graves disease is the causative diagnosis in the patient described, as confirmed by the elevated thyroid-stimulating immunoglobulin result. The patient began treatment with methimazole when overt hyperthyroidism was detected in the early second trimester. Methimazole is the antithyroid drug of choice when treatment is indicated in the second trimester of pregnancy, while propylthiouracil is preferred if medical therapy is required in the first trimester. Although both drugs have been shown to be teratogenic, the severity of birth defects is greater with methimazole. Switching between antithyroid drugs in the middle of pregnancy can precipitate decompensation of control. However, transitioning from propylthiouracil to methimazole in pregnant women who are beyond 16 weeks' gestation can be considered because of the known risk of severe liver toxicity with propylthiouracil. Conversely, discontinuing methimazole and starting propylthiouracil, 50 mg 3 times daily (Answer D), would not be recommended.

When treating hyperthyroidism with antithyroid drugs in pregnancy, the lowest effective dosage should be administered to prevent fetal hypothyroidism. Serum TSH may remain low throughout pregnancy, and antithyroid drugs should not be dosed with the goal of normalizing TSH values. Maternal serum free T_4 or total T_4 should be monitored at least every 4 weeks with the goal of achieving levels at or moderately above the upper limit of the nonpregnant reference range. Total T_4 increases by 5% per week from gestational weeks 7 to 16 and then plateaus. Beginning at 16 weeks, the pregnancy-specific reference range can be determined by multiplying the upper and lower limits of the nonpregnant reference range by 1.5. Spuriously low free T_4 levels can be seen in the latter half of pregnancy with direct free T_4 assays. Pregnancy-specific reference ranges must be used when interpreting free T_4 measurements.

The patient has been taking methimazole 5 mg daily for 4 weeks, and serum total T_4 is now within the pregnancy-specific reference range. The most appropriate management is to continue methimazole at the current dosage (Answer A) and repeat thyroid function tests in 4 weeks.

Advising the patient to increase the methimazole dosage to 10 mg daily (Answer B) or to discontinue methimazole and monitor thyroid function (Answer C) is not recommended. Increasing the methimazole dosage further could lead to fetal hypothyroidism due to the higher sensitivity of the fetal thyroid to antithyroid drugs, while stopping treatment would most likely result in recurrent symptomatic maternal hyperthyroidism.

Thyroidectomy (Answer E) can be considered in the early second trimester (before 23 weeks) in pregnant women with hyperthyroidism who either have allergies or contraindications to antithyroid drugs or in whom sufficient control of hyperthyroidism cannot be achieved. The patient described has well-controlled hyperthyroidism on low-dosage methimazole and thus there is no compelling reason to refer for thyroidectomy now.

Educational Objective
Determine thyroid function test goals during thionamide treatment in a pregnant woman.

Reference(s)

Alexander EK, Pearce EN, Brent GA, et al. 2017 guidelines of the American Thyroid Association for the diagnosis and management of thyroid disease during pregnancy and the postpartum. *Thyroid.* 2017;27(3):315-389. PMID: 28056690

Andersen SL, Olsen J, Wu CS, Laurberg P. Severity of birth defects after propylthiouracil exposure in early pregnancy. *Thyroid.* 2014;24(10):1533-1540. PMID: 24963758

99

ANSWER: E) Add an SGLT-2 inhibitor and reduce her basal insulin dosage

This patient's basal insulin dosage is currently greater than 0.5 units/kg per day. Higher doses of basal have been associated with an increased risk of hypoglycemia and weight gain, but not much further improvement in glycemic control. The frequent hypoglycemia (and fear of these episodes) can become a barrier to continued improvement in glycemic control. This patient is currently fearful of nocturnal hypoglycemia, leading her to reduce her nightly dose of insulin glargine. This most likely has a role in her hemoglobin A_{1c} level being above goal (>7.0% [>53 mmol/mol]). Her blood glucose log shows that her blood glucose concentration frequently drops by more than 100 mg/dL (5.6 mmol/L) while sleeping, with the exception of day 3, where she probably held her dose of insulin glargine (she reports doing so when her bedtime blood glucose level is less than 150 mg/dL [<8.3 mmol/L]). Both her current basal insulin dosage and her blood glucose log suggest she is at a high risk of hypoglycemia, particularly while sleeping.

Moving the time of insulin glargine dosing from bedtime to the morning (Answer A), or splitting the dosing to twice daily, is unlikely to reduce her risk of hypoglycemia. In patients on lower insulin dosages, particularly those who are very insulin sensitive, these maneuvers may be helpful, but in patients receiving much higher doses of basal insulin, such an intervention would be unlikely to have a meaningful impact.

Monnier et al has reported that when the hemoglobin A_{1c} value is less than 8.5% (<69 mmol/mol), the largest contributor to the elevated hemoglobin A_{1c} is postprandial hyperglycemia. This patient demonstrates a consistent step-wise deterioration in glycemic control with progressive meal intake. Accordingly, adding a therapy that may address this aspect of the patient's glycemic profile, such as an SGLT-2 inhibitor, would be a great option, as long as her current issue regarding the increased risk of nocturnal hypoglycemia risk is addressed by simultaneously reducing her dosage of basal insulin therapy (Answer E). Lowering the insulin glargine dosage would certainly be advised, but if this were the only intervention to take place, the patient's progressive rise in serum glucose with each meal would remain an issue that still needs to be addressed. SGLT-2 inhibitors reduce hyperglycemia via blocking the reabsorption of glucose in the proximal tubule, thereby inducing glucosuria. This occurs independent of insulin action. Addition of an SGLT-2 inhibitor would nicely augment this patient's existing regimen.

Increasing the metformin dosage (Answer C) would not be the best option, as this would most likely lower her fasting glucose even further. Likewise, adding a sulfonylurea such as glipizide (Answer B) would further decrease her fasting glucose, which is currently not the primary issue, and this would likely only further worsen her fear of hypoglycemia. While adding a dose of prandial insulin at dinner (Answer D) would help to lower blood glucose near bedtime, without a concurrent reduction in her basal insulin dose, this would most likely increase her risk of nocturnal hypoglycemia.

Educational Objective

Identify patients with type 2 diabetes mellitus who are overtreated with basal insulin (>0.5 units/kg per day) and would benefit from added therapy to address postprandial hyperglycemia.

Reference(s)

Reid T, Gao L, Gill J, et al. How much is too much? Outcomes in patients using high-dose insulin glargine. *Int J Clin Pract.* 2016;70(1):56-65. PMID: 26566714

Monnier L, Lapinski H, Colette C. Contributions of fasting and postprandial plasma glucose increments to the overall diurnal hyperglycemia of type 2 diabetic patients: variations with increasing levels of HbA(1c). *Diabetes Care.* 2003;26(3):881-885. PMID: 12610053

Shapiro ET, Van Cauter E, Tillil H, et al. Glyburide enhances the responsiveness of the beta-cell to glucose but does not correct the abnormal patterns of insulin secretion in noninsulin-dependent diabetes mellitus. *J Clin Endocrinol Metab.* 1989;69(3):571-576. PMID: 2503533

Hinnen DA. Therapeutic options for the management of postprandial glucose in patients with type 2 diabetes on basal insulin. *Clin Diabetes.* 2015;33(4):175-180. PMID: 26487791

Stenlöf K, Cefalu WT, Kim KA, et al. Efficacy and safety of canagliflozin monotherapy in subjects with type 2 diabetes mellitus inadequately controlled with diet and exercise. *Diabetes Obes Metab.* 2013;15(4):372-382. PMID: 23279307

List J, Woo V, Morales E, Tang W, Fiedorek FT. Sodium-glucose cotransport inhibition with dapagliflozin in type 2 diabetes. *Diabetes Care.* 2009;32(4):650-657. PMID: 19114612

100 ANSWER: C) hCG

This man has acquired anterior pituitary dysfunction, with postpubertal hypogonadotropic hypogonadism. He has proven prior fertility, and his modest reduction in testicular size and azoospermia is explained by his longstanding testosterone treatment. While he may respond to hCG monotherapy (Answer C) (which is, among the options given, the best initial treatment), addition of recombinant FSH may become necessary.

While testosterone replacement corrects all features androgen deficiency, it does not maintain, and indeed suppresses, spermatogenesis. Exogenous testosterone suppresses FSH, which acts on the seminiferous tubules to induce and maintain spermatogenesis. Exogenous testosterone fails to achieve the high testicular testosterone concentrations that are present in eugonadal men due to testicular steroidogenesis. High intratesticular testosterone concentrations are, in conjunction with FSH, necessary prerequisites for normal spermatogenesis. Therefore, testosterone treatment should not be started in men desiring paternity.

Because of low cost and ease of administration, testosterone replacement is the usual long-term treatment for men with hypogonadotropic hypogonadism who do not currently desire paternity. Testosterone treatment has not been reported to compromise future fertility. Men must be informed that while future paternity is possible, this needs to be planned, as induction of spermatogenesis can take many months. They should also be informed that testosterone treatment is not a reliable contraceptive.

In this man, the best initial treatment, apart from stopping exogenous testosterone, is hCG, a long-acting LH analogue. This treatment will stimulate testicular testosterone production, leading to physiologic intratesticular testosterone (concentrations 100 times that in the peripheral circulation) and, at the same time, maintain circulating testosterone concentrations in the normal range, thus avoiding symptomatic androgen deficiency. Monotherapy with hCG is often sufficient for stimulation of spermatogenesis in men with acquired postpubertal hypogonadism, especially with proven prior fertility. Given that the seminiferous tubules account for almost 90% of the total testicular volume, testicular size is an important surrogate of fertility potential. Men with congenital hypogonadotropic hypogonadism, especially if there is failure of pubertal onset (evidenced by testicular volume ≤3 mL), or a history of cryptorchidism will generally not respond to hCG alone and early combination therapy with FSH should be considered.

Patients can be self-taught to administer hCG (intramuscularly or subcutaneously) 3 times per week. Sperm concentrations typically take at least 4 to 6 months to increase with hCG monotherapy. While local protocols differ slightly, serum testosterone is usually measured every 1 to 2 months, and the hCG dosage is adjusted to maintain total testosterone concentrations in the normal range. Sperm count is measured monthly and if the count remains less than 5 to 10 million/mL despite normal serum testosterone for 3 to 6 months, recombinant FSH (Answer B) or human menopausal gonadotropin (hMG, a somewhat cheaper source of FSH) (Answer E) is added. If men can afford early initiation of combination therapy, this might lead to a more rapid induction of spermatogenesis. However, FSH or hMG (which contains little LH) alone is not effective for the stimulation for spermatogenesis because neither stimulates Leydig cells, so they do not achieve adequate intratesticular testosterone concentrations. Moreover, they fail to maintain circulating testosterone concentrations and can lead to symptomatic androgen deficiency.

Clomiphene (Answer A), a selective estrogen receptor modulator, acts as an estradiol antagonist at the hypothalamic-pituitary unit. By counteracting estradiol-mediated central negative feedback, a selective estrogen receptor modulator can increase gonadotropin concentrations (and secondarily testosterone) in men with functional suppression of the central gonadal axis. However, in this man, clomiphene will not work in the setting of hypogonadism due to the presence of organic central pathology. Moreover, long-term safety data for clomiphene are lacking, and it is not FDA approved for the treatment of male infertility.

GnRH (Answer D) can stimulate spermatogenesis, but it requires pituitary responsiveness. GnRH only works if the hypogonadism is due to hypothalamic disease but not if it is due to pituitary pathology. To successfully stimulate gonadotropin secretion, GnRH requires administration in a pulsatile fashion, necessitating administration by a pump delivering 2 hourly boluses connected to a subcutaneous needle. This treatment is expensive and available only in specialized centers. Overall, given the rarity of hypogonadotropic hypogonadism, there are no definitive controlled studies demonstrating the superiority of one particular hormonal treatment in the stimulation of spermatogenesis, let alone with respect to pregnancy outcomes.

Educational Objective
Initiate appropriate therapy to induce spermatogenesis in a man with postpubertal acquired hypogonadotropic hypogonadism due to pituitary failure.

Reference(s)

Anawalt BA. Approach to male infertility and induction of spermatogenesis. *J Clin Endocrinol Metab.* 2013;98(9);3532-3542. PMID: 24014811

Prior M, Stewart J, McEleny K, Dwyer AA, Quinton R. Fertility induction in hypogonadotropic hypogonadal men. *Clin Endocrinol (Oxf).* 2018;89(6):712-718. PMID: 30194850

101

ANSWER: D) Taper off hydrocortisone and initiate an oral contraceptive

Congenital adrenal hyperplasia (CAH) due to 21-hydroxylase deficiency and pathogenic variants in the *CYP21A2* gene is one of the most common autosomal recessive diseases. More severe enzyme deficiency results in classic CAH with adrenal insufficiency and ambiguous genitalia in females. Nonclassic CAH, which is not associated with adrenal insufficiency, is more common than classic CAH. Among white populations, the prevalence of nonclassic CAH may be as high as 1 in 1000 to 1 in 100. The prevalence is highest among persons of Hispanic, Yugoslav, and Ashkenazi Jewish ancestry.

Nonclassic CAH can present in childhood, as in this vignette, with precocious puberty and accelerated bone age. Adolescent and adult female patients might be diagnosed during an evaluation for hyperandrogenism, oligomenorrhea, and/or infertility. It is recommended that all women being evaluated for the diagnosis of polycystic ovary syndrome have a screening 17-hydroxyprogesterone measurement to exclude the diagnosis of nonclassic CAH, ideally timed to the follicular phase if menses are regular. Whereas in classic CAH, glucocorticoid and mineralocorticoids are required to replace deficiency, the goal of glucocorticoid treatment in childhood/adolescence in patients with nonclassic CAH is to stop further pubertal development to optimize growth potential and lower androgen excess. This must be accomplished while also avoiding iatrogenic glucocorticoid excess.

The standard 250-mcg cosyntropin-stimulation test results in the table demonstrate that this patient has normal baseline ACTH and cortisol and normal adrenal reserve with cortisol concentrations above 18 μg/dL (496.6 nmol/L) 60 minutes after stimulation. This clarified for the patient that she indeed has nonclassic CAH and does not require both glucocorticoids and mineralocorticoids to replace deficiency. A 17-hydroxyprogesterone concentration above 1000 ng/dL (>30.3 nmol/L) at both 30- and 60-minute time points confirms the diagnosis of nonclassic CAH.

The management of hirsutism in women with nonclassic CAH is the same as management of hirsutism in women without CAH. They do not require glucocorticoids because they are more likely to experience weight gain and even glucose intolerance at the dosages needed to suppress androgens. Once female patients go through puberty, the first-line recommended therapy for hirsutism is the same as in premenopausal women who are not planning to conceive: oral contraceptives (Answer A). Oral contraceptives suppress LH secretion and ovarian androgen production while also increasing hepatic production of SHBG, which lowers serum free androgen concentrations. In this case, since the patient has evidence of sufficient adrenal function and is not trying to conceive, she does not require hydrocortisone replacement. The best next step in her management would be to first taper off hydrocortisone to potentially limit the effect on weight gain and then to initiate an oral contraceptive (Answer D) to address the hirsutism.

In the past, the reverse diurnal rhythm (in this case, hydrocortisone, 5 mg in the morning and 10 mg at bedtime) was thought to better suppress the rise in morning ACTH that leads to increases in 17-hydroxyprogesterone, androstenedione, and DHEA-S androgens, which cause symptoms of hyperandrogenism or interfere with fertility. However, studies have not shown that this approach is any better than standard hydrocortisone replacement therapies. As already mentioned, this patient does not require hydrocortisone. Thus, changing to a normal diurnal pattern (Answer E) is not necessary. Similarly, the switch from hydrocortisone to dexamethasone (Answer C) is also not necessary and is more likely to cause weight gain and worsening insulin resistance, although it might decrease androgens more than hydrocortisone.

She does have impaired fasting glucose or prediabetes, so metformin (Answer B) could be considered for off-label use to prevent diabetes (based on the Diabetes Prevention Program studies). Metformin has been shown to significantly reduce the incidence of type 2 diabetes by 31% over 15 years, while lifestyle changes have been shown to reduce the incidence by 58%. However, the best next step is to taper off hydrocortisone and initiate an oral contraceptive.

Educational Objective
Guide the management of nonclassic congenital adrenal hyperplasia in adolescent girls transitioning to adulthood.

Reference(s)

Diabetes Prevention Program Research Group. Long-term effects of lifestyle intervention or metformin on diabetes development and microvascular complications over 15-year follow-up: the Diabetes Prevention Program Outcomes Study. *Lancet Diabetes Endocrinol.* 2015;3(11):866-875. PMID: 26377054

Ng SM, Stepien KM, Krishan A. Glucocorticoid replacement regimens for treating congenital adrenal hyperplasia. *Cochrane Database Syst Rev.* 2020;3:CD012517. PMID: 32190901

Carmina E, Dewailly D, Escobar-Morreale HF, et al. Non-classic congenital adrenal hyperplasia due to 21-hydroxylase deficiency revisited: an update with a special focus on adolescent and adult women. *Hum Reprod Update.* 2017;23(5):580-599. PMID: 28582566

Martin KA, Anderson RR, Chang RJ, et al. Evaluation and treatment of hirsutism in premenopausal women: an Endocrine Society clinical practice guideline. *J Clin Endocrinol Metab.* 2018;103(4):1233-1257. PMID: 29522147

102 ANSWER: D) Start teriparatide

Glucocorticoid therapy is associated with significant bone loss, which is most pronounced in the first few months of use, as well as an increased fracture risk. FRAX estimates the 10-year probability of fracture for untreated patients between ages 40 and 90 years, using femoral neck bone mineral density and clinical risk factors including glucocorticoid exposure for more than 3 months at a prednisone dosage of ≥5 mg daily, or equivalent dosages of other glucocorticoids. Other risk factors incorporated in FRAX are age, sex, BMI, personal history of fragility fracture, parental history of hip fracture, current cigarette smoking, alcohol use, and rheumatoid arthritis. FRAX does not account for glucocorticoid dosage. For patients receiving prednisone dosages greater than 7.5 mg daily, the fracture risk generated with FRAX should be increased by a relative 15% for major osteoporotic fracture and 20% for hip fracture. In this patient, a 20% increase in her hip fracture risk places her above the treatment threshold of 3% (2.7% + 0.54 = 3.24%). Hence, recommending no therapy at this time (Answer E) is incorrect. In fact, the 2017 American College of Rheumatology guidelines recommend starting osteoporosis therapy in patients beginning long-term glucocorticoid therapy who are at moderate to high risk of fracture (glucocorticoid-adjusted FRAX 10-year risk of major osteoporotic fracture ≥10% or hip fracture ≥1%).

Both alendronate (Answer C) and teriparatide (Answer D) are approved for the treatment of glucocorticoid-induced osteoporosis. While alendronate may be a good treatment option for patients without upper gastrointestinal pathology, it should be avoided in this patient because of her history of esophageal stricture, making teriparatide the most appropriate treatment option. Furthermore, in an 18-month randomized, double-blind, controlled trial comparing teriparatide with alendronate in 428 women and men with osteoporosis who had received glucocorticoids for at least 3 months (prednisone equivalent of ≥5 mg daily), bone mineral density increased more in patients receiving teriparatide than in those receiving alendronate, and fewer new vertebral fractures occurred in the teriparatide group than in the alendronate group (0.6% vs 6.1%; *P* = .004). Therefore, more aggressive medical therapy with teriparatide should also be considered as a first-line option in patients who have glucocorticoid-induced osteoporosis, even in the absence of contraindications to oral bisphosphonates. However, cost and patient willingness to administer daily injections must be considered. Other approved treatments for glucocorticoid-induced osteoporosis include intravenous zoledronic acid and subcutaneous denosumab, which were not given as options in this vignette.

Measurement of fasting C-telopeptide (Answer A) has not been shown to predict fractures in individual patients with glucocorticoid-induced osteoporosis and is not helpful in this scenario. Finally, ordering a bone density test of the one-third distal radius (Answer B) would be indicated in patients with primary hyperparathyroidism or when the hip and spine cannot be measured, but it is not likely to have a role in this patient's management.

Educational Objective
Recognize that FRAX scores must be appropriately adjusted in glucocorticoid-treated patients and recommend the most appropriate intervention.

Reference(s)

Saag KG, Shane E, Boonen S, et al. Teriparatide or alendronate in glucocorticoid-induced osteoporosis. *N Engl J Med.* 2007;357(20):2028-2039. PMID: 18003959

Buckley L, Guyatt G, Fink HA, et al. 2017 American College of Rheumatology guideline for the prevention and treatment of glucocorticoid-induced osteoporosis. *Arthritis Rheumatol.* 2017;69(8):1521-1537. PMID: 28585373

103

ANSWER: C) Nephrogenic syndrome of inappropriate antidiuresis

The patient has hypo-osmolar hyponatremia with raised urine osmolality and inappropriate urine sodium excretion. Clinical assessment and biochemical markers of volume status (serum urea and creatinine) indicate that the patient is broadly euvolemic (ie, not overtly hypovolemic or hypervolemic). In the presence of normal adrenal and thyroid function, and in the absence of any other obvious cause for hyponatremia, the working diagnosis is one of the syndrome of inappropriate antidiuresis (SIAD), which is most commonly due to inappropriate secretion of arginine vasopressin (antidiuretic hormone).

Importantly, however, serum copeptin, which is a stable surrogate marker of circulating arginine vasopressin, is undetectable in a sample collected at a time when the patient has hypo-osmolar hyponatremia, with high urine osmolality and inappropriate natriuresis. Therefore, although the patient meets the diagnostic criteria for SIAD, it is occurring in the absence of antidiuretic hormone as judged by the very low copeptin level. In this context, the rare disorder of nephrogenic syndrome of inappropriate antidiuresis (NSIAD) (Answer C), due to a constitutive activating pathogenic variant in the gene encoding arginine vasopressin receptor type 2 (*AVPR2*), should be considered, and the patient should be referred to a clinical genetics service.

Arginine vasopressin signaling via its renal G protein–coupled receptor AVPR2 is a central step in salt and water homeostasis. Ligand binding and activation lead to cyclic AMP-mediated recruitment of aquaporin-2 channels to the luminal membrane of the medullary collecting duct, resulting in reabsorption of water with resultant urine concentration. Inactivating pathogenic variants in the *AVPR2* gene are a well-recognized cause of nephrogenic diabetes insipidus, with reduced AVPR2-mediated transactivation resulting in diminished cAMP production and aquaporin translocation.

NSIAD resulting from constitutive activation of AVPR2 was first described by Feldman and colleagues in 2005. It has traditionally been considered an X-linked recessive condition, with a variable phenotype in males: some present in infancy (hypotonia, irritability, vomiting and/or seizures); others do not become symptomatic until adulthood, if at all. For the most part, female carriers are usually asymptomatic and identified during familial cascade screening. However, a small number of symptomatic cases have been reported.

Although citalopram (Answer A) has been linked with SIAD, it is mediated by inappropriate ADH release (ie, it is a cause of SIADH) and is most commonly seen in older women. The low serum copeptin levels therefore mean that a trial off citalopram therapy is very unlikely to resolve hyponatremia in this patient.

Similarly, although porphyria (Answer D) (in particular, acute intermittent porphyria) should always be considered in the differential diagnosis of recurrent unexplained hyponatremia in a young patient, it is also typically due to inappropriate ADH release. Screening for urine porphobilinogen during an acute episode would therefore most likely be negative.

Ectopic ADH secretion (eg, from a bronchogenic carcinoma or, less commonly, other neuroendocrine tumor [eg, pulmonary/bronchial carcinoid]) (Answer E) should always be considered in a patient with SIAD; however, the undetectable copeptin level effectively excludes this possibility.

Although the patient has a history of beclomethasone use, there are no other features to suggest hypoadrenalism and the 8-AM cortisol concentration effectively excludes hypocortisolism (Answer B).

Educational Objective

Identify potential causes of the syndrome of inappropriate antidiuresis presenting in a younger patient.

Reference(s)

Feldman BJ, Rosenthal SM, Vargas GA, et al. Nephrogenic syndrome of inappropriate antidiuresis. *N Engl J Med.* 2005;352(18):1884-1890. PMID: 15872203

Powlson AS, Challis BG, Halsall DJ, Schoenmakers E, Gurnell M. Nephrogenic syndrome of inappropriate antidiuresis secondary to an activating mutation in the arginine vasopressin receptor AVPR2. *Clin Endocrinol (Oxf).* 2016;85(2):306-312. PMID: 26715131

Hague J, Casey R, Bruty J, et al. Adult female with symptomatic AVPR2-related nephrogenic syndrome of inappropriate antidiuresis (NSIAD). *Endocrinol Diabetes Metab Case Rep.* 2018;2018. PMID: 29472987

104

ANSWER: C) Partial lipodystrophy

This patient presents with evidence of severe insulin resistance based on her insulin requirements. Severe insulin resistance is defined somewhat arbitrarily as insulin requirements that exceed 2 units/kg or 200 units per day. While many obese patients with metabolic syndrome require high insulin dosages in practice, such requirements in a nonobese person should prompt consideration of syndromic causes of severe insulin resistance, which include lipodystrophy (Answer C), insulin "receptor-opathies," and endocrinopathies such as Cushing syndrome (Answer D) and acromegaly (Answer E). However, specific features of Cushing syndrome such as wide, pigmented striae and "moon facies" are absent in this patient. Similarly, features suggestive of acromegaly (change in hat/ring size, snoring, sweating, prognathism, coarse facial features, "spade hands," or skin tags) are absent, making these diagnoses unlikely.

Type A insulin resistance (Answer B) often presents in childhood and is characterized clinically by severe insulin resistance, acanthosis nigricans, and hyperandrogenism. In contrast, type B insulin resistance (Answer A) is due to insulin-receptor antibodies. Affected persons are usually middle-aged, nonobese black women with acanthosis nigricans, and they often have other rheumatologic conditions. In typical cases of severe insulin resistance, one might expect to see elevated triglyceride levels. But in cases of type B insulin resistance, interestingly, serum triglyceride levels are low, which is not the case in this patient.

The prominent features in this patient are difficult-to-manage diabetes, hypertriglyceridemia, normal BMI, and possibly loss of fat in the legs. This constellation suggests a form of partial lipodystrophy (Answer C). Diagnosis of lipodystrophy is based on history, physical examination, body composition, and metabolic status. Based on the fact that there is selective loss of fat in partial lipodystrophy and that leptin is an adipokine secreted by fat in proportion to fat mass, there is interest in whether levels of leptin could assist in the diagnosis of lipodystrophies. Interestingly, there are no cutoffs for serum leptin levels that are helpful in making the diagnosis. Partial lipodystrophy may be familial or acquired. The latter is associated with low serum complement C3 levels and autoimmune diseases. Identification of partial lipodystrophy is important because complications can include dyslipidemia, hyperandrogenism, coronary artery disease, heart conduction abnormalities, renal dysfunction, and autoimmune disease. Indeed, this patient was subsequently diagnosed with psoriatic arthritis.

Educational Objective
Construct the differential diagnosis for severe insulin resistance.

Reference(s)
Gorden P, Zadeh ES, Cochran E, Brown RJ. Syndromic insulin resistance: models for the therapeutic basis of the metabolic syndrome and other targets of insulin resistance. *Endocr Pract.* 2012;18(5):763-771. PMID: 23047930

Brown RJ, Araujo-Vilar D, Cheung PT, et al. The diagnosis and management of lipodystrophy syndromes: a multi-society practice guideline. *J Clin Endocrinol Metab.* 2016;101(12):4500–4511. PMID: 27710244

105

ANSWER: A) Soybean oil

Current intake of saturated fat in the United Stated accounts for approximately 11% of daily calories. The 2015-2020 Dietary Guidelines for Americans recommend consuming less than 10% of calories from saturated fat for the general population, and the American Heart Association/American College of Cardiology guidelines recommend decreasing it to 5% to 6% to lower cardiovascular risk in individuals with a high LDL-cholesterol concentration. Reducing saturated fat from 14% to 15% of daily calories to 5% to 6% of daily calories lowers LDL cholesterol by 11 to 13 mg/dL (0.28-0.34 mmol/L).

Better effects on lipid profiles are achieved when saturated fat is replaced by polyunsaturated fatty acids, followed by monounsaturated fatty acids and then carbohydrates. Randomized controlled trials show that when dietary saturated fat is replaced by polyunsaturated vegetable oil, the incidence of cardiovascular disease is reduced. Observational studies demonstrate that lower intake of saturated fat and higher intake of polyunsaturated and monounsaturated fat is associated with lower rates of cardiovascular disease, and replacement of saturated fat with refined carbohydrates and sugars is not associated with lower rates of cardiovascular disease.

Saturated fats and oils have high concentrations of lauric, myristic, palmitic, and stearic fatty acids. Monounsaturated fats and oils have mainly oleic fatty acid. Polyunsaturated fats and oils have high concentrations of linoleic and α-linolenic fatty acid. Fats and oils high in saturated fat include coconut oil (Answer B), butter (Answer E), lard palm oil, palm kernel oil (Answer D), and beef tallow.

Polyunsaturated fats are found in high concentrations in corn oil, soybean oil (Answer A), safflower oil high in linoleic acid, and sunflower oil high in linoleic acid (high linoleic acid varieties of oils are uncommon). Monounsaturated fats are found in high concentrations in canola oil, olive oil (Answer C), peanut oil, safflower oil high in oleic acid, and sunflower oil high in oleic acid.

This patient would benefit from using an oil high in polyunsaturated fatty acids (eg, soybean oil [Answer A]).

Educational Objective

Differentiate among the different types of dietary fats and make recommendations based on their effect on cardiovascular disease.

Reference(s)

Eckel RH, Jakicic JM, Ard JD, et al; American College of Cardiology/American Heart Association Task Force on Practice Guidelines. 2013 AHA/ACC guideline on lifestyle management to reduce cardiovascular risk: a report of the American College of Cardiology/American Heart Association Task Force on Practice Guidelines [published correction appears in *J Am Coll Cardiol*. 2014;63(25 Pt B):3027-3028]. *J Am Coll Cardiol*. 2014;63(25 Pt B):2960-2984. PMID: 24239922

Sacks FM, Lichtenstein AH, Wu JHY, et al; American Heart Association. Dietary fats and cardiovascular disease: a presidential advisory from the American Heart Association. *Circulation*. 2017;136(3):e1-e23. PMID: 28620111

106

ANSWER: B) Zoledronic acid

Patients with breast cancer are at risk for osteoporosis based on the presence of either naturally acquired or chemotherapy/surgically-induced menopause, depending on their reproductive status at the time of diagnosis. In addition, the use of aromatase inhibitors, which have been demonstrated to both reduce recurrence risk and improve survival in women with breast cancer, independently increase fracture risk through their profound reduction of systemic estradiol levels. Given this, the assessment of bone mineral density with DXA is critical to help guide skeletal management in these patients. This patient is osteoporotic at the lumbar spine and proximal femur and also has rheumatoid arthritis, which in combination places her at high risk of hip and major osteoporotic fractures. Furthermore, the use of the aromatase inhibitor anastrozole will very likely cause bone loss and further increase her fracture risk. As such, current evidence would support the use of an antifracture therapy in her case. Bisphosphonates have been intensively investigated in women with breast cancer on aromatase inhibitors and have been shown to effectively prevent bone loss in this population. Although definitive data confirming fracture risk reduction are currently lacking, bone mineral density effect (stabilization or improvement) is an acceptable surrogate for fracture risk reduction based on clinical trial results in patients with menopausal osteoporosis. Intravenous zoledronic acid (Answer B) is therefore the best therapy for this patient. In addition, intravenous bisphosphonates are superior to oral bisphosphonates such as alendronate (Answer C) based on existing clinical trial evidence. Intravenous zoledronic acid is preferred for premenopausal women, as it is the only bisphosphonate shown to prevent bone loss in the setting of concomitant therapy with an aromatase inhibitor and GnRH agonist. Bisphosphonates have also been shown to reduce breast cancer recurrence and mortality in postmenopausal women, which provides further support for their use in this patient. Patients are generally treated with bisphosphonates for as long as they remain on aromatase inhibitor therapy, based on the elevated risk of fracture conferred by such therapy.

Denosumab (Answer D), a monoclonal antibody to RANK ligand that is a potent, reversible inhibitor of osteoclast function, also effectively prevents aromatase inhibitor–induced bone loss and has been shown to reduce fracture risk in women with breast cancer on aromatase inhibitor therapy. This patient, however, is on immunosuppressive therapy for her rheumatoid arthritis, which does present concern given that denosumab has been associated with a higher risk of infection, including serious infections, in women with postmenopausal osteoporosis. Additionally, patients are at risk for "rebound" rapid bone loss once denosumab is discontinued, which most likely increases the risk for vertebral fractures based on multiple literature reports. This has not been observed upon cessation of bisphosphonate therapy and is almost certainly due to the long skeletal half-life of these drugs. Denosumab is therefore not the best choice for this particular patient.

Raloxifene (Answer A) is a selective estrogen receptor modulator that is approved for treatment of osteoporosis and prevention of breast cancer in women at high risk. It is, however, a weaker antiresorptive agent and has not been proven to prevent bone loss in women on aromatase inhibitor therapy.

Finally, while teriparatide (Answer E) and the PTHrP analogue abaloparatide are both effective anabolic agents that are proven to reduce the risk of vertebral and nonvertebral fractures, their use is contraindicated in this patient because of her prior radiation therapy. Both drugs have been demonstrated, when given in suprapharmacologic dosages in rats, to increase the risk of osteosarcoma, for which this patient is already at increased risk based on her history of radiotherapy.

Educational Objective
Recommend appropriate treatment in a patient with osteoporosis and breast cancer who is on aromatase inhibitor therapy.

Reference(s)
Hadji P, Aapro MS, Body JJ, et al. Management of aromatase inhibitor-associated bone loss (AIBL) in postmenopausal women with hormone sensitive breast cancer: Joint position statement of the IOF, CABS, ECTS, IEG, ESCEO IMS, and SIOG. *J Bone Oncol*. 2017;7:1-12. PMID: 28413771

107 ANSWER: E) Refer for sleep assessment

This patient is obese and has symptoms that could be consistent with obstructive sleep apnea (OSA): difficulty with concentration while at work, persistent tiredness, and fatigue. A screening questionnaire such as STOP-BANG would deem him to be at high risk, even in the absence of corroboration by a partner noting loud snoring or apneic episodes. In addition, it has been estimated that up to 80% of patients with acromegaly have some degree of OSA at the time of initial presentation, and although a significant proportion demonstrate a marked improvement or complete resolution following successful treatment of acromegaly, an important subgroup has persistent OSA. Referral for a sleep assessment (Answer E) is therefore the most appropriate next step in management.

With good glycemic control, it is unlikely that his symptoms are attributable to his diabetes or its current management. There is no indication therefore to add an SGLT-2 inhibitor (Answer A).

As both the free T_4 and free T_3 levels are already towards the upper end of their respective reference ranges, it is unlikely that a further increase in the levothyroxine dosage (Answer B) would reverse the patient's symptoms.

In a patient with suspected or untreated OSA, additional care should be taken when prescribing testosterone replacement because of the risk of inducing/exacerbating secondary polycythemia (OSA is in itself a recognized cause of secondary polycythemia). Indeed, this patient's hemoglobin and hematocrit levels are already at a degree where, rather than reducing the interval between testosterone injections (Answer C), it would be appropriate to consider increasing the interval or even temporarily suspending replacement while the possibility of OSA is addressed.

There is no indication to reduce the patient's octreotide LAR dosage (Answer D). His acromegaly is currently well controlled.

Educational Objective
Recognize that nonspecific symptoms such as tiredness and fatigue in a patient with hypopituitarism are not always attributable to suboptimal endocrine treatment and may reflect other comorbidities.

Reference(s)
Annamalai AK, Webb A, Kandasamy N, et al. A comprehensive study of clinical, biochemical, radiological, vascular, cardiac, and sleep parameters in an unselected cohort of patients with acromegaly undergoing presurgical somatostatin receptor ligand therapy. *J Clin Endocrinol Metab*. 2013;98(3):1040-1050. PMID: 23393175

Parolin M, Dassie F, Alessio L, et al. Obstructive sleep apnea in acromegaly and the effect of treatment: a systematic review and meta-analysis. *J Clin Endocrinol Metab*. 2020;105(3):1-9. PMID: 31722411

108

ANSWER: D) Medication-induced hemolysis

Hyperglycemia results in nonenzymatic glycation of a number of proteins, including those in red blood cells. The blood test measuring hemoglobin A_{1c} identifies glycation of the N-terminal valine of the hemoglobin β chain. Clinically, it reflects long-term glycemic control (in the preceding 2-3 months). Maintenance of hemoglobin A_{1c} in the optimal range is associated with reduced risk of diabetes-related complications.

A number of clinical variables such as lifespan of the red cell and hemoglobin variants affect the accuracy of hemoglobin A_{1c} measurement. Any feature that prolongs the lifespan of red blood cells raises the hemoglobin A_{1c} level. In patients with iron, vitamin B_{12}, or folate deficiencies, red blood cells are older and hemoglobin A_{1c} values tend to be higher than average glucose levels. In contrast, in patients who are receiving an iron supplement or erythropoietin or have hemolysis for any reason have a resultant shortened red blood cell lifespan, and hemoglobin A_{1c} is lower than expected for average glucose levels. The patient described in this vignette most likely has hemolysis due to the use of dapsone, resulting in discordance between hemoglobin A_{1c} and glucose levels. Thus, medication-induced hemolysis (Answer D) is the most likely explanation. The glucose-6-phosphate dehydrogenase NADPH glutathione pathway is involved in reducing oxidative injury to tissue. Dapsone increases production of reactive oxygen species and can increase hemolysis, especially in patients with glucose-6-phosphate dehydrogenase deficiency. This patient is noted to be pale, so a complete blood cell count would be a reasonable test to order to confirm the suspicion of anemia. The patient's "hypoxia" is also likely due to dapsone. Dapsone causes a larger proportion of iron in hemoglobin to be in the ferric form rather than the ferrous form, resulting in methemoglobinemia. In patients with methemoglobinemia, pulse oximetry has a bias toward reading around 85%, so in patients without hypoxia the reading is inaccurately low and in patients with hypoxia the reading may be inaccurately high.

Genetic variants of hemoglobin (Answer A) can also cause hemoglobin A_{1c} levels to be inaccurate. The assay used and the specific variant determine whether the hemoglobin A_{1c} will be higher or lower than average glucose levels. The National Glycohemoglobin Standardization Program (NGSP) has an online resource at www.ngsp.org that lists variants and assay outcomes. However, if this patient had a genetic variant, the discordance would have been longstanding and not merely over the past year.

In renal insufficiency (Answer B), there is increased carbamylated hemoglobin that can affect hemoglobin A_{1c} levels. In addition, patients in renal failure may be receiving erythropoietin or iron replacement, which can also affect hemoglobin A_{1c} levels. The association between chronic kidney disease and hemoglobin A_{1c} is complex, but in early stages the correlation between hemoglobin A_{1c} and average glucose levels is reasonably good. This patient has stage 1 chronic kidney disease and is unlikely to have such a significant discrepancy between average glucose levels and hemoglobin A_{1c} caused by renal insufficiency alone.

Patients with celiac disease (Answer C) might have iron deficiency anemia that could affect hemoglobin A_{1c}. However, this would result in an elevated hemoglobin A_{1c} level. In addition, this patient appears to be adherent to a gluten-free diet and complications due to celiac disease are unlikely.

Medications such as aspirin can block nonenzymatic glycation of proteins (Answer E) and lower hemoglobin A_{1c} levels. However, this medication was not a recent addition to this patient's regimen and is therefore less likely to be the cause of recent hemoglobin A_{1c} lowering.

Educational Objective
List possible reasons for an inaccurate hemoglobin A_{1c} result.

Reference(s)

Weykamp C. HbA1c: a review of analytical and clinical aspects. *Ann Lab Med.* 2013;33(6):393-400. PMID: 24205486

Pallais JC, Mackool BT, Pitman MB. Case records of the Massachusetts General Hospital: Case 7-2011: 52-year-old man with upper respiratory infection and low oxygen saturation levels. *N Engl J Med.* 2011;364(10):957-966. PMID: 21388314

109

ANSWER: E) TSH measurement in 2 months

Carcinoembryonic antigen (CEA) is normally expressed by mucosal cells. It is metabolized and excreted by the liver. CEA is not a specific biomarker for medullary thyroid carcinoma (MTC), but it is measured in patients with MTC during follow-up. It is overexpressed by a variety of malignancies such as colon/rectum, breast, stomach, pancreas, ovary, and liver. CEA can also be elevated in a number of benign conditions, including in patients who smoke tobacco and in patients with pancreatitis, peptic ulcer disease, heterophilic antibodies, or hypothyroidism. Hypothyroidism has been suggested to affect CEA metabolism or clearance.

The patient in this vignette has MTC. MTC arises from parafollicular cells (C cells), which are different from follicular cells and are not TSH responsive. Therefore, radioiodine scan (Answer A) and radioiodine treatment are not indicated. Simultaneous elevations of serum calcitonin and CEA levels indicate disease progression following total thyroidectomy. This patient's serum calcitonin is undetectable, but his serum CEA level is elevated. In general, a low calcitonin level combined with an elevated CEA level indicates poorly differentiated MTC, but this patient underwent total thyroidectomy 6 weeks earlier. Other causes for elevated CEA should be sought.

Hypothyroidism is one such etiology. Thyroid hormone replacement therapy should be initiated after total thyroidectomy in patients with MTC. TSH should be checked 6 to 8 weeks after the initiation of levothyroxine to ensure that TSH is in the normal range (Answer E). His fatigue and hoarseness occurring several weeks after his thyroidectomy are most likely symptoms of overt hypothyroidism. After normalizing TSH, this patient's CEA level will move into the normal range if his elevated CEA is solely related to hypothyroidism. He does not smoke cigarettes, which can also cause elevated CEA but not to this degree. CEA can be elevated in patients with colon cancer. This patient has a family history of colon cancer, but he had a negative colonoscopy 2 years ago. Therefore, colonoscopy (Answer B) is incorrect. Imaging studies are indicated in patients with MTC who have elevated calcitonin and CEA levels, but in this patient, calcitonin is undetectable and his thyroidectomy happened several weeks ago. No imaging study is indicated now. Neck ultrasonography (Answer C) is usually obtained 3 to 6 months postoperatively. PET-CT (Answer D) is not indicated unless a patient with MTC has a very high calcitonin level (>1000 pg/mL [>292 pmol/L]).

In addition, patients with sporadic MTC should have genetic counseling and testing for *RET* germline pathogenic variants. Once a patient is confirmed to have a *RET* pathogenic variants, first-degree relatives should be offered genetic counseling and genetic testing.

Educational Objective
Explain the effect of hypothyroidism on carcinoembryonic antigen levels.

Reference(s)
Wells SA Jr, Asa SL, Dralle H, et al; American Thyroid Association Guidelines Task Force on Medullary Thyroid Carcinoma. Revised American Thyroid Association guidelines for the management of medullary thyroid carcinoma. *Thyroid.* 2015;25(6):567-610. PMID: 25810047

Sekizaki T, Yamamoto C, Nomoto H. Two cases of transiently elevated serum CEA levels in severe hypothyroidism without Goiter. *Intern Med.* 2018;57(17):2523-2526. PMID: 29109954

110

ANSWER: C) Mitotane-induced elevations in SHBG

This patient has been treated with mitotane for several years, and his mitotane levels have been maintained in the therapeutic range of 14 to 20 μg/mL and at times have exceeded this range. The therapeutic range for mitotane is a general guideline for maximizing antitumor efficacy while minimizing adverse effects and was extrapolated from retrospective studies. Patients with adrenocortical carcinoma may have mitotane levels that are above or below this therapeutic range for a variety of reasons.

Mitotane is used as an adjuvant therapy for high-grade and/or locally advanced adrenocortical carcinoma. It is dosed orally, and the dosage is generally escalated to 3 to 5 g daily (or as tolerated) to achieve the therapeutic range, and then ideally maintained for at least 2 years. Mitotane is associated with several adverse effects, which include gastrointestinal symptoms (nausea, vomiting, diarrhea), fatigue, depression, ataxia, memory loss, and bone marrow suppression. Mitotane can also induce a number of complex endocrinopathies, including adrenal insufficiency, hypothyroidism, and male hypogonadism.

Patients with adrenocortical carcinoma treated with mitotane typically have only 1 adrenal gland, since the other gland has usually been removed during surgery to address the primary tumor. Mitotane can inhibit or destroy the remaining normal adrenal cortex (mitotane may have adrenolytic and/or adrenostatic properties). Therefore, all patients treated with mitotane should receive supplemental maintenance glucocorticoids. Mitotane induces hepatic globulin synthesis and increases the circulating cortisol-binding globulin level. Mitotane also increases CYP3A4 activity, which increases the metabolism of exogenous glucocorticoids. Therefore, supplemental glucocorticoid doses often need to be escalated to supraphysiologic doses to maintain euadrenal status.

Patients treated with mitotane often have low TSH levels. Whether this reflects a sick euthyroid state or direct central suppression is not clear. Further, mitotane increases thyroxine-binding globulin and CYP3A4 activity. Therefore, supplemental doses of levothyroxine must be administered, and the levothyroxine dosage often needs to be substantially higher than what would be expected to maintain a euthyroid state. Total T_4 levels can be high (as often seen in pregnancy) when free T_4 levels are normal.

Men treated with mitotane can develop hypogonadism via several mechanisms. Mitotane may inhibit testicular steroidogenesis and can substantially increase SHBG and CYP3A4 activity. Collectively, this may require treatment with testosterone in symptomatic men, but the dosage necessary to normalize bioavailable testosterone can be quite high. For example, this patient's SHBG concentration was 65.2 µg/mL (1.1-6.7 µg/mL) (SI: 580 nmol/L [10-60 nmol/L]), thus accounting for the very high total testosterone, yet undetectable free testosterone (Answer C). Some studies also suggest that mitotane may impair 5α-reductase activity, thereby further complicating the value of testosterone therapy. The exact mechanism and effects of mitotane on female reproductive hormones are less consistently described.

There are no known circulating antibodies (Answer A) or mitotane metabolites (Answer B) that would cause a high total testosterone and low free testosterone. An aromatase inhibitor (Answer D) would lower the conversion of testosterone to estrogen, but this would not explain the discrepancy between total and free testosterone. Anabolic androgens (Answer E) would either suppress all testosterone measures if not detected by the testosterone assay or increase all testosterone measures if detected by the testosterone assay.

Educational Objective
Describe endocrine consequences of mitotane therapy for adrenocortical carcinoma.

Reference(s)
Vaidya A, Nehs M, Kilbridge K. Treatment of adrenocortical carcinoma. *Surg Pathol Clin.* 2019;12(4):997-1006. PMID: 31672303

111

ANSWER: B) Perform a glucose-suppression test

This patient has a pituitary macroadenoma. Her examination findings are not suggestive of hypercortisolism, and her prolactin is only mildly elevated. Her headaches and hyperhidrosis raise concern for a GH-secreting adenoma. Although she has a normal serum IGF-1 concentration, this does not completely exclude acromegaly. This is particularly true in a woman who is on an oral contraceptive. Oral estrogens, due to the first-pass effect, cause liver resistance to GH. Because most serum IGF-1 comes from the liver, serum IGF-1 can be normal in patients with acromegaly who are on oral estrogen. Accordingly, oral estrogen (and selective estrogen receptor modulators such as clomiphene and tamoxifen) are occasionally used to treat acromegaly. Conversely, patients on GH replacement therapy require a higher dosage of GH to normalize IGF-1 if they are also taking an oral estrogen.

The gold standard to diagnose acromegaly is the oral glucose-suppression test (Answer B), during which serum GH should suppress below 0.4 ng/mL (<0.4 µg/L). This patient underwent a glucose-suppression test (*see table*), which diagnosed acromegaly.

Analyte	Baseline	30 minutes	60 minutes	90 minutes	120 minutes
Glucose	92 mg/dL (SI: 5.1 mmol/L)	113 mg/dL (SI: 6.3 mmol/L)	141 mg/dL (SI: 7.8 mmol/L)	93 mg/dL (SI: 5.2 mmol/L)	117 mg/dL (SI: 6.5 mmol/L)
Growth hormone	5.8 ng/mL (SI: 5.8 µg/L)	5.0 ng/mL (SI: 5.0 µg/L)	5.2 ng/mL (SI: 5.2 µg/L)	4.7 ng/mL (SI: 4.7 µg/L)	4.4 ng/mL (SI: 4.4 µg/L)

Referral to neurosurgery (Answer A) is premature, as the diagnosis of this lesion is not yet established. Performing a dexamethasone-suppression test (Answer C) is not indicated in the absence of signs of hypercortisolism (she has normal blood pressure and low BMI). Additionally, oral estrogen, by increasing cortisol-binding globulin, may cause a false-positive dexamethasone-suppression test result, with incomplete suppression, even in the absence of unregulated ACTH secretion. Measuring prolactin after dilution (Answer D) would be indicated to exclude the "hook effect." This occurs in the presence of giant prolactin-secreting adenomas, when the extremely elevated prolactin levels saturate the assay's antibodies and cause an inaccurately low reading. This adenoma is not as big as those associated with the hook effect. Chromogranin (Answer E) is a protein released from neuroendocrine cells, and its measurement has no role in the differential diagnosis of this pituitary lesion.

Educational Objective
Consider the diagnosis of acromegaly despite a normal IGF-1 concentration in a patient with a pituitary adenoma who is taking an oral contraceptive.

Reference(s)
Melmed S, Casanueva FF, Klibanski A, et al. A consensus on the diagnosis and treatment of acromegaly complications. *Pituitary.* 2013;16(3):294-302. PMID: 22903574

Duarte FH, Jallad RS, Bronstein MD. Estrogens and selective estrogen receptor modulators in acromegaly. *Endocrine.* 2016;54(2):306-314. PMID: 27704479

112 ANSWER: C) Increase the basal rate from 5:30 PM to 12 AM, and change the insulin-to-carbohydrate ratio to 1 to 10 at 8 AM

Maintaining glucose levels in the normal or near-normal glycemic range is important in pregnant women with preexisting diabetes to prevent adverse outcomes in the mother, fetus, and neonate. The exception is in women with hypoglycemia unawareness, for whom less stringent glucose control is warranted.

The American Diabetes Association recommends a hemoglobin A_{1c} target less than 6.0% to 6.5% (<42-48 mmol/mol) in early pregnancy, as observational studies have demonstrated lower rates of adverse fetal outcomes with tighter glucose control. The American College of Obstetricians and Gynecologists recommends a target hemoglobin A_{1c} level less than 6.0% (<42 mmol/mol).

The target glucose values recommended by the American Diabetes Association and the American College of Obstetricians and Gynecologists during pregnancy are as follows:
- Fasting and premeal glucose levels <95 mg/dL (≤5.3 mmol/L)
- 1-hour postprandial glucose levels <140 mg/dL (≤7.8 mmol/L)
- 2-hour postprandial glucose levels <120 mg/dL (≤6.7 mmol/L)

The patient in this vignette has type 1 diabetes and is being treated with an insulin pump and continuous glucose monitoring (CGM). She has hypoglycemia unawareness, and strict glycemic control is warranted as long as she is not having recurrent hypoglycemia.

An international multicenter controlled trial of pregnant women with type 1 diabetes (CONCEPTT trial) randomly assigned patients to use CGM combined with capillary glucose monitoring or capillary glucose monitoring alone during the pregnancy. The women assigned to real-time CGM had a lower hemoglobin A_{1c} level later in pregnancy (–0.19%; P = .021), had more time in the glucose target range (68% vs 61%; P = .034), and less hyperglycemia (27% vs 32%; P = .028) compared with women in the conventional glucose monitoring group. There was no difference in the rates of severe hypoglycemia between the 2 groups. Continuous glucose sensors have not been approved for use during pregnancy in the United States. Despite this, CGM is increasingly being used in pregnancy, even though this is an off-label use.

The patient in this vignette is in the first trimester of pregnancy, when insulin sensitivity is greatest. Patients are more likely to have recurrent hypoglycemia during this time. She appropriately reduced the basal insulin rates 10 days ago. However, further adjustments in the basal rates and insulin-to-carbohydrate ratios should be made.

In reviewing the CGM tracing, the glucose levels are elevated at midnight but rapidly trend down to about 100 mg/dL (5.6 mmol/L) by 3 AM, then continue to fall and reach a nadir in the hypoglycemic range by 6 AM. The glucose levels increase after breakfast and remain elevated until 10 AM, then trend down slightly by the midafternoon. The glucose levels continue to trend down until the evening meal. Hyperglycemia develops after dinner and the glucose levels remain elevated until midnight.

Given these data, making no changes in the basal insulin rates and insulin-to-carbohydrate ratios (Answer A) is inappropriate. Increasing the insulin-to-carbohydrate ratio to 1 unit per 10 g carbohydrate at 8 AM (Answer B) is appropriate, but an additional change in the basal rate should be made in the evening. Decreasing the basal rate from 12 PM to 5:30 PM (Answer E) is not necessary. Increasing the basal rate from 5:30 PM to 12 AM (Answer D) is appropriate, but it is an inadequate step without adjusting the insulin-to-carbohydrate ratio before breakfast. Therefore, the most appropriate step, in addition to lowering the basal rates from 12 AM to 7 AM, is to increase the insulin-to-carbohydrate ratio to 1 unit per 10 g carbohydrate at 8 AM and increase the basal rate from 5:30 PM to 12 AM (Answer C). Making these changes in the insulin rates should improve this patient's glucose levels without increasing the risk for hypoglycemia.

Educational Objective
Set the goals for management of diabetes during pregnancy and analyze trends from glucose monitoring to make appropriate changes in insulin dosages and rates.

Reference(s)
American Diabetes Association. 14. Management of diabetes in pregnancy: standards of medical care in diabetes-2020. *Diabetes Care.* 2020;43(Suppl 1):S183-S192. PMID: 31862757

ACOG Practice Bulletin No 201: pregestational diabetes mellitus. *Obstet Gynecol.* 2018;132(6):e228-e248. PMID: 30461693

Feig DS, Donovan LE, Corcoy R, et al. Continuous glucose monitoring in pregnant women with type 1 diabetes (CONCEPTT): a multicentre international randomised controlled trial. *Lancet.* 2017;390(10110): 2347-2359. PMID: 28923465

113 ANSWER: E) Progressive diaphyseal dysplasia

Bone pain is not an uncommon reason for patients to present to a health care provider, although it is relatively unusual in young individuals. Athletes such as long-distance runners can present with stress fractures of the tibia or femur, but no such history is present in this patient. She also describes upper-extremity pain that is inconsistent with an overuse-related injury. The presence of high bone mass by DXA, as well as the symmetric nature of the radiographic findings, suggests the presence of a hereditary dysplastic bone disease. While several inherited bone disorders can present with bone pain as in this patient, the clinical findings are most consistent with progressive diaphyseal dysplasia (PDD) (Answer E). Also known as Camurati-Engelmann disease, PDD is a craniotubular hyperostotic disease that is due to pathogenic variants in the gene encoding transforming growth factor-β1 (*TGFB1*) that affect binding of the protein to its latency-associated peptide. This disruption is thought to permit exuberant cortical bone formation in the diaphyseal regions of the long bones, lower more commonly than upper, although other sites such as the scapula and pelvis can also be involved. Patients with PDD typically present in childhood or adolescence with complaints of lower-extremity pain and fatigue, and it is typically accompanied by limping or a wide-based, waddling gait. Affected patients are usually tall and may have a large head with prominent forehead, as well as thin limbs that are palpably widened and tender. Pertinent laboratory measurements, including calcium, phosphate, alkaline phosphatase, and PTH, are typically normal. Plain radiographs show pathognomonically thickened cortices of the long bones with sparing of the epiphyseal regions and typically the metaphyseal regions as well. Technetium ^{99}Tc whole-body bone scintigraphy reveals increased uptake in the involved skeletal areas. There is no proven treatment for PDD, although symptoms may remit as patients age into adulthood. Low doses of corticosteroids given on alternate days may provide some relief from bone pain and weakness, presumably by suppressing abnormal osteoblast bone formation. Losartan may also have some benefit based on an unclear mechanism of action, although adverse effects may limit its use.

Other genetically acquired metabolic bone disorders can also present with bone pain and abnormal radiographs, although the clinical findings in this patient are not supportive of these conditions specifically. Hypophosphatasia (Answer A) is a form of inherited osteomalacia that is due to pathogenic variants in the gene encoding tissue nonspecific alkaline phosphatase (*ALPL*) that is responsible for cleavage of pyrophosphate to inorganic phosphate molecules. Accumulation of pyrophosphate in the skeletal matrix inhibits bone mineralization and leads to osteomalacia, bone pain, and lower-extremity fractures in adult patients with hypophosphatasia, as well as causes femoral diaphyseal fractures that can mimic the atypical femoral fractures that are rarely seen with bisphosphonates. Patients with hypophosphatasia, however, have frankly low alkaline phosphatase levels, which are not present in this patient.

X-linked hypophosphatemic rickets (Answer D), due to pathogenic variants in the *PHEX* gene (phosphate regulating endopeptidase homolog X-linked), cause osteomalacia with poor longitudinal growth, lower-extremity bowing, bone pain, and fractures. X-linked hypophosphatemia is due to altered catabolism of FGF-23 with resultant excessive phosphaturia, reduced calcitriol levels, and hypophosphatemia. Affected patients may have increased bone mineral density, particularly at the lumbar spine, due to osteosclerosis. Hypophosphatemia, however, is absent in this patient. Dental pathology, namely excessive and premature tooth loss, which is a hallmark of both hypophosphatasia and x-linked hypophosphatemia, is not present in this patient. Her normal calcium and PTH levels rule out the presence of primary hyperparathyroidism (Answer B), which causes cortical bone loss diffusely throughout the skeleton and not symmetric cortical thickening as in this patient. Finally, although Paget disease of bone (Answer C) can result in higher bone mineral density focally and may be inherited in up to 20% of patients, a symmetric pattern of bone involvement and normal alkaline phosphatase level rule out this diagnosis.

Educational Objective
Diagnose high bone density due to progressive diaphyseal dysplasia.

Reference(s)
Kim YM, Kang E, Choi JH, Kim GH, Yoo HW, Lee BH. Clinical characteristics and treatment outcomes in Camurati-Engelmann disease: a case series. *Medicine (Baltimore)*. 2018;97(14):e0309. PMID: 29620655

114

ANSWER: A) Vitamin B$_{12}$ measurement

Reduced serum levels of vitamin B$_{12}$ in the setting of metformin treatment has been noted on the basis of cross-sectional studies since the early 1970s. Within the last decade, the association between reduced serum vitamin B$_{12}$ levels and metformin treatment has been noted in prospective placebo-controlled trials for treatment durations of at least 4 years. In a secondary analysis of the DPPOS study (Diabetes Prevention Program Outcomes Study), there was a 13% increased risk of vitamin B$_{12}$ deficiency per year of metformin use as an associated increase in homocysteine levels. The concurrence of neuropathy strengthens this association, but vitamin B$_{12}$ deficiency was seen in the absence of anemia. Therefore, the American Diabetes Association recommends that screening for vitamin B$_{12}$ deficiency (Answer A) should be considered in patients taking metformin for a long duration. Whether low serum vitamin B$_{12}$ levels are associated with true deficiency is controversial, although the finding of high homocysteine levels suggests that this may be the case. The mechanism for this effect is thought to be metformin interfering with vitamin B$_{12}$-intrinsic factor absorption in the terminal ileum. If the patient is symptomatic, treatment of vitamin B$_{12}$ deficiency can be administered via the parenteral route with 1000 mcg weekly until the deficiency is resolved. This can be followed by a regimen of 1000 mcg once monthly. For patients in whom dietary deficiency is the cause, the treatment can be oral vitamin B$_{12}$ treatment with 1000 mcg daily. If there is concern about vitamin B$_{12}$ absorption, as is the case with metformin use, then higher dosages of 2000 mcg daily may be needed.

This patient is already on moderate-intensity statin therapy. Given his age and 10-year risk of atherosclerotic cardiovascular disease (>20%), a high-intensity statin would be reasonable. While fasting lipid profiles (Answer B) are recommended annually, this would not likely affect management at this time.

Routine screening for coronary artery disease (Answers C and E) in asymptomatic individuals does not improve outcomes, as long as other risk factors are being managed.

There is no evidence that treatment with vitamin D in patients without risk factors for fracture is of any benefit or that vitamin D benefits glycemic management. Therefore, monitoring circulating vitamin D levels (Answer D) is not necessary.

Educational Objective
Screen for vitamin B$_{12}$ deficiency in patients on longstanding metformin therapy.

Reference(s)

American Diabetes Association. 3. Prevention or delay of type 2 diabetes: standards of medical care in diabetes-2020. *Diabetes Care*. 2020;43(Suppl 1):S32-S36. PMID: 31862746

Aroda VR, Edelstein SL, Goldberg RB, et al; Diabetes Prevention Program Research Group. Long-term metformin use and vitamin B12 deficiency in the diabetes prevention program outcomes study. *J Clin Endocrinol Metab*. 2016;101(4):1754-1761. PMID: 26900641

de Jager J, Kooy A, Lehert P, et al. Long term treatment with metformin in patients with type 2 diabetes and risk of vitamin B-12 deficiency: randomised placebo controlled trial. *BMJ*. 2010;340:c2181. PMID: 20488910

115 ANSWER: E) Transdermal estradiol and micronized progesterone

This patient discontinued oral contraceptives to confirm that they were the cause of elevated total cortisol due to increased cortisol-binding globulin. Her total cortisol and urinary free cortisol normalized. As a consequence of discontinuing oral contraceptives, she developed symptoms of menopause with an FSH concentration in the menopausal range. Menopause is defined by the last menstrual period after 1 year or an FSH concentration of 25 mIU/mL or greater (≥25 IU/L). In women older than 45 years, the menopausal transition is highly likely in the presence of irregular menstrual cycles and symptoms of estrogen deficiency such as vasomotor hot flashes with sleep disturbance or genitourinary syndrome of menopause (vulvovaginal atrophy with vaginal dryness and dyspareunia or sexual dysfunction). The menopausal transition is on average 4 years until the final menstrual period. Most women with menopausal symptoms who seek medical therapy for menopausal symptoms are in perimenopause or early menopause (late 40s to 50s).

Although there are alternative therapies for vasomotor symptoms, none are as effective as estrogen. When the Women's Health Initiative found significant adverse outcomes of hormone replacement therapy (HRT) in postmenopausal women older than 60 years, there was a significant decline in HRT for prevention but also for symptomatic women. However, subsequent studies in younger women in their 50s, within 10 years of their last period and with estradiol rather than conjugated estrogens used in the Women's Health Initiative, have not documented the same increase in breast cancer risk, venous thrombosis, and cardiovascular events. Women in the most symptomatic age group (late 40s to 50s) can be reassured that the absolute risk of complications for healthy, young postmenopausal women taking HRT for up to 5 years is very low if there are no contraindications to HRT. Although the primary indication for HRT should be relief of symptoms significantly impacting quality of life and well-being and not for prevention of disease, HRT can decrease postmenopausal bone loss with additional data to support a decrease in cardiovascular events and mortality in women younger than 60 years.

If a woman has a personal history of breast cancer, cardiovascular disease, venous thromboembolic event, or stroke or if a woman is at moderate or high risk for these complications, alternatives can be suggested. Paroxetine (Answer A) at the dosage of 7.5 mg daily is an FDA-approved treatment for hot flashes with studies showing that this low dosage can decrease vasomotor symptoms. Other off-label treatments shown to be effective include selective serotonin reuptake inhibitors at lower dosages than those used to treat psychiatric conditions (citalopram, escitalopram), serotonin-norepinephrine reuptake inhibitors (venlafaxine [Answer D], desvenlafaxine), gabapentinoids (gabapentin and pregabalin), and clonidine.

This patient is not sexually active, so she does not need to restart the combined oral contraceptive pill (Answer B). A menopausal woman who is sexually active could continue contraception until age 55 years and could consider lower-dosage estradiol in the combined oral contraceptive pill and progestins with lower potential thrombotic risk such as norethindrone and norgestimate. To best limit potential cardiovascular risk in an obese woman with elevated blood pressure, transdermal estradiol would be preferred since it has not been shown to increase C-reactive protein and other acute-phase proteins that could promote vascular inflammation compared with oral estradiol (Answer C), presumably through a first-pass hepatic effect. Therefore, the combination of transdermal estradiol with micronized progesterone (Answer E) to prevent endometrial hyperplasia would be the best treatment option for this patient. Weight gain during the menopausal transition is common because of changing metabolism with estrogen deficiency. However, weight loss is not anticipated with hormone replacement alone without significant lifestyle changes.

Educational Objective

Diagnose and treat menopausal hot flashes.

Reference(s)

Stuenkel CA, Davis SR, Gompel A, et al. Treatment of symptoms of the menopause: an Endocrine Society clinical practice guideline. *J Clin Endocrinol Metab.* 2015;100(11):3975-4011. PMID: 26444994

The NAMS 2017 Hormone Therapy Position Statement Advisory Panel. The 2017 hormone therapy position statement of the North American Menopause Society. *Menopause.* 2017;24(7):728-753. PMID: 28650869

116 ANSWER: E) McCune-Albright syndrome

The young woman in this vignette presents with asymptomatic expansile bone lesions, and her bone scan shows multiple areas of increased uptake involving the right-sided ribs, thoracic vertebral bodies, pelvis, and right calcaneus, compatible with polyostotic fibrous dysplasia. In the setting of a history of precocious puberty and "coast of Maine" café-au-lait skin lesions, these clinical manifestations are consistent with a diagnosis of McCune-Albright syndrome (Answer E). McCune-Albright syndrome is caused by postzygotic (somatic) activating pathogenic variants in the *GNAS* gene, encoding the α-subunit of the stimulatory G protein. Other manifestations of McCune-Albright syndrome include thyrotoxicosis, gigantism or acromegaly, and Cushing syndrome. McCune-Albright syndrome is not inherited; germline occurrences of this pathogenic variant would presumably be lethal.

Multiple endocrine neoplasia type 1 (Answer A) is caused by inactivating pathogenic variants in the *MEN1* tumor suppressor gene, which lead to an autosomal dominant predisposition to tumors of the parathyroid glands, anterior pituitary, and enteropancreatic endocrine cells.

Carney complex (Answer B) is a rare multiple endocrine neoplasia syndrome characterized by distinctive lentiginous pigmented lesions of the skin and mucosal surfaces, cardiac and noncardiac myxomatous tumors, and multiple endocrine abnormalities most frequently due to tumors of the adrenal and pituitary glands or testicular tumors. Thyroid nodules occur in up to 75% of patients with Carney complex and typically develop early in life; however, patients are generally euthyroid. Thyroid cancer (papillary and follicular carcinoma) develops in less than 10% of affected patients. Carney complex is most frequently associated with inactivating pathogenic variants in the protein kinase A type I α regulatory subunit gene (*PRKAR1A*) and is inherited in an autosomal dominant fashion.

Neurofibromatosis type 1 (Answer C) is also an autosomal dominant genetic disorder. It is caused by inactivating pathogenic variants in the *NF1* tumor suppressor gene, which encodes the protein neurofibromin. The hallmarks of neurofibromatosis type 1, also known as von Recklinghausen disease, are multiple café-au-lait macules and neurofibromas. These macules tend to have smooth borders resembling the "coast of California," as opposed to the jagged "coast of Maine" borders typically seen in McCune-Albright syndrome. Other clinical manifestations include iris hamartomas (aka Lisch nodules), optic pathway gliomas, and gastrointestinal stromal tumors. Patients with neurofibromatosis type 1 are at an increased risk of developing soft-tissue sarcomas and, rarely, pheochromocytomas. Bony abnormalities in neurofibromatosis type 1 include pseudoarthrosis and sphenoid bone dysplasia, as well as short stature, scoliosis, nonossifying fibromas, and osteoporosis.

Finally, von Hippel-Lindau disease (Answer D) is an inherited, autosomal dominant syndrome manifested by a variety of benign and malignant tumors. It is caused by inactivating pathogenic variants in the *VHL* tumor suppressor gene. Clinical manifestations of this condition include hemangioblastomas, pheochromocytomas, renal cell carcinomas, pancreatic tumors, endolymphatic sac tumors of the middle ear, and papillary cystadenomas of the epididymis and broad ligament.

Educational Objective

Identify the features of polyostotic fibrous dysplasia and diagnose McCune-Albright syndrome.

Reference(s)

Chapurlat RD, Orcel P. Fibrous dysplasia of bone and McCune-Albright syndrome. *Best Pract Res Clin Rheumatol.* 2008;22(1):55-69. PMID: 18328981

117

ANSWER: E) Start insulin

Immune checkpoint inhibitors are small molecules that are present on immune cells and modulate their function. In recent years, antibodies that inhibit the activity of some of these checkpoints such as cytotoxic T-lymphocyte–associated protein 4 (CTLA-4), programmed death-1 (PD-1) or its ligand PD-L1, have been increasingly used in the treatment of malignancies. Immune checkpoint inhibitors are associated with toxicities that can affect a number of organs systems. Adverse effects include often irreversible damage to the endocrine glands.

Endocrine dysfunction typically occurs weeks to months after the initial dose of immune checkpoint inhibitor therapy. Hypophysitis, thyroid dysfunction, hyperglycemia (insulin deficiency), primary testicular dysfunction and primary adrenal insufficiency have been observed. Risk of adverse effects appears to be based on the agent used, and CTLA-4 inhibitors are more likely to be associated with hypophysitis, while PD-1 inhibitors are associated with thyroid dysfunction and diabetes.

Immune checkpoint inhibitor–related diabetes is a rare but potentially life-threatening complication, almost always seen with use of PD-1 and PD-L1 inhibitors such as atezolizumab. β-Cell destruction leads to insulin deficiency, and these patients will not have positive autoantibodies. A review article of patients who developed hyperglycemia on PD-1 and PD-L1 inhibitors noted that 70% of these patients went on to develop diabetic ketoacidosis. Clinical features of immune checkpoint inhibitor–induced diabetes are similar to those of another entity called fulminant diabetes and include the following: rapid onset of hyperglycemia, high likelihood of diabetic ketoacidosis, and near-normal hemoglobin A_{1c} levels at the time of presentation.

When a patient is diagnosed with immune checkpoint inhibitor–related diabetes, diabetic ketoacidosis should be ruled out or managed. Because the mechanism for hyperglycemia is insulin deficiency, the patient should be started on insulin (Answer E) to treat blood glucose elevations. Lifestyle change (Answer A), metformin (Answer B), glimepiride (Answer C), or a GLP-1 receptor agonist (Answer D) is incorrect because none of these treatment options addresses insulin deficiency. This patient should be counseled about the risk of diabetic ketoacidosis, its signs and symptoms, and the management plan. He would also benefit from seeing a nutritionist to learn how to count carbohydrates and administer mealtime insulin accurately.

Educational Objective
Explain the risk of fulminant diabetes with use of immune checkpoint inhibitors.

Reference(s)
Chang LS, Barroso-Sousa R, Tolaney SM, Hodi FS, Kaiser UB, Min L. Endocrine toxicity of cancer immunotherapy targeting immune checkpoints. *Endocr Rev.* 2019;40(1):17-65. PMID: 30184160

Imagawa A, Hanafusa T, Miyagawa J, Matsuzawa Y. A novel subtype of type 1 diabetes mellitus characterized by a rapid onset and absence of diabetes related antibodies. *N Engl J Med.* 2000;342(5):301-307. PMID: 10655528

118

ANSWER: E) Stop testosterone therapy

This man was inappropriately prescribed testosterone treatment based on nonspecific symptoms and a single testosterone measurement that was modestly low (relative to reference ranges based on healthy young men). It is not stated whether pretreatment testosterone was drawn in the afternoon or after food intake, both of which can reduce serum testosterone by up to 30%. Of note, reference ranges are based on morning samples drawn in the fasting state. Endocrine Society guidelines recommend that if there is clinical suspicion of androgen deficiency, the clinical impression should be confirmed biochemically by documenting at least 2 low total testosterone concentrations, drawn in the morning, in the fasted state. Testosterone should not be measured during an intercurrent illness, as such illness can lead to temporary gonadal axis suppression. If testosterone is repeatedly and unequivocally low, additional investigations are required to determine the etiology of the hypogonadism. The diagnostic workup must be performed before testosterone treatment is commenced, as exogenous testosterone will make interpretation of additional investigations (eg, gonadotropins) impossible.

In this man, a trial of testosterone therapy, despite consistently achieving "therapeutic" serum testosterone concentrations (ie, in the midnormal reference range) over 12 months, did not lead to sustained improvement of his nonspecific symptoms. A trial of 3 to 6 months is generally sufficient to determine whether sexual and subjective symptoms are testosterone responsive. Other effects of testosterone, such as effects on muscle or bone mass, may not achieve full effect until after several years of treatment. The initial improvement in his nonspecific symptoms is consistent with a placebo response, which is well documented. For example, in the Testosterone Trials, the largest randomized controlled trials of testosterone therapy in men to date, there was a marked improvement in fatigue in both the placebo and testosterone groups, but the between-group difference was not significant (*see figure*). There is good evidence that testosterone therapy is overprescribed. In one US Veterans Affairs database study of more than 110,000 men, only 3.1% of those prescribed testosterone received this treatment in full compliance with Endocrine Society testosterone therapy clinical practice guidelines. Of note, the Endocrine Society guidelines are less stringent than the US FDA recommendations, which restrict testosterone treatment to men with established organic hypogonadism due to medical disease of the hypothalamic-pituitary-testicular axis. Consistent with testosterone overuse, observational studies have reported that less than 20% of men initiating testosterone therapy continue the treatment for longer than 6 months. In this man, testosterone treatment should not have been initiated and should now be stopped (Answer E). The risk of iatrogenic gonadal axis suppression is very low. In one randomized controlled trial of 100 men receiving testosterone therapy for 12 months, in the months after cessation, men did not report hypogonadal symptoms, nor was there evidence that serum testosterone decreased below pretrial concentrations. Gonadal axis suppression after cessation of exogenous androgens is usually only seen with supraphysiologic dosing, for example in trials using testosterone as a male contraceptive, or more typically following anabolic steroid misuse. Nevertheless, the patient should be seen 3 months after testosterone cessation. Testosterone gel is short acting, and in this patient, the serum testosterone after 3 months off testosterone (sample drawn in the morning and in the fasted state) was 328 ng/dL (11.4 nmol/L), which is commensurate with his age and being overweight.

Effect of Testosterone Treatment on Vitality in the Testosterone Trials

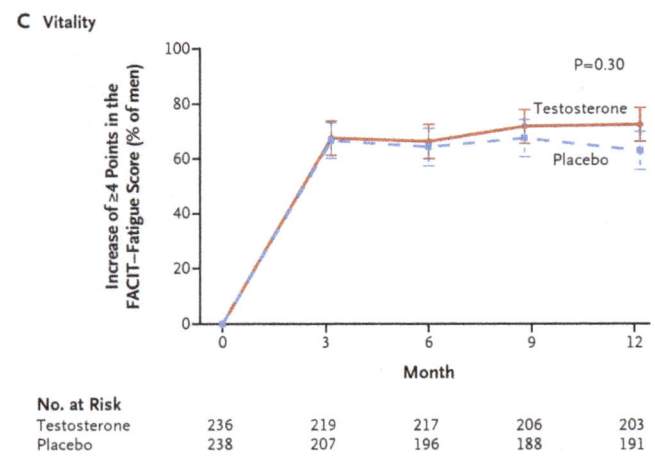

Reprinted from Snyder PJ, Bhasin S, Cunningham GR, et al; Testosterone Trials Investigators. Effects of testosterone treatment in older men. *N Engl J Med.* 2016;374(7):611-624.

Setting aside the fact that testosterone treatment was started inappropriately, there was no sustained improvement despite achieving midnormal serum testosterone concentrations for a sufficient duration of time. Therefore, increasing the transdermal dosage (Answer A) or switching to intramuscular testosterone (Answer B) is inappropriate.

Aromatase inhibitors (Answer C) and selective estrogen receptor modulators (Answer D) decrease endogenous estradiol production and action and are sometimes used on a trial basis for male gynecomastia (especially if painful), although no high-level evidence for benefit is available. Some anabolic steroid misusers also use such agents to reduce gynecomastia, an adverse effect of anabolic steroids. It is possible that in this man, the gynecomastia was triggered by the testosterone gel. Adding an aromatase inhibitor or selective estrogen receptor modulator is inappropriate. Simply stopping testosterone therapy may resolve the gynecomastia.

Educational Objective

List appropriate indications for testosterone treatment and determine when to stop inappropriate testosterone therapy.

Reference(s)

Bhasin S, Brito JP, Cunningham GR, et al. Testosterone therapy in men with hypogonadism: an Endocrine Society clinical practice guideline. *J Clin Endocrinol Metab.* 2018;103(5):1715-1744. PMID: 29562364

Snyder PJ, Bhasin S, Cunningham GR, et al; Testosterone Trials Investigators. Effects of testosterone treatment in older men. *N Engl J Med.* 2016;374(7):611-624. PMID: 26886521

Jasuja GK, Bhasin S, Reisman JI, Berlowitz DR, Rose AJ. Ascertainment of testosterone prescribing practices in the VA. *Med Care.* 2015;53(9):746-752. PMID: 26196850

Ng Tang Fui M, Hoermann R, Zajac JD, Grossmann M. The effects of testosterone on body composition in obese men are not sustained after cessation of testosterone treatment. *Clin Endocrinol (Oxf).* 2017;87(4):336-343. PMID: 28561278

119

ANSWER: A) Perform left adrenalectomy without adrenal venous sampling

This patient has primary aldosteronism and an incidentally discovered adrenal mass, which is concerning for a primary adrenal malignancy or pheochromocytoma. The radiographic characteristics of an adrenal mass are critical in evaluating whether the mass is benign or potentially malignant. Reassuring features that are suggestive of a benign adrenal mass include round and uniform shape, homogenous appearance, high lipid content (such as low attenuation on unenhanced CT [<10 Hounsfield units] or loss of signal on out-of-phase sequencing on MRI), and high contrast washout on delayed contrast CT imaging (absolute washout on delayed imaging of 50%-60%). Small size (generally <4 cm) is usually reassuring, but it is not a reliable feature. Features that raise concern for a malignant process include larger size (generally >4 or 6 cm), irregular shape or contour, heterogeneous content, calcifications, low lipid content on CT or MRI, and poor washout on delayed contrast CT imaging. A benign pheochromocytoma may have poor lipid content and poor washout on delayed contrast CT imaging, but it generally presents with a round contour and shape and with substantial elevations in metanephrines.

The initial characteristics of this patient's mass (size, shape, and lipid content) are not reassuring. The CT attenuation characteristics are the most specific findings: the high unenhanced attenuation (>10 Hounsfield units) in combination with poor absolute washout (<50%) should raise concern for adrenocortical carcinoma or pheochromocytoma. A functional pheochromocytoma is effectively excluded on the basis of normal plasma metanephrines and the presence of primary aldosteronism.

Adrenocortical carcinomas can secrete adrenocortical hormones. Most adrenocortical carcinomas produce some degree of glucocorticoids and androgens, and a minority may also secrete mineralocorticoids. In this case, the combination of clear primary aldosteronism (high aldosterone and suppressed renin activity in the context of hypertension and hypokalemia) and an adrenal mass that has features suggestive of malignancy should raise immediate concern that this is an aldosterone-producing adrenocortical carcinoma. The first-line and only curative therapy for adrenocortical carcinoma is surgical resection (Answer A).

Adrenal venous sampling (Answers B and E) would be preferred for reliable localization if the adrenal mass appeared lipid rich and benign and the patient were open to surgical therapy, because a unilateral mass does not exclude the possibility of bilateral or contralateral primary aldosteronism. When adrenal venous sampling is pursued, it is generally advised that mineralocorticoid receptor antagonists be stopped in advance to prevent normalization of the contralateral gland in the setting of unilateral primary aldosteronism. However, one study has shown that if used in low doses, mineralocorticoid receptor antagonists may not interfere with the final adrenal venous sampling interpretation.

Licorice ingestion can cause a mineralocorticoid excess syndrome. Glycyrrhizic acid can inhibit 11β-steroid dehydrogenase type 2, thereby permitting cortisol to activate the mineralocorticoid receptor. Patients who consume sufficient amounts of licorice to induce this effect may present with hypertension, hypokalemia, and suppression of aldosterone and renin. Although this patient is aware of some licorice root consumption in her tea, the amount is most likely insufficient to have contributed to her presentation (or may be an incidental fact unrelated to the current presentation) given that her aldosterone values remain elevated despite hypokalemia and hypertension. Thus, recommending that she stop drinking licorice-containing tea (Answers C and D) is not necessary; however, doing so may improve her blood pressure to some degree.

The most optimal way to improve this patient's survival and quality of life is to proceed directly to surgical left adrenalectomy. This patient did undergo adrenalectomy, and pathologic examination revealed an adrenocortical carcinoma. Postoperatively, her hypertension, hypokalemia, and primary aldosteronism resolved.

Educational Objective

Evaluate an incidentally discovered adrenal mass in a patient with primary aldosteronism.

Reference(s)

Funder JW, Carey RM, Mantero F, et al. The management of primary aldosteronism: case detection, diagnosis, and treatment: an Endocrine Society clinical practice guideline. *J Clin Endocrinol Metab.* 2016;101(5):1889-1916. PMID: 26934393

Fassnacht M, Arlt W, Bacos I, et al. Management of adrenal incidentalomas: European Society of Endocrinology clinical practice guideline in collaboration with the European Network for the Study of Adrenal Tumors. *Eur J Endocrinol.* 2016;175(2):G1-G34. PMID: 27390021

Vaidya A, Hamrahian A, Bancos I, Fleseriu M, Ghayee HK. The evaluation of incidentally discovered adrenal masses. *Endocr Pract.* 2019;25(2):178-192. PMID: 30817193

120

ANSWER: A) Thiamine

Micronutrients are essential factors that participate in various metabolic processes and biochemical pathways. Micronutrients include trace elements, essential minerals, water-soluble vitamins, and fat-soluble vitamins. After bariatric surgery, patients are at risk for micronutrient deficiency due to impairment in micronutrient absorption, aversion to specific foods, or exacerbation of a deficiency that existed before surgery. Postoperatively, patients should take a multivitamin that includes B vitamins and minerals (either once or twice daily) and calcium and vitamin D daily. Menstruating women should also take extra elemental iron (50-100 mg daily).

Key features in this vignette include the patient's symptoms (episodes of emesis, paresthesias, balance problems, and fatigue) and physical examination findings (dry mucous membranes; dry skin; absence of edema, nystagmus, or asterixis) and when the symptoms presented in relation to her surgery.

Given her recent surgery and intermittent emesis, she is at high risk of having thiamine deficiency (Answer A). Thiamine (vitamin B_1), a water-soluble vitamin, is a cofactor within several metabolic pathways. Early thiamine deficiency results in peripheral neuropathy, muscle weakness, nausea, vomiting, gait ataxia, and edema, while severe thiamine deficiency can result in Wernicke-Korsakoff syndrome, which includes ophthalmoplegia, nystagmus, confabulation, short-term memory loss, hallucinations, and psychosis. Thiamine levels are maintained in the normal range through dietary sources, as only a small amount is synthesized by the enterocolic bacteria. When intake is inadequate, thiamine stores usually deplete after 18 to 20 days. Food sources of thiamine include yeast, legumes, pork, rice, and cereals. Patients with mild thiamine deficiency should add 100 mg of oral thiamine daily to their supplements. If the patient does not tolerate the oral supplement because of persistent emesis, the recommendation is to start 100 mg of intramuscular thiamine daily.

Patients with iron deficiency (Answer B) present with microcytic anemia, dysphagia, fatigue, palpitations, brittle nails, angular cheilosis, koilonychia, and hair loss. Ruling out sources of bleeding is important, especially if the patient is a man or a nonmenstruating woman. Food sources of iron include meats, fortified cereals, and beans. Iron deficiency is treated with elemental iron, 200-300 mg daily.

Folate is a water-soluble vitamin that is essential in carbon and amino acid metabolism and DNA synthesis. Signs and symptoms of folic acid deficiency (Answer C) include fatigue, megaloblastic anemia, diarrhea, cheilosis, glossitis, and cognitive impairment. Food sources of folate include green leafy vegetables, fruits, cereals, grains, nuts, and meats. Patients with a deficiency should take 1 mg of folic acid daily. Also, patients should be encouraged to abstain from drinking alcohol, as it impedes folate absorption.

Patients with cobalamin deficiency (Answer D) present with megaloblastic anemia, fatigue, palpitations, muscle weakness, numbness, paresthesia, and mood disorders. Cobalamin deficiency is common in reduced gastric acid states, and its stores usually deplete after 3 to 5 years. Food sources of cobalamin include liver, milk, fish, and meat. Cobalamin deficiency is treated with 1000 mcg of vitamin B_{12} administered intramuscularly daily until the deficiency is corrected, after which the regimen is 1000 mcg monthly.

Measurement of methylmalonic acid and homocysteine helps distinguish between cobalamin and folate deficiency. Patients with vitamin B_{12} deficiency have normal levels of homocysteine and elevated levels methylmalonic acid. Patients with folate deficiency have normal levels of methylmalonic acid and elevated levels of homocysteine.

Copper, a trace metal, participates in neurotransmitter synthesis, respiratory oxidation, and iron absorption. Early symptoms of copper deficiency (Answer E) include hypopigmentation of hair, skin, and nails; painful neuropathy; myelopathy; optic neuropathy; and poor wound healing. Affected patients also develop hypochromic anemia, neutropenia, and pancytopenia. Advanced symptoms of copper deficiency include gait abnormalities. Food sources of copper include meats, fish, poultry, beans, peas, and lentils. Patients with copper deficiency should add 2 mg of copper (either citrate or gluconate) per day to their supplements.

Educational Objective
Identify symptoms of thiamine deficiency.

Reference(s)

Parrott J, Frank L, Rabena R, Craggs-Dino L, Isom KA, Greiman L. American Society for Metabolic and Bariatric Surgery integrated health nutritional guidelines for the surgical weight loss patient 2016 update: micronutrients. *Surg Obes Relat Dis.* 2017;13(5):727-741. PMID: 28392254

Via MA, Mechanick JI. Nutritional and micronutrient care of bariatric surgery patients: current evidence update. *Curr Obes Rep.* 2017;6(3):286-296. PMID: 28718091

Bal BS, Finelli FC, Shope TR, Koch TR. Nutritional deficiencies after bariatric surgery. *Nat Rev Endocrinol.* 2012;8(9):544-556. PMID: 22525731

ENDOCRINE SELF-ASSESSMENT PROGRAM 2021

Part III

This question-mapping index groups question topics according to the 8 umbrella sections of ESAP (Adrenal, Bone-Calcium, Diabetes, Lipids-Obesity, Pituitary, Reproduction [Female], Reproduction [Male], and Thyroid). Relevant **question numbers** follow each topic.

ADRENAL

CALCIUM-BONE

DIABETES

LIPIDS-OBESITY

www.ingramcontent.com/pod-product-compliance
Lightning Source LLC
Chambersburg PA
CBHW050454200326
41458CB00014B/5175